The ANTI-INFLAMMATORY DIET COOKBOOK FOR BEGINNERS

A Complete Guide to Lose Weight Quickly, to Heal the Immune System and Restore Overall Health with A 4 Weeks Meal Plan + 400 Healthy Recipes

Zoe S. Brown

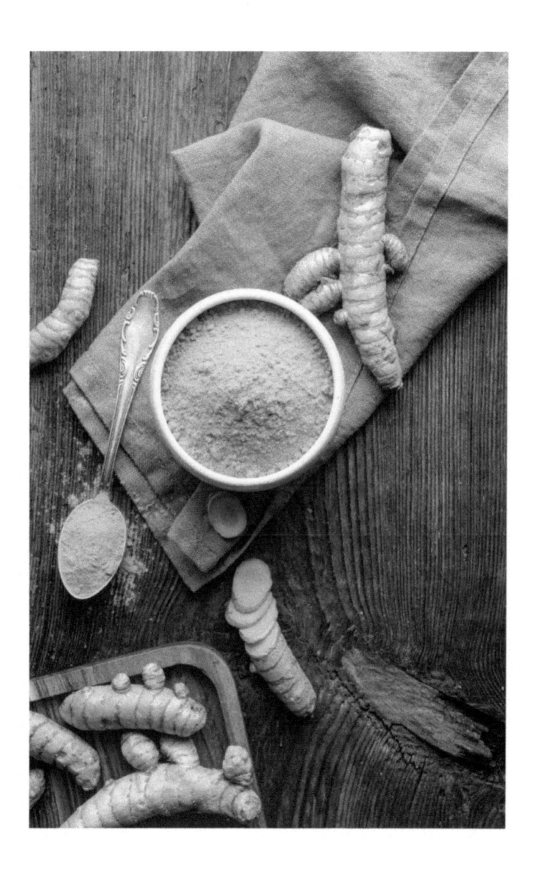

Table of Contents

Introduction
What is an Anti-Inflammatory Diet?

Inflammation plays an important role in your body, but the difference between "good" and "bad" inflammation can sometimes be confusing. There is "good" inflammation. This is the natural reaction your body goes through to help heal and protect you from influences that can harm your well-being.

The problem comes when inflammation is triggered and continues to occur. This is called "chronic" inflammation, and this kind of "bad" inflammation is what causes negative health side effects. It is possible to suffer from inflammation for a couple of weeks to several years. The longer and more severe the chronic inflammation, the more serious the side effects can be for you. It can even lead to death! Luckily for you, there are several steps you can take to minimize the amount of inflammation in your body so you can support and improve your overall health.

When your body is injured, infected, or is ill inflammation jumps in to save the day. The purpose of inflammation is to prevent these things from occurring or minimize the effect something like this could have on your body if it was unprotected. White blood cells are triggered in response to an "outside" invader or influence that threatens the balance in your body.

In addition to the white blood cells, your inflammation response produces immune cells and other substances like cytokines all to help ward off infection. When inflammation first occurs, you can often feel and see the response in your body. The area of injury or infection can become painful, warm, or red. But when inflammation is constant, it may not be as obvious. And when inflammation is silently attacking your own body as if it were a foreign invader, you create an opportunity for serious diseases such as cancer, fatty liver disease, heart issues, and type-2 diabetes.

If you suffer from obesity or constant stress in your life, chances are you also suffer from chronic inflammation. The habits you reenact every day are one of the best determining factors for the likelihood of chronic inflammation in your body. The way you live your life and eat foods determine most cases of chronic inflammation in the United States.

The Western diet is high in things like high-fructose corn syrup and refined sugars, both of which are known inflammation instigators for extended periods of time. "Empty" carbs and processed foods are also linked to chronic inflammation and are prevalent in the American diet. Eating these foods often have been linked over and over again in scientific studies to the increased risk of developing insulin resistance, type-2 diabetes, and obesity. More studies have shown a link between carbs and processed foods to chronic inflammation. Other inflammation culprits include a sedentary lifestyle, use of tobacco, and overuse of alcohol.

Your diet is one of the best methods for reducing inflammation in your body, and it is one of the easiest (and cheapest) methods you can control. Some foods have been linked to the reduction of inflammation, while others are known to exacerbate the problems you are experiencing. The general rule in any diet designed to help reduce inflammation is to eat more foods you know will help fight inflammation and stay away as often as possible from the foods that are known to cause it. This means eating more whole foods on a daily basis and staying away from refined or processed foods.

To go even further, consider choosing whole foods that also give you a dose of antioxidants to help fight off and reduce the number of free radicals bouncing around in your body. Free radicals, like inflammation, are a natural response to support your well-being, but when they are not controlled and limited, they can lead to a variety of health issues. One of the most dangerous health concerns of excessive free radicals is the increase in chronic inflammation.

Foods with a lot of antioxidants help naturally control your level of free radicals, and a lot of these foods are found in most anti-inflammatory meal plans. What makes an anti-inflammatory diet different than other options, like a low-carb diet, is that it supports the proper nutrition your body needs for optimal functioning. It is not about losing weight, but rather gaining your health back.

Anti-inflammatory diets mix in antioxidant-rich foods through "good" fats, proteins, and carbs in every meal and snack. You also will focus on proper vitamins, minerals, fiber, and water consumption. It is considered a lifestyle, meaning most anti-inflammatory diet plans include recommendations for not just eating, but sleeping and physical activity as well.

How to Follow an Anti-Inflammatory Lifestyle

To truly change and live a healthy life, you need to change more than just the food you eat. The extra things you do are what assist you in reaching and maintaining your goals. The following list is full of recommendations for living and loving the life of anti-inflammation:

• Sleep well each night. Your well-being is directly impacted by the amount and the quality of sleep you get each evening. The time you take to rest your mind and body at night is the time your body takes to inventory itself and reboot your system. This period of rest is also the time your body begins to naturally reduce inflammation you do not need. If you do not allow your body to take this important time, you slow down and can even stop the process. It does not matter how well you are doing regarding the food you are putting into your body, if you do not give it the chance to heal at night, you are just spinning your wheels, metaphorically speaking.

• Make your body work often. Every day you need to move your body moderately for approximately 20 minutes. Notice this says, "move your body," and not "exercise." You do not need to go for a run or lift weights to check this off your to-do list every day. Instead, you need to do things like walk for five minutes after dinner or parking further away, so you have to walk a long distance to work or home. Breaking up the 20 minutes into five-minute intervals is an easy way to sneak in your daily requirement. When you begin to do this, you also help reduce the risk of various diseases along with inflammation.

• Take supplements when needed, especially if you are having trouble figuring out your meals. When you begin changing what you eat it can be overwhelming. You need to balance carbs, proteins, fats, minerals, vitamins, etc. and that is a lot to tackle, especially if you have never done it before. To help you make empowered choices and to silence the negative voices, consider adding a supplement to your daily routine. This way you know you are getting the nutrients you need until you figure out your plate.

A good multi-vitamin is great for the transition period you will go through when learning about foods you like and that work well together to give you a nice balanced meal full of all the good stuff you need. In addition, you can add in supplements like curcumin and omega-3 fatty acids to make sure you get these in your diet until you figure out whole food sources. It is important to recognize that supplements are not intended to be something you take for the long-term or as a permanent part of your health plan. They are simply a transitional tool until you find your plan that fulfills all your dietary needs through whole foods. Supplements can have a place during the big changes, but make sure to "retire" them when you get a handle on your foods.

When you do make the change to the anti-inflammatory diet, a host of benefits accompany the feeling of empowerment and health. A sample of the benefits you can potentially enjoy are:

1. Improved energy levels and mood.
2. Better triglyceride, blood sugar, and cholesterol levels.
3. Reduced markers in your blood for inflammation.
4. Lowered obesity, heart disease, type-2 diabetes, depression, and cancer risk for development.
5. Enhanced treatment for diseases like autoimmune diseases. This includes arthritis, lupus, and irritable bowel syndrome.

To generalize the results, chronic inflammation is significantly reduced when you change your lifestyle to support anti-inflammation, including changing your diet. This lowered chronic inflammation is what helps lower the risk of developing additional serious diseases as well as help heal others you may already be suffering from. Inflammation is the result of your diet, lifestyle, and environment. When you change up these key areas of your like to control your well-being and health, you can expect to see a big difference.

Unfortunately, the Western diet is dominated by unhealthy food choices and relationships. This means Americans and those who eat a Western diet are more at risk than other cultures for developing chronic inflammation. Men are also at more a risk than women are. Chronic inflammation is directly linked to heart disease, which is currently the number one killer in the United States. By changing the quality of your life and making good choices regarding your body's nutritional intake, you take great steps in lengthening your lifespan and the quality of that life.

The "How" of the Anti-inflammatory Diet

The focus of this lifestyle is on plants. It encourages you to consume mostly plants that offer specific chemicals known to reduce the body's inflammation levels naturally. The reason this diet focuses on plants is due to their organic ability to produce various beneficial chemicals for the human body. One of the chemicals most plants produce that is so good for your body is called phytochemicals. These are important chemicals for plant function, and while certain phytochemicals are poisonous for the human body, others are vital.

For example, you most likely can name several plants you recognize should be eaten regularly, while there are specific berries or mushrooms you know you need to be cautious of in the wild because they can be dangerous to your health if you eat them. Because of the amazing natural abilities of plants to thrive and protect themselves with these phytochemicals, you should not be caught off guard when you learn these plants you can eat safely are some of the best foods you can eat.

This natural protection from plants for your organs and cells is what makes the anti-inflammatory diet so unique. Many contemporary diet plans encourage whole foods and a plant focus, but while they may avoid the subject of inflammation, most of the time the benefits they list for consuming these foods is because of their anti-inflammatory properties. The protection these plants offer to your body against all levels of chronic inflammation is vital to your overall health and longevity.

Yes, not all inflammation should be counteracted. When you are fighting a cold or ingest a toxin, inflammation is a natural response you need to rely upon. If you have an injury, damaged cells send out a specific chemical to your blood vessels so fluid can be leaked into the tissue around the injury site. The swelling of the tissue is what protects the body from a spreading injury and provides an isolated space for the damaged area to heal.

The swelling side effect alerts your immune system that the area requires specific cells that need to clean up the damaged cells or even to come in and kill the infected cells. It is when your body sends inflammation-triggering cells to locations that do not heal, or tissue is swollen and inflamed for a long time that your body begins to malfunction. This is when more diseases can manifest in the body, and you are no longer equipped to fight them off. You are too busy fighting yourself!

Most of the research published discusses the footprints or biomarkers of the body's inflammation. Some of these "footprints" include C-reactive proteins, or CRP, and cytokines. These are chemicals that travel in your bloodstream and act as a sort of signaling device for inflammation that is occurring in the body. Foods known to lower these markers are also known as anti-inflammatory foods. The markers are lower from eating these foods because the chronic inflammation in your body is lower.

When you lower your inflammation, you lower your risk of developing a variety of deadly and painful diseases. Some doctors may still consider the positive effects the anti-inflammatory diet has on inflammation as "controversial," but no doctor can deny that a healthy diet can positively impact your overall health, including lowering your inflammation and risk of certain diseases. And the anti-inflammatory diet definitely is a lifestyle that falls in the "healthy" category!

When you are choosing foods for your anti-inflammatory diet plan, make sure you are selecting foods for their properties associated with lowering inflammation rather than because they have a specific nutrient in them that are known to lower inflammation. You want to choose foods that are going to give you the most "bang for your buck." You want foods that are going to support your body and satisfy your hunger and taste buds. This requires you to choose foods that contain a high level of healthy fat and beneficial phytochemicals, are plant-based and are a whole food.

Beans, nuts, whole grains, and specific spices and herbs are a few of the primary foods you want to consume. These types of foods should not alarm you; they are the food types that often make the top of most healthy eating diet plans. Another healthy chemical that these foods offer is called "flavonoids." This is a compound found in many plant-based foods that are known for helping lower inflammation levels.

Other chemicals certain foods offer to help lower inflammation are omega-3 fatty acids, often found in oily fish, and fiber. And while these foods perform wonders for your health and the number you see on the scale, they are not magic pills that will have you dropping several dress sizes overnight while curing all your ailments. You have to give these healthy foods a chance to work their magic. This means adopting and sticking to the anti-inflammatory diet for an extended period of time in order to truly enjoy the benefits it has to offer you.

The Mediterranean Diet - A Good Example of Eating to Lower Inflammation

Not all diets or meal plans fit all people, but there are a few dietary guidelines that are good for almost every person and definitely worth considering. Any adaptation of the anti-inflammatory diet fits this description, but the "Mediterranean Diet," is a commonly mentioned anti-inflammatory plan you should look into. The foundational principles rest in the anti-inflammatory guidelines for healthy eating, but also specify the types and frequency of consuming various fish. In addition, it gives you room to enjoy a little wine, too! If it works for you and your life, when you follow the diet based on the cultures living along the Mediterranean Sea, you can have a small glass of red wine a day and still be "following the rules!"

All anti-inflammatory diets introduce the foundational concepts of avoiding pro-inflammation foods like unhealthy fats and refined foods while consuming a large number of anti-inflammatory foods like fruits, vegetables, fish, and whole grains. The presentation and preparation of these foods are what make each one distinct. A significant part of this includes the size of the portions during each meal. In most anti-inflammatory diets, including the Mediterranean Diet, portion sizes are very specific. You will learn more about this later in the book.

The primary components of the Mediterranean Diet are:
•   Meals are a social event and should be enjoyed in the company of friends and family often. This also includes the preparation and clean-up of a meal.
•   Pour yourself a small glass of red wine a few times a week. Drinking red wine in moderation is approved on the Mediterranean Diet, but you do not have to do this if you do not want to or should not drink alcohol at all.
•   Two times a week make sure you eat lean poultry and oily fish.
•   If you must eat red meat, do not eat it more than two times a month. Try not to eat it at all!
•   Season your food with spices and various herbs instead of other, unhealthy seasoning options.
•   Choose healthy fats, like extra virgin olive oil, over unhealthy options, like butter.

When you follow an anti-inflammatory diet like this, you do not have to give up alcohol or bread completely, but you do have to consume them in moderation and with empowerment. Sometimes you will be advised against these "treats" altogether, while others will be more lenient on your consumption of them. Make sure you listen to your body and your team of professionals, as well as allow yourself the permission to eat with empowerment.

Dietary Causes of Inflammation

Chronic inflammation is just the beginning of a life spent trying to resist more major conditions like diabetes and heart disease. Inflammation definitely increases as people get older, but it can also be made worse by obesity and poor diet. When people constantly consume a poor diet filled with inflammation-causing foods then they are just feeding the inflammation and not their bodies. Many foods are known to cause inflammation in the human body.

Artificial and Alternative Sweeteners – Many people turn to these to eliminate their dependence on sugar, which is known to cause problems in people with chronic inflammation. Unfortunately, artificial and alternative sweeteners, with one exception, are no better for your body than real sugar is. Saccharin does not appear to have the same inflammatory effects on the body that artificial and alternative sweeteners do. Those often cause insomnia, fatigue, mood swings, joint pain, abdominal pain, muscle aches, headache, and vomiting, and nausea. They may also cause skin rashes and inflammation of the skin. All of these conditions will contribute to chronic inflammation.

Saturated Fats and Trans Fats – Hydrogenated oil, which is made by using hydrogen to turn liquid unsaturated fat into solid fat, causes inflammation. Hydrogenated oil contains trans-fat, which in addition to causing inflammation, will also cause your good cholesterol to decrease and your bad cholesterol to increase. Hydrogenated oils appear in abundance in vegetable shortening, coffee creamer, refrigerator dough, potato chips, fried foods, ready-made baked goods such as crackers, cookies, and pie crusts, and margarine.
Saturated fat is found in red meat, cheese, coconut oil, palm oil, and butter. Besides causing or adding to inflammation, fats that are saturated can also cause other diseases to develop in your body. You will also find saturated fat at various levels in pork, milk, and the skin of poultry.

Carbohydrates – Some carbs lead to increased inflammation, and some carbs do not. The carbohydrate food group encompasses a wide variety of foods. A carbohydrate is a compound that contains cellulose, starch, and sugar. Carbs fill up milk, vegetables, fruit, and grains. They are found in muffins, bread, sweet rolls, cookies, and cakes. Carbs are either classified as simple or complex. The simple carbs group, also known as refined carbs, includes the sugary treats and processed baked goods, and those are the ones that cause inflammation. Complex carbs such as vegetables and fruits do not.

Processed Foods – This food group includes and food that is processed, fully or partially. This includes fast food, pre-made dinners, cold cereal, bread and pastries, processed meats, and convenience foods such as ready-made meals or microwave meals.

Many different triggers can cause inflammation. Some are not as easy to control as your dietary choices are. The best way to control or eliminate inflammation in your body is by eating a diet of foods that do not cause inflammation and will help to fight inflammation from other sources.

Food to Eat That Fight Inflammation

In this chapter, we will discuss all the foods and drinks you can eat on the anti-inflammatory diet and why they are good for you.

Omega-3 fatty acids are responsible for building and growing your body. They are a good source of fatty acids to have. Omega-3 curbs inflammation. You can find Omega 3 and sausage like olive oil, walnuts, pumpkin seeds, hemp seeds, chia, and flax seeds. Algal oil is a great supplement to take to increase your omega- 3 fatty acids in your diet as well.

Other great sources of omega-3 fatty acids are fish that is super oily and super fatty like fatty sardines, mackerel, tuna, and salmon. When possible, opt for the wild version of fish and not the farm ones for more intense results.

Dark leafy plants that help stop inflammation are broccoli, red cabbage, spinach, kale, asparagus, and rainbow swiss chard. They are good sources of vitamin K which help with your chronic inflammatory diseases. You can even throw in collards that contain vitamin E. Vitamin E protects your cells from substances that want to cause inflammation. To take it to the next level, even try spirulina, celery, and chlorella which can lower cholesterol, too.

Blueberries, strawberries, blackberries, oranges, cherries, and raspberries all contain polyphenols that prevent inflammation. If you are ever craving sugar, they're all so great to have because they are low in sugar. These berries are also a good source of quercetin which fights inflammation and can even help prevent cancer. Also, do not forget about the acai berry which is another great food to have.

Maca is a great hormone regulator. This is often taken as a powder and it has lots of anti-inflammatory characteristics. Try to make it a staple in your diet like having it in or putting it in a smoothie.

Ginger is great for those suffering from arthritis especially osteoarthritis and rheumatoid arthritis and migraine headaches. The active component in ginger known as 6 - gingerol l is one of the major properties that prevent inflammation.

Turmeric's active property called curcumin exemplifies many anti-inflammatory characteristics. It is great for arthritis, diabetes, and cancer. Because turmeric can be difficult for the body to absorb, a lot of people try to take it, in fact, to help ease absorption. The more turmeric your body can absorb, the more it can help you prevent inflammation. If you are concerned about the yellow staining turmeric when you cook, you can opt for a curcumin supplement instead.

Sweet potatoes and butternut squash plus other foods rich in beta-carotene are excellent sources of inflammation-fighting properties.
Cacao is best added to a smoothie, and if you want the sugar version, opt for dark chocolate. Cacao has over 300 compounds that help prevent inflammation. Do not forget about this wonderful food in your anti-inflammatory diet meal plans.

Coffee contains polyphenols that help prevent inflammation. To get the most out of coffee, try to choose a lighter roast and be sure to brew your coffee without a coffee filter. The best part about having coffee in your diet is it does not have to be caffeinated. A decaf cup of coffee contains just as many polyphenols as a caffeinated cup of coffee. If you do not like coffee at all, then you want to check out green or white tea because they contain just as many polyphenols. Green and white tea also contain catechins, another powerful property that fights inflammation.

Pineapple is another grapefruit to have because of bromelain. Bromelain helps your body prevent unnecessary inflammation. It also contains vitamin B1, potassium, magnesium, and vitamin C.

Beans have lots of fiber, which is an important nutrient in fighting inflammation. Any type of bean is good for you, and they all prevent inflammation!

Bone broth contains minerals your body can absorb like magnesium, silicon, phosphorus, sulfur, and calcium which all help reduce joint pain arthritis and inflammation.
Whole grains like brown rice whole wheat bread and unrefined grains and oatmeal contain lots of fiber which can help your inflammation. If you do not have gluten sensitivity, feel free to eat whole grains, but watch how much you eat to prevent unwanted weight.

Nuts, like walnuts, almonds, and cashews, etc., contain healthy fat that stops inflammation. Avocados, coconut, and olive oil are also good sources of healthy fats. These fats prevent unwanted weight gain as well. Celery also prevents inflammation and fights bacterial infections. It is an excellent source of potassium, as well as antioxidants and vitamins.

Water is an excellent source of hydration! It helps to flush toxins out of your system that can cause inflammation. So drink up! Drink as much water as you can.

Food to Avoid

There are lots of foods that do not help with your chronic inflammation. This chapter highlights them, even the sneaky ones you may not notice in the food you are eating every day.

Alcohol overworks your liver. The anti-inflammatory advises you to drink as little alcohol as possible. This prevents your liver from having to work overtime, which causes internal inflammation.

Sugar is a tricky product to avoid because it is usually in everything that we eat! When you eat sugar, it releases cytokines or proteins in your body that trigger inflammation. When looking for sugar, pay close attention to words that end in the three letters 'ose.' High Fructose syrup is a very important word to look out for! Junk food like cookies and sodas are very important to limit.

Aspartame is an FDA-approved product that is an artificial sweetener that gives you no nutrients in your body. Many people react negatively to it. If your body reacts negatively towards this product, it will cause inflammation since your body recognizes it as a foreign product. When you are looking for sugar in products you are buying, be sure to watch out for aspartame. Good luck since it is in over 4,000 products!

White flour is found in white potatoes and rice, bread, crackers and rolls, French fries and instant mash potatoes. When you eat white flour products, they release advanced glycation. End products in these can cause inflammation. To prevent inflammation, it is best to avoid these products.

Processed foods are foods that are already prepared and require limited cooking. Foods in this category include soups and sauces in cans, pre-cooked freezer meat, microwavable dinners, and deli meat. These foods typically contain a lot of sugar, salt, and trans-fats. Avoid heavily processed foods, like microwavable dinners, packaged deli meats, and high-sodium canned soups and sauces. These foods are likely to contain added trans-fats, sodium, and sugars.

Omega-6 fatty acids are a necessity for your body to go through the natural growth and development cycle. For the natural growth and development cycle to be successful, your body needs a normal balance of fatty acids that are omega-3 and omega-6. When you eat too many omega-6 fatty acids, it throws your balance off and triggers inflammation in your body. The issue is that omega-6 fatty acids are found everywhere! They are in lots of salad dressings, mayonnaise, and most cooking oils. A major way to avoid omega-6 is to give up fried food, which is found in lots of fast food.

Mono-sodium glutamate (MSG) is typically found in soup mixes, salad dressings, deli meats in Asian Foods, and soy sauce. This additive affects your liver's health and causes chronic inflammation. Try to avoid it.

Trans fats and partially hydrogenated oils are the same thing. Trans fats raise your LDL cholesterol (low-density lipoprotein cholesterol) levels. Too much LDL cholesterol can cause inflammation of your heart and heart disease. Do not buy it at all if you want to remain inflammation free.

Saturated fats can cause heart disease and make your arthritis inflammation worse! Saturated fats cause inflammation of your fat tissue. Guess what the biggest sources of saturated fats are? It is pizza and cheese! You can also get saturated fats from red meat. If you must have meat, choose the leanest cuts like sirloin, loin or ground. Then trim off as much fat as you can before cooking. Also, for the cheese and dairy lovers, go for low-fat dairy.

Salt can cause tissue inflammation! It is found in lots of junk food and many people tend to over salt their food. When you are cooking, try to use other herbs and spices besides salt to season your food and watch your inflammation go down.

Gluten is found in whole grains like barley, rye, wheat or casein. It is also found in some dairy products. For those that have arthritis, eliminating gluten can be helpful. If you notice that when you eat gluten, you have inflammation and pain, you could also be at risk for celiac disease. Once you give up gluten, you can determine if it is a trigger for your inflammation. Then proceed based on your results. If gluten does not bother you, feel free to eat whole grains. However, to take your anti-inflammatory diet to the next level, you can replace your whole grains with high-quality carbs like carrots, squash and sweet potatoes.

Anti-Inflammatory Diet, Sport And Life Style

When it comes to any lifestyle shift, it is necessary to have a plan. Not having a plan can leave you frustrated and broke, especially when it comes to diet. Changing your eating plan affects different parts of your life. You will need to consider your bank account, available time, allergens, your preferences, and the preferences and dietary needs of those in your family - assuming you do not live alone. You will also need to find the types of food to include in your anti-inflammatory diet and which not to.

By combining all this information, you can successfully develop a plan that clears your path to decreased inflammation. There isn't just one anti-inflammatory diet. There is quite a number to choose from. The Sears's Zone diet, Dr. Hyman's Detox, Dr. Weil's Paleo Diet, and the Whole 30 are considered to be highly anti-inflammatory.

However, the most research-backed anti-inflammatory diet is the traditional Mediterranean diet that focuses on fruits, whole grains, vegetables, legumes, fish rich in omega-3, and olive oil. A beginner is advised to follow a well-balanced, generally healthy diet, which includes anti-inflammatory nutrients and learn to reshape the diet plan according to the acquired knowledge of how each food affects them.

The anti-inflammatory benefits come from the synergistic effect of foods consumed together as well as those gotten from individual foods. Even small changes in a person's diet can play a massive role in improving one's health.

Therefore, it is vital to focus on goals that are yours and making them as achievable as possible. For example, eating an extra serving of legumes or fruits at breakfast or lunch is key to helping someone make lasting dietary changes that will help reduce inflammation and enhance overall health. However, based on your past medical history, your diet may need to be modified along with the types of anti-inflammatory foods you should consume.

It would be wise to speak with a dietitian before embarking on this journey. I honestly think there isn't too much thought that needs to be put into starting this diet because it is relatively easy. Just make healthy food choices and find recipes you might enjoy, because just like any diet, if you do not like it, you will not last very long in it. Please, do remember that you do not have to be 100% perfect.

Take it easy, and kiss it. By which I mean Keep It Stupid Simple. Unless you are under some type of medically specific diet rules, if you're at a friend's wedding, please have a piece of cake. Life is too short, and its meant to be enjoyed. Some people think diets have to be all or nothing, which makes them fail to see it through to the end because anything that prevents eating from being a fun activity is considered stressful.

So, when you're ready to go to the grocery stores, be sure to have a list of healthy whole foods that you would like. You should try looking for some recipes that seem tasty first. There are thousands online. Also, when you go out to eat, many restaurants make nutritional info available on the menu or sell a lot of whole foods. Feel free to ask restaurants how they prepare foods you're interested in, and if need be, request if you would like your item prepared a certain way or with ingredients you want.

Long-term changes take some time to stick, and you need to cut yourself some slack during this process. Do not feel sad if you do not notice any changes over a short period because sustainable lifestyle changes do not happen overnight. Rome wasn't built in a day, am I right? You should also be ready to eliminate the foods that are inflammatory and likely doing your body more harm than good.

Also, be prepared because time-consuming preparation is vital, and you will need a lot of preparation time in the kitchen since you will be cooking foods from scratch in a bid to eat nutrient-rich whole foods. It's also normal to experience some or all of the withdrawal symptoms that can happen while your body removes the toxicity and rebalances nutritionally. These withdrawal symptoms can include headaches, fatigue, nausea, abdominal discomfort, and mood swings, among other things. If you can, speak with a health coach or nutritionist for guidance, support, and medical advice. Most importantly, savor the journey, lovelies. Good health is definitely worth it.

Why It Can Be So Hard

Anti-inflammatory dieting is a safe practice that has been found to reduce inflammation, depression, and anxiety. Evidence suggests that experienced practitioners of this diet also underwent certain changes at the genetic and molecular levels that could lead to lower chances of cognitive impairment and endless beneficial health effects. So tough! But despite its many advantages, a lot of people, especially beginners, call it quits when they hit obstacles in their practice.

But to succeed, it is imperative that you understand that in all honesty, the anti-inflammatory is way more than just eating healthy, tasty foods. At its core, it is an active training of the mind to increase mindfulness, concentration, and resiliency - qualities that are in short supply these days, unfortunately. And this kind of training needs effort and commitment, not to mention the patience you'll need to put in if you really want to condition your mind.

What many beginners do not realize is that finding solutions to problems that we encounter in our practice is also part of the journey. If we can overcome the obstacles that stop us from being healthier, our minds also become better focused and more resilient to external and internal factors in the process.

Obstacles and how to overcome them:

• I can't just stop thinking. So, you're supposed to be focusing on your anti-inflammatory journey, but your mind keeps moving off to everything else but what you should be focused on! Or you might find you're giving yourself this obsessive, incessant pep talk that just makes you more anxious and unsettled and covers everything about everything, except, of course, your diet. What can I do?

Breath counting is a very effective method to calm down an overactive mind. All you need to do is count every breath cycle. One inhale followed by one exhale is a complete breath cycle, which means you will count a number right after every exhale. If you want, you can also count at each inhale instead. It doesn't matter. Keep counting to 15, and then start from the top again. Try not to lose count.

The idea behind this method is simple. By busying the mind with a simple task, the tendency to wander off is relatively reduced. "But what if my mind adapts to this game so well that it is now able to count and think at the same time?" It means it is time to change the rules of the game to trick your mind again. You could always count backward. 10, 9, 8, 7, 6, 5, 4, 3, 2, 1. Or you could even count only even numbers 2, 4, 6, 8, 10, 12.... 24. Just play with this.

• There is no time! "My schedule always seemed to be packed to the hilt every single day, and I can't seem to get any time for food preparation. Even when I get some free time, there is always something that pops up and seems more important, making my diet very inconsistent."

Is this you? Yes? What can I do? Do well to pay yourself first before you throw your money on anything else. This is a vital rule to keep in mind when it comes to making time for your new diet. Before you are thrown into the drama of the day, invest at least 10 minutes of your time into a well-prepared healthy meal. Allow nothing to distract you from this, and make it known to the people living with you, if any, the sacredness of this you-time. This may mean you have to wake up 10 minutes earlier than usual. But hey, good investment, right?

• I can't seem to be relaxed and focused You might be familiar with this scenario: once you get home after a highly stressful day at work, you figure a cup of green tea and some fresh fruits will be helpful. So, you start to take off your work clothes, making a mental note to go and prepare those things, but despite your efforts, you just cannot seem to relax per normal. Instead, you end up getting more stressed out and even agitated, wondering why in the world you can't just seem to calm down. What can I do? Personally, I can say it's very difficult to cook when the mind is very hyper, like in the case of a very stressed out person, or someone currently dealing with a panic attack.

Because the mind is so caught up in its own web of thoughts, it will not be able to focus on the recipes or any ingredient except whatever it is obsessed with at the moment. To get out of that agitated state of mind, it would be better to expend its energies and relax through some external means, such as listening to music, taking a walk, or talking with someone. We must have at least one reliable external solace we can turn to when we need to cool off in times of great stress or anxiety

Other Common Difficulties.

• Getting Enough Omega-3s. Balancing the ratio between your Omega 3 and Omega 6 is critical to keeping systemic inflammation at bay. What I mean is, when your Omega-6 levels exceed your Omega-3 levels, systemic inflammation will drastically increase, and with it, the secondary side effects of inflammation. There are way more foods rich in Omega-6 fatty acids than omega-3. And somehow, we have to make sure to include Omega 3 in our diet to maintain the necessary 1:2 balance between the two.

Omega 3's are found in plant products, but more often than not, they are accompanied by even higher levels of Omega-6, meaning plants aren't exactly useful for omega-3 supplementation. However, there is one plant-based source with very high Omega 3s and low-Omega 6s. Flaxseeds. The issue is that there are several types of Omega 3 fatty acids, and the kind found in flaxseeds must be metabolized by the body into different forms before it can be utilized. Err... the body is not very good at this. Research has shown that only around 1-3% of the flaxseeds you eat eventually get metabolized. This means you will have to consume somewhere around 35 grams of flaxseeds for your body to get 1g of usable Omega 3's.

• Too much fruit is bad. Sounds completely absurd, doesn't it? The anti-inflammatory diet is centered around fresh fruits, so how come we can't eat 'too much of one of the only things we can eat? Popular opinion is that fruit is generally perceived to be healthy, but recent studies suggest otherwise. Fruits are basically a glorified natural high-fructose snack. Back in the day, fruit provided reasonable amounts of vitamins and minerals.

Today, grocery stores are filled with fruit grown in over-farmed, depleted soils and have a tiny fraction of the nutrition that fruit usually should. Even worse, fruit brings with it loads of fructose, which recent studies have shown is not good for the body. Fructose is a reactive molecule that binds with bodily proteins to form a substance called Advanced Glycation End Products (AGEs). AGEs cause something called cross-linking in collagen, the body's basic connective tissue.

Cross-linking decreases the flexibility of collagen, creating several problems including but not limited to stiff joints, damaged DNA, and aging skin. Fructose has also been linked to insulin resistance, obesity, and even decreased brain function. When we eat fructose, the body doesn't absorb it like with most other nutrients. Fructose is sent to the liver to be processed and turned into glycogen or fat.

• Plant toxins. Most of the time, eating a lot of veggies is a beneficial thing to do, seeing as it contains a lot of nutrients, including the anti-inflammatory ones. But studies have shown that there are a handful of plants out there that contain very little levels of natural toxins that can be harmful if ingested in large quantities. Seeing that the anti-inflammatory diet consists of a lot of these foods, this can particularly be a cause for concern. Do not blame the plants. They are living organisms, and like all living organisms, they have their own defense mechanisms. The toxins they produce naturally are a defense mechanism against being over-eaten by insects in their niche. Usually, when we consume these foods sparingly, our body is able to weed out the toxins, and as a result, they never accumulate and cause problems. However, when they become major constituents of a diet, they become ingested several times a week. That is an entirely different matter because the body cannot clear them out that fast, and they tend to accumulate and can disrupt digestion, cause inflammation, and change hormonal functions. The plants in this category are:

• Legumes, because they contain phytic acid and tannins
• Quinoa, because they also contain phytic acid, tannins, and saponins.
• Some nuts contain tannins and phytic acid
• Kale and some cruciferous plants contain oxalates and goitrogens
• Rice is believed to contain arsenic
• Corn and wheat contain phytic acid, gluten, and mycotoxins.

Anti-inflammatory recipes

BREAKFAST

1) Mushroom Frittata

PREPARATION TIME: 10 minutes
COOKING TIME: 30 minutes
SERVINGS: 4
INGREDIENTS:
¼ cup coconut milk, unsweetened
6 eggs
1 yellow onion, chopped
4 ounces white mushrooms, sliced
2 tablespoons olive oil
2 cups baby spinach
A pinch of salt and black pepper
DIRECTIONS:
Heat up a pan with the oil over medium-high heat, add the onion, stir and cook for 2-3 minutes. Add the mushrooms, salt and pepper, stir and cook for 2 minutes more. In a bowl, mix the eggs with salt and pep-per, stir well and pour over the mush-rooms. Add the spinach, mix a bit, place in the oven and bake at 360 degrees F for 25 minutes. Slice the frittata and serve it for breakfast.
Enjoy!
Nutrition: calories 200, fat 3, fiber 6, carbs 14, protein 6

2) Almond Breakfast Crepes

PREPARATION TIME: 10 minutes
COOKING TIME: 10 minutes
SERVINGS: 4
INGREDIENTS:
2 eggs
1 teaspoon vanilla extract
½ cup almond milk, unsweetened
½ cup water
2 tablespoons agave nectar
1 cup coconut flour
3 tablespoons coconut oil, melted

DIRECTIONS:
In a bowl, whisk the eggs with the vanilla extract, almond milk, water and agave nectar. Add the flour and 2 tablespoons oil gradually and stir until you obtain a smooth batter. Heat up a pan with the rest of the oil over medium heat, add some of the batter, spread into the pan and cook the crepe until it's golden on both sides then transfer to a plate. Repeat with the rest of the batter and serve the crepes for breakfast.
Enjoy!
Nutrition: calories 121, fat 3, fiber 6, carbs 14, protein 6

3) Millet Muffins

PREPARATION TIME: 10 minutes
COOKING TIME: 15 minutes
SERVINGS: 12
INGREDIENTS:
¼ cup coconut oil, melted
1 egg
½ teaspoon vanilla extract
1 teaspoon baking powder
1½ cups organic millet, cooked
½ cup coconut sugar
Cooking spray
DIRECTIONS:
In a blender, blend the melted coconut oil with the egg, vanilla extract, baking powder, millet and sugar. Grease a muffin tray with cooking spray and divide the millet mix into each cup. Place the muffins in the oven and bake at 350 degrees F for 30 minutes. Let the muffins cool and then serve!
Enjoy!
Nutrition: calories 167, fat 4, fiber 7, carbs 15, protein 6

4) Kale and Pears Smoothie

PREPARATION TIME: 10 minutes
COOKING TIME: 0 minutes
SERVINGS: 5
INGREDIENTS:
10 kale leaves
5 bananas, peeled and cut into chunks

2 pears, chopped
5 tablespoons almond butter
5 cups almond milk
DIRECTIONS:
In your blender, mix the kale with the bananas, pears, almond butter and almond milk, pulse well, divide into glasses and serve for breakfast.
Enjoy!
Nutrition: calories 267, fat 11, fiber 7, carbs 15, protein

5) **Apple Muesli**

PREPARATION TIME: 10 minutes
COOKING TIME: 0 minutes
SERVINGS: 4
INGREDIENTS:
2 apples, peeled, cored and grated
1 cup rolled oats
3 tablespoons flax seeds
1¼ cups coconut cream
1¼ cups coconut water
½ cup goji berries
2 tablespoons chopped mint
3 tablespoons raw honey
DIRECTIONS:
In a bowl, mix the apples with the oats, flax seeds, coconut cream, coconut water, goji berries, mint and honey. Stir well, divide into smaller bowls and serve for breakfast.
Enjoy!
Nutrition: calories 171, fat 2, fiber 6, carbs 14, protein 5

6) **Veggie Mix**

PREPARATION TIME: 10 minutes
COOKING TIME: 10 minutes
SERVINGS: 2
INGREDIENTS:
½ cup chopped yellow onions
½ cup chopped red bell pepper
A pinch of garlic powder
A pinch of salt and black pepper
1 tablespoon olive oil
2 eggs
DIRECTIONS:

Heat up a pan with the oil over medium-high heat, add the onions, stir and cook for 1-2 minutes. Add the bell pepper, garlic powder, salt and pepper then stir and cook for 3 minutes more. Add the eggs, stir and cook until the eggs are done, about 1-2 minutes. Divide everything between plates and serve. Enjoy!
Nutrition: calories 221, fat 6, fiber 6, carbs 14, protein 11g

7) **Sweet Potato Cakes**

PREPARATION TIME: 10 minutes
COOKING TIME: 10 minutes
SERVINGS: 6
INGREDIENTS: 1 cup coconut flour
2 tablespoons brown rice flour
½ tablespoon ground flax seed
1 teaspoon baking soda
A pinch of salt and black pepper
1 small yellow onion, chopped
2 garlic cloves, minced
1 small sweet potato, peeled and grated
2½ cups chopped kale - 3 eggs
3 tablespoons olive oil
DIRECTIONS: In a bowl, add the coconut flour with the rice flour, flax seed, baking soda, salt, pepper, eggs, onion, garlic, sweet potato and kale stir well. Shape medium cakes out of this mix, you should get about 6 cakes. Heat up a pan with the olive oil over medium-high heat then add the cakes and cook them for about 4-5 minutes on each side. Divide them between plates and serve them for breakfast. Enjoy!
Nutrition: calories 211, fat 4, fiber 7, carbs 14, protein 7

8) **Green Salad with Pine Nuts**

PREPARATION TIME: 10 minutes
COOKING TIME: 0 minutes
SERVINGS: 2
INGREDIENTS:
1 cucumber, sliced
2 handfuls cherry tomatoes, halved

1 avocado, peeled, pitted and cubed
1 red bell pepper, cubed
A handful basil, torn
A handful parsley, chopped
1 tablespoon olive oil
¼ cup pine nuts, toasted
A pinch of salt and black pepper
DIRECTIONS:
In a salad bowl, mix the cucumber with the cherry tomatoes, avocado, bell pepper, basil, parsley, salt, pepper, oil and pine nuts. Toss the mix together then divide between plates and serve for breakfast.
Enjoy!
Nutrition: calories 181, fat 4, fiber 4, carbs 11, protein 5

9) Bean Sprout Breakfast Salad

PREPARATION TIME: 10 minutes
COOKING TIME: 2 minutes
SERVINGS: 2
INGREDIENTS:
1½ cups mixed bean sprouts, soaked for 12 hours and drained
1/3 cup tomato, cubed
1/3 cup carrot, grated
1 cucumber, sliced
½ cup yellow onion, chopped
10 mint leaves, chopped
1 tablespoon olive oil
1 tablespoon chaat masala
1 tablespoon lemon juice
A pinch of salt and black pepper
DIRECTIONS:
Heat up a pan with the oil over medium-high heat, add the bean sprouts, toss and cook for 1 minute. Add the tomato, carrot, cucumber, onion, mint, chaat masala, lemon juice, salt and pepper then toss and cook for 1-2 minutes more. Divide into bowls and serve for breakfast.
Enjoy!
Nutrition: calories 177, fat 2, fiber 6, carbs 15. protein 6

10) Fruit and Veggie Mix

PREPARATION TIME: 10 minutes
COOKING TIME: 0 minutes
SERVINGS: 3
INGREDIENTS: 1 cup baby spinach, torn
6 lettuce leaves, torn
1 peach, chopped
1 mango, cubed
1 cucumber, sliced
10 strawberries, halved
1 tablespoon hemp seeds
1 tablespoon tahini paste
1 tablespoon lime juice
1 tablespoon coconut water
1 teaspoon dates, chopped
½ teaspoon spirulina powder
DIRECTIONS:
In a bowl, mix the tahini paste with the lime juice, water, dates and spirulina, stir well. In a separate salad bowl, mix the spinach with the lettuce, peach, mango, cucumber, strawberries and hemp seeds. Toss the salad together then add the salad dressing and toss again. Serve for breakfast. Enjoy!
Nutrition: calories 143, fat 2, fiber 4, carbs 30, protein 4

11) Rosemary Oats

PREPARATION TIME: 10 minutes
COOKING TIME: 15 minutes
SERVINGS: 2
INGREDIENTS:
½ cup almond milk, unsweetened
½ cup water - ½ cup oats
½ teaspoon coconut oil, melted
½ cup chopped onion
½ cup sliced white mushrooms
½ cup chopped collard greens
½ cup chopped tomato
½ tablespoon chopped rosemary
A pinch of salt and black pepper
DIRECTIONS: Heat up a pan with the coconut oil over medium-high heat. Add the onion, stir and cook for 1-2 minutes. Add the mushrooms, the collard greens, tomato, rosemary, salt and pepper, stir and cook for

5 minutes more then take off the heat. Heat up a small pot with the almond milk and the water over medium heat. Add the oats, stir and cook for 4-5 minutes. Add the collard greens mix to the pan with the oats, stir and cook for 5 minutes more. Divide into bowls and serve for breakfast. Enjoy!
Nutrition: calories 211, fat 3, fiber 6, carbs 15, protein 7

12) Garlic Swiss Chard Bowls

PREPARATION TIME: 10 minutes
COOKING TIME: 5 minutes
SERVINGS: 4
INGREDIENTS:
1 bunch Swiss chard, chopped
1 garlic clove, minced
2 teaspoons olive oil
1 cup quinoa, cooked
½ cup cherry tomatoes, halved
1 carrot, shredded
1 roasted red pepper, cubed
1 green onion, chopped
A pinch of salt and black pepper
2 teaspoons lemon juice
4 eggs, fried
DIRECTIONS: Heat up a pan with the olive oil over medium-high heat, add the chard, stir and cook for 1-2 minutes. Add the garlic, tomatoes, carrot, red pepper, onions, salt and pepper, toss and cook for 2 minutes more. Add the quinoa and the lemon juice, toss, cook for 1 minute, divide into bowls, top each bowl with a fried egg and serve for breakfast. Enjoy!
Nutrition: calories 211, fat 2, fiber 4, carbs 15, protein 6

13) Veggie Bowls

PREPARATION TIME: 10 minutes
COOKING TIME: 1 hour
SERVINGS: 2
INGREDIENTS: 1½ cups black barley
4 cups water - 2 cups blueberries
1 fennel bulb, shaved
1 bunch watercress

1 orange, peeled and cut into segments
1 small red onion, sliced
¼ cup walnuts
1 avocado, peeled, pitted and cubed
For the dressing:
½ cup orange juice
¼ cup olive oil
1 small red onion, chopped
2 tablespoons red vinegar
1 tablespoon raw honey
1 teaspoon bee pollen
A pinch of salt and black pepper
DIRECTIONS: Put the barley in a small pot, add the water and bring it to a simmer, Cook for 1 hour, drain and let the mix cool down before putting it in a salad bowl. Add the blueberries, fennel, watercress, orange, 1 red onion, avocado and walnuts and toss. In another bowl, whisk together the orange juice with the oil, onion, vinegar, honey, bee pollen, salt and pepper. Pour over the salad and serve for breakfast. Enjoy!
Nutrition: calories 216, fat 11, fiber 7, carbs 15, protein 5

14) Chili Veggie Bowls

PREPARATION TIME: 10 minutes
COOKING TIME: 0 minutes
SERVINGS: 2
INGREDIENTS:
½ cup quinoa, cooked
1 scallion, chopped
1 sweet potato, peeled, cooked and cubed
1 bunch broccolini, steamed
2 carrots, shredded
¼ cup pomegranate seeds
A handful bean sprouts, soaked for 12 hours, drained
1 teaspoon sesame seeds
1 tablespoon olive oil
2 tablespoons orange juice
1 teaspoon coconut aminos
1 teaspoon sesame oil
1 teaspoon chili paste
1 teaspoon white vinegar
DIRECTIONS:
In a bowl, whisk the sesame oil with the orange juice, aminos, chili paste and vinegar.

In a separate salad bowl, mix the scallion with the quinoa, sweet potato, broccolini, carrots, pomegranate seeds, bean sprouts, sesame seeds and olive oil. Add the chili mix and toss the salad together then serve for breakfast.

Enjoy!

Nutrition: calories 171, fat 2, fiber 6, carbs 11, protein 5

15) Colorful Veggie Mix

PREPARATION TIME: 10 minutes
COOKING TIME: 0 minutes
SERVINGS: 4
INGREDIENTS:
1½ cups coconut cream
½ cup coconut milk
2 tablespoons olive oil
2 teaspoons white vinegar
1 garlic clove, minced
1 teaspoon chopped dill
¼ cup chopped parsley
1 handful chives, chopped
1 jalapeno, chopped
1 cup quinoa, cooked
1 cup beans sprouts, soaked for 12 hours and drained
2 cups cherry tomatoes, halved
1½ cups sliced cucumbers
2 avocados, peeled, pitted and cubed
A handful basil, chopped
1 tablespoon crushed almonds
A pinch of salt and black pepper
DIRECTIONS:
In a salad bowl, mix the quinoa with the bean sprouts, tomatoes, cucumbers, avocados, basil, almonds, salt and pepper. In a separate bowl, whisk the oil with the vinegar, garlic, coconut milk and cream, dill, parsley, chives and jalapeno. Add the dressing to your salad, toss and serve for breakfast.

Enjoy!

Nutrition: calories 199, fat 4, fiber 8, carbs 15, protein 4

16) Sweet Mediterranean Veggie Mix

PREPARATION TIME: 10 minutes
COOKING TIME: 30 minutes
SERVINGS: 4
INGREDIENTS:
2 zucchinis, cubed
1 eggplant, cubed
2 cups quinoa, cooked
1 tablespoon olive oil
½ teaspoon smoked paprika
A pinch of chili powder
1 tablespoon lemon juice
A pinch of salt and black pepper
1 tablespoon chopped oregano
4 cups baby arugula, torn
For the sauce:
½ cup sesame seeds paste
2 tablespoons lemon juice
1 teaspoon red wine vinegar
1 garlic clove, minced
1 teaspoon real maple syrup
¾ teaspoon harissa paste
½ teaspoon smoked paprika
½ teaspoon ground cumin
¾ cup water
DIRECTIONS:
Spread the zucchinis and the eggplant on a lined baking sheet and season with ½ teaspoon smoked paprika, chili powder, salt, pepper, and ½ tablespoon oil. Toss the veggies to coat in the seasoning then bake in the oven at 400 degrees F for 30 minutes. Cool the veggies down, put them in a salad bowl and add the oregano, baby arugula, quinoa, ½ tablespoon oil and lemon juice. Mix together briefly. In another bowl, whisk together the sesame paste with 2 tablespoons lemon juice, vinegar, garlic, maple syrup, harissa paste, ½ teaspoon smoked paprika, cumin and water. Pour the dressing over the salad, toss and serve for breakfast.

Enjoy!

Nutrition: calories 226, fat 5, fiber 7, carbs 16, protein 7g

17) **Breakfast Pizza**

PREPARATION TIME: 10 minutes
COOKING TIME: 20 minutes
SERVINGS: 4
INGREDIENTS:
5 oz chorizo, chopped
4 oz Parmesan, grated
½ teaspoon basil
1 cup almond flour
4 tablespoons butter
½ teaspoon salt
½ teaspoon paprika
5 oz Mozzarella, sliced
1 tomato, diced
DIRECTIONS:
In the mixing bowl, mix up together almond flour with butter, and salt.
Knead the soft dough.
Roll it up to get the shape of the pizza crust. Line the tray with the baking paper and transfer the dough on it.
Sprinkle it with the diced tomato and basil.
Add paprika and chorizo.
Then make the later of Mozzarella cheese and Parmesan.
Preheat the oven to 370F.
Place the tray with pizza inside and cook it for 20 minutes or until the pie crust is light brown.
Then cut the pizza into servings.
Nutrition: calories 498, fat 41, fiber 1, carbs 5.2, protein 29.5

18) **Zucchini and Egg Breakfast Bowl**

PREPARATION TIME: 10 minutes
COOKING TIME: 2 hours
SERVINGS: 4
INGREDIENTS:
2 zucchinis, cut with a spiralizer
1 small avocado, pitted, peeled and chopped
2 tablespoons water
4 tablespoons olive oil
2 sweet potatoes, peeled and cubed
2 tablespoons chopped green onion
2 garlic cloves, minced

2 eggs, whisked
A pinch of salt and black pepper
DIRECTIONS: Heat up a pan with the oil over medium-high heat. Add the green onion and garlic, a pinch of salt and pepper then stir and cook for 2-3 minutes. Transfer the mix to your slow cooker. Add zucchinis, water, potatoes and whisked eggs, toss, cover and cook on High for 2 hours. Divide the mix into bowls, top each with some avocado pieces and serve for breakfast. Enjoy!
Nutrition: calories 211, fat 2, fiber 5, carbs 16, protein 5

19) **Eggs Benedict**

PREPARATION TIME: 7 minutes
COOKING TIME: 10 minutes
SERVINGS: 2
INGREDIENTS:
2 eggs
2 oz bacon, sliced
1 tablespoon butter
½ teaspoon ground black pepper
1 pinch salt
1 cup water for cooking
DIRECTIONS:
Pour water in the saucepan and add salt. Close the lid and cook it until it starts to boil. Meanwhile, Place sliced bacon in the skillet and roast it for 1 minute over the medium heat from each side. Sprinkle the cooked bacon with the ground black pepper and transfer on the serving plates. Beat the eggs in the boiled water gently to not damage them. Cook the eggs for 3-4 minutes over the medium heat or until the egg white will get white color.
Transfer the cooked eggs over the bacon with the help of the ladle.
Sprinkle the eggs with the spices if desired.
Nutrition: calories 269, fat 22, fiber 0.1, carbs 1.1, protein 16.2

20) **Mushroom Frittata**

PREPARATION TIME: 10 minutes
COOKING TIME: 30 minutes

SERVINGS: 6
INGREDIENTS:
6 eggs, whisked
1 cup mushrooms, sliced
1 oz fresh parsley, chopped
3 oz Parmesan, grated
½ teaspoon ground black pepper
1 teaspoon paprika
1 teaspoon turmeric
½ cup broccoli, chopped
1 tablespoon butter
¾ cup of water
DIRECTIONS:
Place butter in the pan.
Add mushrooms and sprinkle them with the ground black pepper.
Cook the mushrooms for 5 minutes over the medium heat. Stir them from time to time.
Add broccoli and mix up. Add water and close the lid.
Saute the vegetables for 10 minutes.
Then add whisked eggs, chopped parsley, Parmesan, paprika, turmeric, and mix it up.
Close the lid and cook the frittata for 15 minutes or place in the oven and cook for 10 minutes at 375F.
Chill the cooked frittata to the room temperature and cut into the servings.
Nutrition: calories 135, fat 9.5, fiber 0.7, carbs 2.6, protein 10.9

21) Stuffed Avocado

PREPARATION TIME: 10 minutes
SERVINGS: 4
INGREDIENTS:
2 avocado, halved, pitted
8 oz smoked salmon, chopped
1 teaspoon fresh dill, chopped
½ teaspoon garlic powder
4 tablespoons ricotta cheese
DIRECTIONS:
Mix up together ricotta cheese, dill, and chopped smoked paprika.
Then remove the flesh from the avocado and finely chop it.
Ad dit in the cheese mixture and stir.
Fill the avocado halves with ricotta cheese and transfer on the serving plates.

Nutrition: calories 295, fat 23.3, fiber 6.8, carbs 9.8, protein 14.2

22) Croque Madame

PREPARATION TIME: 10 minutes
COOKING TIME: 10 minutes
SERVINGS: 2
INGREDIENTS:
½ cup cottage cheese
2 teaspoons ground flax meal
5 eggs, whisked
½ teaspoon salt
1 tablespoon coconut oil
½ white onion, diced
2 oz Cheddar cheese, sliced
DIRECTIONS:
In the mixing bowl, mix up together cottage cheese, ground flax meal, eggs, and salt.
Add diced onion and stir it well.
Toss coconut oil in the skillet and melt it.
Then with the help of the ladle pour the egg mixture in the hot coconut oil. Shake the skillet gently to make the shape of the pancake.
Cook the meal for 3 minutes from each side over the medium-high heat.
Repeat the same steps with all the egg mixture. You should get 4 egg pancakes.
Then place slices Cheddar into 2 egg pancakes and cover them with the remaining egg pancakes.
Transfer croque madame on the serving plates.
Nutrition: calories 404, fat 29.1, fiber 1.3, carbs 6.7, protein 29.5

23) Breakfast Chai Latte

PREPARATION TIME: 5 minutes
COOKING TIME: 5 minutes
SERVINGS: 4
INGREDIENTS:
2 tablespoons chai tea
3 cups of water
1 cup heavy cream, whipped
DIRECTIONS:

Boil water and put chai tea in it. Close the lid and let it rest for 10 minutes.

Then strain the water and pour it in the serving cups.

Add whipped cream and stir gently.

Nutrition: calories 104, fat 11.1, fiber 0, carbs 0.8, protein 0.6

24) Cauliflower-Meat Skillet

PREPARATION TIME: 10 minutes
COOKING TIME: 25 minutes
SERVINGS: 4
INGREDIENTS:
1 cup ground beef
1 cup cauliflower florets
1 teaspoon chili flakes
½ cup heavy cream
1 white onion, diced
1 tablespoon olive oil
½ teaspoon salt
½ teaspoon ground black pepper
DIRECTIONS:
Place the ground beef in the pan and sprinkle it with the chili flakes, ground black pepper, and salt.

Add olive oil and mix up the mixture. Close the lid and cook it for 10 minutes.

Meanwhile, finely chop the cauliflower florets and add them in the ground beef mixture.

Mix up well and add the onion.

Then add heavy cream and stir the meal.

Preheat oven to 365F and place the pan with a meal inside.

Cook it for 15 minutes or until cauliflower is cooked.

Nutrition: calories 165, fat 13.2, fiber 1.3, carbs 4.5, protein 7.7

25) Broccoli Muffins

PREPARATION TIME: 10 minutes
COOKING TIME: 10 minutes
SERVINGS: 6
INGREDIENTS:
6 tablespoons almond flour

1/3 cup broccoli, chopped
6 eggs, whisked
½ teaspoon salt
3 teaspoons butter
DIRECTIONS:
Spread the muffin molds with the butter.

After this, mix up together almond flour, whisked eggs, and salt in the mixing bowl.

Add chopped broccoli and stir gently with the help of the spoon.

Then pour the egg mixture in the prepared muffin molds.

Preheat the oven to 365F.

Place the molds of the muffin in the preheated oven and cook them for 10 minutes.

The muffins are cooked when they are solid.

Remove them from the oven and chill little before serving.

Nutrition: calories 241, fat 20.3, fiber 3.1, carbs 6.7, protein 11.7

26) Kale Egg Ramekins

PREPARATION TIME: 10 minutes
COOKING TIME: 20 minutes
SERVINGS: 4
INGREDIENTS:
4 eggs
3 oz Mozzarella, shredded
1 cup kale, chopped
½ teaspoon cayenne pepper
½ teaspoon salt
1 teaspoon butter
DIRECTIONS:
Place butter in the skillet and melt it.

Add chopped kale and salt. Mix up the mixture and close the lid.

Saute the kale for 5 minutes over the medium heat.

Then transfer the kale in the ramekins. Add shredded Mozzarella cheese.

Beat the eggs over Mozzarella and sprinkle with the cayenne pepper.

Cover the ramekins with foil.

Preheat the oven to 375F.

Place the ramekins in the train and transfer in the preheated oven.

Cook the breakfast for 15 minutes.

Nutrition: calories 140, fat 9.1, fiber 0.3, carbs 3, protein 12.1

27) Avocado Eggs in Bacon

PREPARATION TIME: 10 minutes
COOKING TIME: 15 minutes
SERVINGS: 6
INGREDIENTS:
1 avocado, peeled, pitted
6 bacon slices
2 eggs, boiled, chopped
1 tablespoon heavy cream
½ teaspoon salt
1 teaspoon white pepper
1 tablespoon coconut oil
DIRECTIONS:
Mash the avocado and mix it up with chopped eggs.
After this, heavy cream, salt, and white pepper. Mix it up again.
Make 6 balls from the mixture and wrap each ball in the slices bacon.
Secure the bacon balls with the toothpick.
Place coconut oil in the skillet and melt it.
Transfer the avocado balls in the skillet and roast them for 1 minute from each side.
Meanwhile, preheat oven to 365F.
Transfer the skillet with bacon balls in the oven and cook for 10 minutes.
Nutrition: calories 221, fat 19.1, fiber 2.3, carbs 3.6, protein 9.6

28) Morning Fritters

PREPARATION TIME: 10 minutes
COOKING TIME: 10 minutes
SERVINGS: 4
INGREDIENTS:
1 zucchini, grated
1 egg, whisked
4 tablespoons almond flour
½ teaspoon ground coriander
¼ teaspoon salt
1 teaspoon olive oil
½ carrot, grated
DIRECTIONS:

In the mixing bowl, mix up together grated zucchini and carrot.
Add the whisked egg, almond flour, ground coriander, and salt. Mix the mixture up.
Then preheat the skillet well and pour olive oil.
With the help of two spoons make medium size fritters and transfer them in the pre-heated skillet.
Cook them for 2 minutes from each side.
Dry the fritters with the help of the paper towel and transfer on the serving plates.
Nutrition: calories 197, fat 16.4, fiber 3.7, carbs 8.5, protein 8

29) Egg Muffins

PREPARATION TIME: 10 minutes
COOKING TIME: 15 minutes
SERVINGS: 2
INGREDIENTS:
4 eggs, whisked
1 bell pepper, chopped
1 tablespoon coconut flour
1 tablespoon sour cream
½ teaspoon chili flakes
DIRECTIONS:
In the mixing bowl, mix up together eggs, chopped bell pepper, coconut flour, sour cream, and chili flakes.
Then pour the liquid into the non-sticky muffin molds.
Preheat oven to 365F.
Place the muffin molds in the oven and cook for 15 minutes.
Chill the cooked muffins little and remove them from the molds.
Nutrition: calories 173, fat 10.5, fiber 2.3, carbs 8, protein 12.4

30) Brussel Sprout Eggs

PREPARATION TIME: 10 minutes
COOKING TIME: 20 minutes
SERVINGS: 4
INGREDIENTS:
1 cup Brussel Sprouts
1 red onion, sliced

1 tablespoon coconut oil
½ teaspoon ground black pepper
¾ teaspoon sumac
½ cup almond milk
4 eggs

DIRECTIONS:

Cut Brussel sprouts into halves and place in the pan.

Add sliced red onion, coconut oil, and ground black pepper.

Cook the vegetables on medium-high heat for 5 minutes. Stir them from time to time.

Then sprinkle the vegetables with sumac. Add almond milk and stir it. Close the lid.

Saute the vegetables for 10 minutes more.

Then beat the eggs over the vegetables and cook for 5 minutes.

Let the cooked meal chill little before serving.

Nutrition: calories 182, fat 15, fiber 2.2, carbs 6.7, protein 7.3

31) Coconut Porridge

PREPARATION TIME: 5 minutes
COOKING TIME: 15 minutes
SERVINGS: 2
INGREDIENTS:

1 tablespoon coconut shred
2 eggs, beaten
3 tablespoon butter
3 tablespoons coconut flour
½ cup coconut cream

DIRECTIONS:

Whisk the eggs and transfer them in the saucepan.

Ad coconut shred, butter, coconut flour, and coconut cream. Mix up the mixture until smooth.

Close the lid and saute it on the low heat for 15-20 minutes.

When the mixture gets porridge texture it is cooked. Transfer the meal in the serving plates.

Nutrition: calories 423, fat 39.5, fiber 6.2, carbs 11.1, protein 9.5

32) Avocado Smoothie

PREPARATION TIME: 10 minutes
SERVINGS: 2
INGREDIENTS:

1 avocado, pitted
½ cup of coconut milk
1 teaspoon chia seeds
1 scoop protein powder
½ teaspoon Erythritol

DIRECTIONS:

Remove the flesh from the avocado with the help of the spoon and transfer it in the food processor.

Add coconut milk, chia seeds, protein powder, and Erythritol.

Blend the mixture until smooth and homogenous.

Pour the cooked smoothie in the serving glasses.

Nutrition: calories 421, fat 35.9, fiber 9.3, carbs 16.1, protein 14.9

33) Seafood Omelette

PREPARATION TIME: 8 minutes
COOKING TIME: 15 minutes
SERVINGS: 2
INGREDIENTS:

¼ cup heavy cream
4 eggs, whisked
6 oz shrimps, peeled
¼ teaspoon salt
½ teaspoon ground black pepper
1 teaspoon butter
1 teaspoon dried dill
½ teaspoon ground coriander

DIRECTIONS:

Chop the shrimps roughly and place them in the pan.

Add butter and cook them for 3 minutes over the medium-high heat.

Then add salt, ground black pepper, dried dill, and ground coriander.

In the mixing bowl, mix up together whisked eggs with heavy cream.

Pour the liquid over the shrimps and stir gently.

Close the lid and set the heat on Low.
Cook the omelet for 10 minutes.
Cut it into servings.
Nutrition: calories 298, fat 17.7, fiber 0.2, carbs 3, protein 30.9

34) Breakfast Beef Casserole

PREPARATION TIME: 15 minutes
COOKING TIME: 45 minutes
SERVINGS: 6
INGREDIENTS:
1 cup broccoli florets
½ cup cauliflower florets
8 oz Parmesan, grated
1 cup heavy cream
1 tablespoon butter
8 oz beef brisket, chopped
1 white onion, sliced
1 teaspoon coconut oil
3 tablespoon pork rind
½ teaspoon ground black pepper
1 teaspoon dried dill
DIRECTIONS:
Rub the casserole mold with butter.
Mix up together chopped beef brisket, ground black pepper, and dried dill.
Transfer the meat in the casserole mold and flatten it to get the layer.
Then place the layer of broccoli over it.
Sprinkle with ¼ part of all Parmesan.
After this, add sliced onion and cauliflower florets.
Sprinkle the casserole with the pork rind and remaining Parmesan.
Add heavy cream and cover the casserole with foil. Secure the edges of the mold and pin the foil to make small holes.
Preheat the oven to 365F.
Put the casserole in the preheated oven and cook it for 45 minutes.
Then let the casserole rest for 10-15 minutes and transfer it in the serving plates.
Nutrition: calories 333, fat 22.7, fiber 1.1, carbs 5.3, protein 28.6

35) Winter Fruit Salad

PREPARATION TIME: 10 minutes
COOKING TIME: 0 minutes
SERVINGS: 6
INGREDIENTS:
4 persimmons, cubed
4 pears, cubed
1 cup grapes, halved
1 cup apples, peeled, cored and cubed
¾ cup pecans halved
1 tablespoon olive oil
1 tablespoon peanut oil
1 tablespoon pomegranate flavored vinegar
2 tablespoons agave nectar
DIRECTIONS:
In a salad bowl, mix the persimmons with the pears, grapes, apples, and pecans. In another bowl, mix the olive oil with the peanut oil, vinegar and agave nectar. Whisk well then pour over the salad, toss and serve for breakfast.
Enjoy!
Nutrition: calories 125, fat 3, fiber 6, carbs 14, protein 8

36) Rhubarb Vanilla Muffins

PREPARATION TIME: 10 minutes
COOKING TIME: 25 minutes
SERVINGS: 8
INGREDIENTS:
½ cup almond meal
2 tablespoons crystallized ginger
¼ cup coconut sugar
1 tablespoon linseed meal
½ cup buckwheat flour
¼ cup brown rice flour
2 tablespoons powdered arrowroot
2 teaspoon gluten-free baking powder
½ teaspoon fresh grated ginger
½ teaspoon ground cinnamon
1 cup rhubarb, sliced
1 apple, cored, peeled and chopped
1/3 cup almond milk, unsweetened
¼ cup olive oil
1 free-range egg
1 teaspoon vanilla extract

DIRECTIONS:
In a bowl, mix the almond meal with the crystallized ginger, sugar, linseed meal, buckwheat flour, rice flour, arrowroot powder, grated ginger, baking powder, and cinnamon and stir. In another bowl, mix the rhubarb with the apple, almond milk, oil, egg, and vanilla and stir well. Combine the 2 mixtures, stir well, and divide into a lined muffin tray. Place in the oven at 350 degrees F and bake for 25 minutes. Serve the muffins for breakfast.
Enjoy!

37) **Cocoa Buckwheat**

38) **Granola**

PREPARATION TIME: 10 minutes
COOKING TIME: 45 minutes
SERVINGS: 6
INGREDIENTS:
2 cups oats
1 cup buckwheat
1 cup sunflower seeds
1 cup pumpkin seeds
1½ cups dates, pitted and chopped
1 cup apple puree
6 tablespoons coconut oil
5 tablespoons cocoa powder
1 teaspoon fresh grated ginger
DIRECTIONS:
In a large bowl, mix the oats with the buckwheat, sunflower seeds, pumpkin seeds, dates, apple puree, oil, cocoa powder and ginger then stir really well. Spread on a lined baking sheet, press well and place in the oven at 360 degrees F for 45 minutes. Leave the granola to cool down, slice and serve for breakfast.
Enjoy!
Nutrition: calories 161, fat 3, fiber 5, carbs 11, protein 7

Mains

39) Chicken Salad

PREPARATION TIME: 10 minutes
COOKING TIME: 10 minutes
SERVINGS: 4
INGREDIENTS:
2 sweet potatoes, baked
A drizzle of olive oil
1 yellow onion, chopped
12 ounces mushrooms, chopped
2 garlic cloves, minced
½ teaspoon dried thyme
3 cups chicken, already cooked and shredded
2 cups baby spinach

40) Zucchini Mix

PREPARATION TIME: 10 minutes
COOKING TIME: 20 minutes
SERVINGS: 4
INGREDIENTS:
¼ cup olive oil
2 zucchinis, cut into small rounds
1 red bell pepper, cut into thin strips
1 yellow onion, cut into medium wedges
1 eggplant, cubed
A pinch of ground turmeric
A pinch of salt and black pepper
1 tablespoons capers
10 cherry tomatoes, halved

41) Spicy Cauliflower Stew

PREPARATION TIME: 10 minutes
COOKING TIME: 35 minutes
SERVINGS: 2
INGREDIENTS:
1 teaspoon ground coriander
½ teaspoon ground turmeric
A pinch of cayenne pepper
½ teaspoon garam masala
2 cups vegetable stock
A pinch of salt and black pepper
1 teaspoon lemon juice
DIRECTIONS:

A pinch of salt and cayenne pepper
A splash of balsamic vinegar
DIRECTIONS:
Cut potatoes in half lengthwise, scoop out the flesh, chop it and put in a bowl. Heat up a pan with the oil over medium-high heat. Add onion, potato flesh, garlic, mushrooms, thyme, chicken, salt and cayenne pepper, toss, cook for 10 minutes, take off heat and transfer to the bowl with the sweet potato flesh. Add the spinach and the vinegar, toss and serve.
Enjoy!
Nutrition: calories 260, fat 2, fiber 8, carbs 17, protein 11

2 tablespoons pine nuts
1 tablespoons raisins
1 bunch basil, chopped
DIRECTIONS:
Heat up a pan with the oil over medium-high heat, add the onion, salt, pepper and turmeric, mix and cook for 5 minutes. Add the zucchini, bell pepper and eggplant, mix and cook for 5 minutes more. Add the capers, tomatoes, pine nuts and raisins, mix and cook for 10 minutes over medium heat. Add the basil, stir, cook for another minute more. Divide into bowls and serve for lunch.
Enjoy!
Nutrition: calories 162, fat 3, fiber 4, carbs 12, protein 7
½ teaspoon olive oil
1 small cauliflower head, florets separated
½ teaspoon cumin seeds
½ cup red onion, chopped
2 tomatoes, chopped
1 teaspoon fresh grated ginger
4 garlic cloves, minced
In your blender, add the tomatoes with garlic, onions, ginger, salt, pepper, garam masala, cayenne, coriander and turmeric and pulse really well. Heat up a pot with the oil over medium heat, add the tomato mix, stir and sauté for 15 minutes. Add cauliflower, stock, salt, pepper, lemon juice and cumin,

stir, cover and simmer over medium heat for 20 minutes. Divide into bowls and serve. Enjoy!
Nutrition: calories 200, fat 6, fiber 7, carbs 10, protein 8

43)Green Bean Mix

PREPARATION TIME: 10 minutes
COOKING TIME: 25 minutes
SERVINGS: 4
INGREDIENTS:
2 tablespoons olive oil
2 carrots, chopped
1 yellow onion, chopped
1 sweet potato, cubed
14 ounces green beans
2 garlic cloves, minced
14 ounces canned tomatoes, chopped
1 cup corn
5 cups water
A pinch of salt and black pepper
1 tablespoon chopped cilantro
DIRECTIONS:
Heat up a pan with the oil over medium heat, add onion, stir and cook for 5 minutes. Add carrots, sweet potato, green beans, garlic, to-matoes, corn, salt, pepper and water, stir, cover and cook over medium heat for 20 minutes Add the cilantro, stir, divide into bowls and serve.
Enjoy!
Nutrition: calories 201, fat 5, fiber 5, carbs 8, protein 11

44) Chickpea Stew

PREPARATION TIME: 10 minutes
COOKING TIME: 50 minutes
SERVINGS: 4
INGREDIENTS:
1 teaspoon olive oil
1 cup chickpeas, soaked for 4 hours and drained
4 garlic cloves, minced
1 small yellow onion, chopped
1 green chili pepper, chopped
1-inch fresh ginger, grated

42)

1 teaspoon ground coriander
½ teaspoon ground cumin
½ teaspoon sweet paprika
2 tomatoes, chopped
1½ cups water
A pinch of salt and black pepper
3 cups spinach leaves
1 tablespoon lemon juice
1 cup coconut milk, unsweetened
DIRECTIONS:
Heat up a pot with the oil over medium heat, add garlic, ginger, chili and onion. Stir and cook for 5 minutes. Add tomatoes, cumin, paprika, coriander, chickpeas, water, salt and pepper to the pot. Stir, bring to a simmer and cook for 45 minutes. Add spinach, lemon juice and coconut milk, stir and cook for 10 minutes more. Divide into bowls and serve.
Enjoy!
Nutrition: calories 250, fat 7, fiber 6, carbs 9, protein 12

45)Spicy Eggplant Stew

PREPARATION TIME: 10 minutes
COOKING TIME: 15 minutes
SERVINGS: 3
INGREDIENTS:
½ teaspoon cumin seeds
1 tablespoon coriander seeds
½ teaspoon mustard seeds
5 eggplants, cubed
2 tablespoon coconut, shredded, unsweet-ened
1 teaspoon fresh grated ginger
2 garlic cloves, minced
1 green chili pepper, chopped
A pinch of cayenne pepper
A pinch of ground cinnamon
½ teaspoon ground cardamom
½ teaspoon ground turmeric
A pinch of salt and black pepper
1 teaspoon lime juice

1 cup vegetable stock
1 tablespoon chopped parsley
DIRECTIONS:
Heat up a pan over medium-high heat and add the cumin, coriander, mustard seeds, coconut, ginger, garlic, chili pepper, cayenne, cinnamon, cardamom, turmeric, salt and pepper. Stir and cook for 5-6 minutes. Transfer to a food processor and pulse. Transfer to a pot and heat up over medium heat. Add the stock, the eggplant, lime juice and the parsley. Mix and cook over medium heat for 30 minutes. Divide into bowls and serve.
Enjoy!
Nutrition: calories 300, fat 4, fiber 7, carbs 8, protein 9

46) **Beans and Cauliflower Stew**

PREPARATION TIME: 10 minutes
COOKING TIME: 1 hour
SERVINGS: 4
INGREDIENTS:
1 cup black beans, soaked for 12 hours and drained
4 garlic cloves, minced
1 yellow onion, chopped
½ teaspoon garam masala
1-inch fresh grated ginger
½ teaspoon ground coriander
½ teaspoon cayenne pepper
1 teaspoon ground turmeric
2 cups unsweetened coconut shredded
2 tomatoes, pureed
1 ½ cups cauliflower florets
2 cups veggie stock
A pinch of salt and black pepper
1 teaspoon olive oil
½ teaspoon cumin seeds
DIRECTIONS:
Heat up a pot with the oil over medium heat. Add cumin, onion, ginger and garlic, stir and cook for 5 minutes. Add the beans, coriander, cayenne pepper, turmeric, coconut, tomatoes, cauliflower, salt, pepper and stock.

Stir, cover the pot, cook over medium heat for 1 hour, divide into bowls and serve.
Enjoy!
Nutrition: calories 219, fat 8, fiber 8, carbs 12, protein 8

47) **Squash and Chickpea Stew**

PREPARATION TIME: 10 minutes
COOKING TIME: 1 hour
SERVINGS: 2
INGREDIENTS:
2 cups chickpeas, soaked overnight and drained
2 cups veggie stock
1 butternut squash, cubed
1 teaspoon olive oil
½ cup red onion, chopped
½ teaspoon cumin seeds
4 garlic cloves minced
1 green chili, chopped
½ inch fresh grated ginger
½ teaspoon garam masala
¼ teaspoon ground turmeric
1 teaspoon lime juice
2 tomatoes chopped
A pinch of salt and black pepper
A pinch of cayenne pepper
1 cup spinach
1 tablespoon chopped cilantro
DIRECTIONS:
Heat up a pot with the oil over medium heat. Add cumin, chili, garlic, ginger and onions, stir and sauté them for 5 minutes. Add turmeric, garam masala, lime juice, spinach, tomato, stir and cook for 5 minutes. Add chickpeas, stock, salt, pepper, cayenne, squash, stir, simmer over medium heat for 45 minutes. Add the spinach and the cilantro, mix and cook for 5 minutes more than divide into bowls and serve.
Enjoy!
Nutrition: calories 281, fat 6, fiber 4, carbs 8, protein 12

48) **Black Beans Chili**

PREPARATION TIME: 10 minutes
COOKING TIME: 1 hour and 15 minutes
SERVINGS: 6
INGREDIENTS:
1 red bell pepper, chopped
2 teaspoons olive oil
2 yellow onions, chopped
6 garlic cloves, minced
1 green bell pepper, chopped
24 ounces canned black beans, drained
6 cups veggie stock
1 tablespoon cocoa powder
2 tablespoons chili powder, mild
2 teaspoons ground cumin
½ teaspoon chipotle powder
2 teaspoons smoked paprika
30 ounces canned tomatoes, chopped
1/3 cup quinoa
1½ cups corn
A pinch of salt and black pepper
DIRECTIONS:
Heat up a pot with the oil over medium heat. Add onions, stir and cook them for 5 minutes. Add red peppers, green bell peppers, garlic, stock, beans, cocoa powder, chili powder, cumin, chipotle powder, paprika and tomatoes. Stir everything together, cover and cook over medium heat for about 50 minutes. Add quinoa, corn, salt and pepper, stir, cook for 10-15 minutes more then divide into bowls and serve.
Enjoy!
Nutrition: calories 300, fat 2, fiber 10, carbs 15, protein 11

49) **Black Bean and Corn Soup**

PREPARATION TIME: 10 minutes
COOKING TIME: 1 hour
SERVINGS: 6
INGREDIENTS:
1 yellow onion, chopped
1 pound black beans, soaked for a few hours and drained
2 teaspoons ground cumin
6 cups veggie stock
12 ounces corn
¼ teaspoon chipotle powder
1 cup salsa
DIRECTIONS:
Pour the stock into a pot and heat over medium. Add the onion, the beans, cumin, corn, chipotle powder and salsa, mix, bring to a boil and cook for 1 hour. Ladle into bowls and serve.
Enjoy!
Nutrition: calories 224, fat 2, fiber 12, carbs 10, protein 17

50) **Barley Soup with Mushrooms**

PREPARATION TIME: 10 minutes
COOKING TIME: 1 hour and 10 minutes
SERVINGS: 4
INGREDIENTS:
2 yellow onions, chopped
¼ cup pearl barley
4 cups veggie stock
6 ounces brown mushrooms, halved
A pinch of salt and black pepper
3 garlic cloves, minced
2 teaspoons chopped thyme
12 ounces cabbage, shredded
½ teaspoon smoked paprika
½ teaspoon hot paprika
4 cups water
16 ounces canned black beans, drained and rinsed
1 tablespoon lemon juice
DIRECTIONS:
In a pot, mix stock with the barley. Stir, bring to a simmer over medium heat and cook for 30 minutes. Add mushrooms, cabbage, smoked paprika, hot paprika, garlic, onions, salt, pepper, thyme, beans, lemon juice and water. Stir, cover the pot, cook over medium heat for 40 minutes more. Ladle into bowls and serve.
Enjoy!
Nutrition: calories 100, fat 0, fiber 7, carbs 19, protein 5

51) **Spicy Sweet Potato Soup**

PREPARATION TIME: 10 minutes
COOKING TIME: 35 minutes
SERVINGS: 4
INGREDIENTS:
2 tablespoons olive oil
4 garlic cloves, minced
1 yellow onion, chopped
2 tablespoons chopped cilantro
1 small red chili, chopped
2 teaspoons ground cumin
A pinch of salt and black pepper
1 teaspoon sweet paprika
1 teaspoon coriander seeds
1 pound sweet potatoes, cubed
3 cups water
Juice of ½ lime
10 ounces canned black beans, drained and rinsed
2 cups tomatoes, chopped
A handful parsley, chopped
DIRECTIONS:
Heat up a pot with the oil over medium heat then add the onion, stir and cook for 5 minutes. Add chili, garlic, salt, pepper, cilantro, cumin, coriander, paprika, sweet potatoes, tomatoes, black beans, water and lime juice. Stir, bring to a simmer and cook for 30 minutes. Add parsley, ladle into bowls and serve.
Enjoy!
Nutrition: calories 203, fat 5, fiber 4, carbs 7, protein 8

52) **Beet and Carrot Soup**

PREPARATION TIME: 10 minutes
COOKING TIME: 45 minutes
SERVINGS: 4
INGREDIENTS:
2 tablespoons olive oil
1 yellow onion, chopped
A pinch of salt and black pepper
1 carrot, grated
2 beets, grated
1 small green cabbage, shredded
4 garlic cloves, minced

3 tablespoons apple cider vinegar
10 porcini mushrooms, dried
1½ tablespoons tomato paste
5 cups water
1 tablespoons chopped parsley
DIRECTIONS:
Heat up a pot with the oil over medium heat, add onion, stir and cook for 5 minutes. Add beets, carrot, garlic, cabbage, mushrooms, tomato paste, vinegar, salt, pepper and water. Stir, bring to a boil and cook over medium heat for 40 minutes. Add parsley, stir, ladle into bowls and serve.
Enjoy!
Nutrition: calories 300, fat 5, fiber 9, carbs 8, protein 7

53) **Spicy Chicken and Zucchini Meatballs**

PREPARATION TIME: 10 minutes
COOKING TIME: 10 minutes
SERVINGS: 4
INGREDIENTS:
1 cup shredded zucchini
2 pounds ground chicken
2 tablespoons harissa
1 garlic clove, minced
¼ cup chopped green onions
1 egg
2 tablespoons balsamic vinegar
1 tablespoon maple syrup
A pinch of salt and black pepper
DIRECTIONS:
In a bowl, mix chicken with zucchini, green onions, egg, garlic clove, harissa, balsamic vinegar, salt, pepper and maple syrup, stir well and shape into medium meatballs. Heat up a pan with the oil over medium heat, add the meatballs and cook them for 5 minutes on each side. Divide between plates and serve for lunch with a side salad.
Enjoy!
Nutrition: calories 200, fat 2, fiber 2, carbs 14, protein 12

54) Crispy Cod

PREPARATION TIME: 10 minutes
COOKING TIME: 15 minutes
SERVINGS: 2
INGREDIENTS:
1 egg white
½ cup red quinoa, already cooked
2 teaspoons whole wheat flour
4 teaspoons lemon juice
½ teaspoon smoked paprika
3 teaspoons olive oil
2 medium black cod fillets, skinless and boneless
1 red plum, pitted and chopped
2 teaspoons raw honey
¼ teaspoon black peppercorns, crushed
2 teaspoons parsley
¼ cup water
DIRECTIONS:
In a bowl, whisk together 1 teaspoon lemon juice with egg white, flour and ¼ teaspoon paprika. Put quinoa in a bowl and mix it with 1/3 of egg white mix. Put the fish into the bowl with the remaining egg white mix, toss to coat, then dip the fish in quinoa mix and also toss to coat. Heat up a pan with 1 teaspoon oil over medium heat and add peppercorns, honey and plum. Stir, bring to a simmer and cook for 1 minute. Add the rest of the lemon juice, the rest of the paprika and the water to the pan, stir well and simmer for 5 minutes. Add parsley, stir, take the sauce off the heat and set aside for now. Heat up a pan with the rest of the olive oil over medium heat, add the coated fish cook for 3 minutes. Move the fish to a lined sheet tray and bake in the oven at 400 degrees F for 10 minutes more. Divide between plates, drizzle the plums sauce all over and serve.
Enjoy!
Nutrition: calories 324, fat 1, fiber 2, carbs 17, protein 22

55) Greek Sea Bass Mix

PREPARATION TIME: 10 minutes
COOKING TIME: 22 minutes
SERVINGS: 2
INGREDIENTS:
2 sea bass fillets, boneless
1 garlic clove, minced
5 cherry tomatoes, halved
1 tablespoon chopped parsley
2 shallots, chopped
Juice of ½ lemon
1 tablespoon olive oil
8 ounces baby spinach
Cooking spray
DIRECTIONS:
Grease a baking dish with cooking oil then add the fish, tomatoes, parsley and garlic. Drizzle the lemon juice over the fish, cover the dish and place it in the oven at 350 degrees F. Bake for 15 minutes and then divide between plates. Heat up a pan with the olive oil over medium heat, add shallot, stir and cook for 1 minute. Add spinach, stir, cook for 5 minutes more, add to the plate with the fish and serve.
Enjoy!
Nutrition: calories 210, fat 3, fiber 6, carbs 10, protein 24

56) Creamy Asparagus Soup

PREPARATION TIME: 10 minutes
COOKING TIME: 0 minutes
SERVINGS: 2
INGREDIENTS:
8 ounces white mushrooms
12 asparagus spears, trimmed
1 avocado, pitted and peeled
A pinch of salt and white pepper
1 yellow onion, peeled and chopped
3 cups water
DIRECTIONS:
In your blender, add the mushrooms with asparagus, avocado, onion, water, salt and pepper. Pulse well, divide into soup bowls and serve right away. Heat if desired.
Enjoy!
Nutrition: calories 176, fat 3, fiber 9, carbs 16, protein 9

57) **Garlic Mushroom Cream**

PREPARATION TIME: 10 minutes
COOKING TIME: 0 minutes
SERVINGS: 2
INGREDIENTS:
2 tablespoons coconut aminos
1 tablespoon lime juice
A pinch of sea salt and white pepper
1 cup white mushrooms
1 garlic clove, peeled
1 small yellow onion, chopped
2 cups cashew milk, unsweetened
DIRECTIONS:
In your blender, mix mushrooms with garlic, onion, cashew milk, salt, pepper, lime juice and coconut aminos and pulse really well. Divide into soup bowls and serve right away. Enjoy!
Nutrition: calories 191, fat 2, fiber 6, carbs 14, protein 7

58) **Tomato Cream with Celery**

PREPARATION TIME: 10 minutes
COOKING TIME: 0 minutes
SERVINGS: 2
INGREDIENTS:
3 sun-dried tomato sliced
2 celery stalks, chopped
3 big tomatoes, chopped
½ teaspoon powdered onion
2 basil springs, chopped
½ teaspoon garlic powder
1 small avocado, pitted and peeled
A pinch of sea salt and white pepper
DIRECTIONS:
In your blender, add the tomatoes with celery, onion powder, garlic powder, basil, avocado, salt and pepper and pulse really well. Add sun-dried tomatoes and blend again until smooth. Divide into soup bowls and serve. Enjoy!
Nutrition: calories 167, fat 11, fiber 9, carbs 14, protein 4

59) **Grape Gazpacho**

PREPARATION TIME: 5 minutes
COOKING TIME: 0 minutes
SERVINGS: 4
INGREDIENTS:
1 cup white grapes, seedless and halved
1 teaspoon sesame oil
2 cups almond milk, unsweetened
1 small cucumber, chopped
A pinch of salt and white pepper
1 tablespoon chives, chopped for garnish
Ice cubes for serving
DIRECTIONS:
In your blender, mix grapes with cucumber, almond milk, sesame oil, salt and pepper. Pulse really well. Divide into soup bowls, add ice cubes, sprinkle chopped chives all over and serve.
Enjoy!
Nutrition: calories 152, fat 2, fiber 4, carbs 7, protein 6

60) **Mushroom and Tomato Cream**

PREPARATION TIME: 3 hours and 10 minutes
COOKING TIME: 0 minutes
SERVINGS: 3
INGREDIENTS:
1 yellow onion
1 tablespoon agave nectar
1 tablespoon balsamic vinegar
4 tablespoons extra-virgin olive oil
1 teaspoon olive oil
12 ounces mushrooms, sliced
1 tomato, chopped
1 avocado, pitted, peeled and roughly chopped
1 garlic clove, minced
A pinch of salt and black pepper
1½ cups water
DIRECTIONS:
In a bowl, mix mushrooms with agave, vinegar, garlic, salt, pepper and 3 tablespoons olive oil. Toss well then transfer this to your dehydrator and dehydrate the mushrooms

for 3 hours. Pour the mushrooms in your blender, add onion, 1 tablespoon oil, tomato, avocado, salt, pepper and the water. Pulse very well until smooth. Divide into soup bowls, drizzle 1 teaspoon oil on top and serve.
Enjoy!
Nutrition: calories 199, fat 4, fiber 6, carbs 14, protein 7

61) <u>Veggie Tangine</u>

PREPARATION TIME: 10 minutes
COOKING TIME: 35 minutes
SERVINGS: 6
INGREDIENTS:
2 tablespoons olive oil
1 yellow onion, chopped
1 parsnip, chopped
2 garlic cloves, minced
1 teaspoon cumin, ground
½ teaspoon fresh grated ginger
½ teaspoon ground cinnamon
A pinch of salt and cayenne pepper
3 tablespoons tomato paste
2 sweet potatoes, peeled and cubed
2 purple potatoes, peeled and cubed
2 bunches baby carrots, peeled
1-quart veggie stock
2 tablespoons lemon juice
2 cups chopped kale
¼ cup chopped cilantro
DIRECTIONS:
Place a pot with the oil over medium heat, add the onion, stir and sauté for 5 minutes. Add the parsnip, toss and cook for 3 minutes more. Add the garlic, ginger, cumin, salt, cayenne, cinnamon and tomato paste, toss and cook for 2 minutes. Add baby carrots, purple potatoes sweet potatoes and stock. Mix well and cover the pot, reduce heat to medium-low and cook for 20 minutes. Add lemon juice and kale, mix and cook for 1-2 minutes. Divide into bowls and serve with chopped cilantro on top.
Enjoy!
Nutrition: calories 212, fat 7, fiber 7, carbs 12, protein 7

62) <u>Shrimp Stir-Fry</u>

PREPARATION TIME: 10 minutes
COOKING TIME: 10 minutes
SERVINGS: 4
INGREDIENTS:
¼ cup coconut aminos
2 tablespoons raw honey
2 teaspoons sesame oil
2 tablespoons hemp seeds
2 tablespoons olive oil
1 pound shrimp, peeled and deveined
1 yellow onion, chopped
1 red bell pepper, sliced
1 yellow squash, peeled and cubed
4 ounces shiitake mushrooms, sliced
2 garlic cloves, minced
2 cups rainbow chard
DIRECTIONS:
In a bowl, mix the aminos with the honey, sesame oil and hemp seeds. Heat up a pan with the olive oil over medium-high heat, add the onion, stir and cook for 2 minutes. Add the bell pepper, squash, mushrooms and garlic, stir and cook for 5 minutes. Add the shrimp and the coconut aminos then mix, cook for 4 minutes more, take off heat and add the chard. Mix well and divide everything into bowls and serve.
Enjoy!
Nutrition: calories 211, fat 6, fiber 4, carbs 11, protein 8

63) <u>Black Rice with Hemp Seeds Mix</u>

PREPARATION TIME: 10 minutes
COOKING TIME: 10 minutes
SERVINGS: 4
INGREDIENTS:
2 carrots, chopped
2 tablespoons coconut oil
1 yellow onion, chopped
1 bunch scallions, sliced
2 garlic cloves, minced
1 cup sliced snap peas
1 tablespoon fresh grated ginger
3 cups black rice, cooked

2 teaspoons sesame oil
3 tablespoons coconut aminos
1 teaspoon sriracha
2 eggs, whisked
1 tablespoon hemp seeds
DIRECTIONS:
Heat up a pan with the coconut oil over medium heat then add the onion, carrots and scallions. Stir and cook for 5 minutes. Add the garlic, snap peas and ginger. Stir and cook for 2 minutes more. Add the rice, aminos, the sriracha and sesame oil, stir and cook for 2 minutes. Add the eggs, mix and cook until they are done (about 1-2 minutes. Divide into bowls, sprinkle hemp seeds on top and serve.
Enjoy!
Nutrition: calories 182, fat 2, fiber 9, carbs 21, protein 11

64) **Chard Soup**

PREPARATION TIME: 10 minutes
COOKING TIME: 30 minutes
SERVINGS: 4
INGREDIENTS:
1 yellow onion, chopped
2 tablespoons olive oil
2 carrots, chopped
2 garlic cloves, minced
1 teaspoon ground cumin
½ teaspoon ground ginger
½ teaspoon ground turmeric
½ teaspoon red chili flakes
A pinch of salt and black pepper
15 ounces canned tomatoes, chopped
1 cup red lentils
2 quarts veggie stock
1 bunch chard, roughly chopped
DIRECTIONS:
Heat up a pot with the oil over medium heat. Add the onion and carrot, stir and cook for 7 minutes. Add chili flakes, garlic, cumin, ginger, turmeric, salt and pepper, stir and cook for 1 more minute. Add tomatoes, stir and cook for another 5 minutes. Add the lentils and stock, stir, bring to a boil, reduce heat to medium-low and simmer for 10 minutes.

Add the chard, toss, cook for 5 minutes, ladle into bowls and serve.
Enjoy!
Nutrition: calories 181, fat 4, fiber 4, carbs 9, protein 11

65) **Lemony Lentil Soup**

PREPARATION TIME: 10 minutes
COOKING TIME: 1 hour and 20 minutes
SERVINGS: 6
INGREDIENTS:
1½ cups carrots, sliced
1 tablespoon olive oil
1 yellow onion, chopped
1½ cups chopped celery
3 garlic cloves, minced
A pinch of salt and black pepper
4 teaspoons fresh grated ginger
32 ounces veggie stock
2 teaspoons ground turmeric
2 cups green lentils, rinsed
Juice of 3 small lemons
Zest of ½ lemon, grated
DIRECTIONS:
Heat up a pot with the oil over medium heat and add the celery, carrots, onion, a pinch of salt and pepper. Mix together and sauté for 5 minutes. Add the ginger and the garlic, stir and cook for 1 minute more. Add the lentils, stock and turmeric. Stir, reduce heat to low, cover the pot and cook for 45 minutes. Add lemon juice and lemon zest, stir and cook the soup for 30 minutes more. Ladle into bowls and serve.
Enjoy!
Nutrition: calories 271, fat 8, fiber 11, carbs 16, protein 8

66) **Veggie and Egg Burrito Bowls**

PREPARATION TIME: 10 minutes
COOKING TIME: 8 minutes
SERVINGS: 1
INGREDIENTS:
¼ cup spinach leaves, torn

1 tablespoon black olives, pitted and chopped
1 tablespoon chopped red bell pepper
1 teaspoon olive oil
3 cherry tomatoes, halved
2 eggs, whisked
1 tablespoon chopped parsley
Avocado mayonnaise for serving
DIRECTIONS:
Heat up a pan with the olive oil over medium-high heat. Add olives, bell pepper, tomatoes and spinach, stir and cook for 3 minutes. Add the eggs, stir and cook until everything is done (about 1-2 minutes. Divide into bowls, sprinkle with parsley, top with avocado mayonnaise and serve. Enjoy!
Nutrition: calories 217, fat 18, fiber 2, carbs 6, protein 14

67) Turkey Burgers

PREPARATION TIME: 10 minutes
COOKING TIME: 10 minutes
SERVINGS: 4
INGREDIENTS:
1 pound turkey meat, ground
1 shallot, minced
1 tablespoon olive oil
1 small jalapeno pepper, minced
2 teaspoons lime juice
Zest of 1 lime, grated
Salt and black pepper to the taste
1 teaspoon turmeric powder
DIRECTIONS:
In a bowl, mix the turkey meat with shallot, jalapeno, lime juice, lime zest, salt, pepper and turmeric stir well and shape medium burgers out of this mix. Heat up a pan with the oil over medium-high heat, add the turkey burgers, cook them for about 5 minutes on each side, divide between plates and serve for lunch.
Enjoy!
Nutrition: calories 200, fat 12, fiber 5, carbs 12, protein 7

68) Turkey Soup

PREPARATION TIME: 10 minutes
COOKING TIME: 40 minutes
SERVINGS: 4
INGREDIENTS:
4 shallots, chopped
3 carrots, chopped
1 pound ground turkey
Salt and black pepper to the taste
1 red bell pepper, chopped
5 cups vegetable stock
1½ cups cauliflower florets, chopped
4 cups kale, chopped
2 tablespoons coconut oil, melted
15 ounces canned tomatoes, chopped
DIRECTIONS:
Heat up a pot with the oil over medium-high heat. Add shallots, cauliflower, bell pepper and carrots, stir and cook for 10 minutes. Add ground turkey, stir and cook for 8 more minutes. Add tomatoes, salt, pepper, kale and stock. Stir, bring to a boil, cover, cook for 15 minutes then ladle into bowls and serve Enjoy!
Nutrition: calories 210, fat 1, fiber 5, carbs 14, protein 6

69) Poached Cod

PREPARATION TIME: 10 minutes
COOKING TIME: 25 minutes
SERVINGS: 4
INGREDIENTS:
4 cod fillets, skinless
3 garlic cloves, minced
1 yellow onion, chopped
Salt and black pepper to the taste
2 tablespoons olive oil
2 tablespoons chopped tarragon
¼ cup chopped parsley
Juice of 1 lemon
1 lemon, sliced
1 tablespoon chopped thyme
4 cups water
DIRECTIONS:
Heat up a pan with the oil over medium-high heat, Add onion and garlic, stir and cook for

3 minutes. Add salt, pepper, tarragon, parsley, thyme, water, lemon juice and lemon slices, stir and bring to a gentle boil. Add cod, cook for 15 minutes, drain and serve with a side salad.

Enjoy!

Nutrition: calories 173, fat 3, fiber 4, carbs 9, protein 12

70) Chicken and Kale Soup

PREPARATION TIME: 10 minutes
COOKING TIME: 15 minutes
SERVINGS: 6
INGREDIENTS:
1 bunch kale, chopped
Salt and black pepper to the taste
2 quarts vegetable stock
1 cup cooked shredded chicken
3 carrots, chopped
1 tablespoon chopped parsley
1 cup white mushrooms, sliced
DIRECTIONS:
Heat up a pot with the stock over medium heat, add carrots, mushrooms, chicken, kale, salt and pepper. Stir the soup, bring to a simmer and cook for 15 minutes. Ladle into bowls and serve for lunch.

Enjoy!

Nutrition: calories 210, fat 7, fiber 2, carbs 10, protein 8

71) Cod and Fennel

PREPARATION TIME: 10 minutes
COOKING TIME: 15 minutes
SERVINGS: 4
INGREDIENTS:
4 cod fillets, boneless
Salt and black pepper to the taste
Juice of ½ lemon
2 fennel bulbs, sliced
1 tablespoon coconut oil, melted
1 tablespoon olive oil
DIRECTIONS:

Heat up a pan with the coconut oil over medium-high heat. Add fennel slices, season with salt and pepper, mix, cover, cook for 10 minutes and divide between plates. Heat up a pan with the olive oil over medium-high heat, add fish fillets and season with salt and pepper. Cook for 3 minutes, flip and cook for 2 more minutes. Serve next to the fennel and drizzle the lemon juice all over the plate before serving.

Enjoy!

Nutrition: calories 200, fat 2, fiber 4, carbs 10, protein 8

72) Broccoli Soup

PREPARATION TIME: 10 minutes
COOKING TIME: 25 minutes
SERVINGS: 4
INGREDIENTS:
4 leeks, chopped
2 tablespoons olive oil
1 yellow onion, chopped
Salt and black pepper to the taste
1½ pounds broccoli florets, chopped
3 shallots, chopped
¼ apple, chopped
1-quart vegetable stock
½ teaspoon ground turmeric
1 teaspoon ground curry
1 cup coconut milk, unsweetened
DIRECTIONS:
Heat up a soup pot with the oil over medium heat and add onions, leeks and shallots. Stir and cook for 6 minutes. Add apple, broccoli and stock, turmeric, curry powder, salt and pepper and stir. Cook over medium heat for 20 minutes. Transfer mix to a blender, add coconut milk, pulse well, divide into bowls and serve.

Enjoy!

Nutrition: calories 210, fat 8, fiber 6, carbs 10, protein 7

73) Cauliflower Cream

PREPARATION TIME: 10 minutes

COOKING TIME: 50 minutes
SERVINGS: 4
INGREDIENTS:
3 pounds cauliflower, florets separated
1 yellow onion, chopped
1 tablespoon coconut oil
A pinch of salt and black pepper
2 garlic cloves, minced
2 carrots, chopped
3 cups vegetable soup
½ cup coconut milk, unsweetened
A pinch of nutmeg
A pinch of cayenne pepper
A handful parsley, chopped
DIRECTIONS:
Heat up a pot with the oil over medium-high heat, add carrots, onion and garlic then stir and cook for 5 minutes. Add cauliflower and stock, stir, bring to a boil, reduce heat, cover, cook for 45 minutes. Transfer the soup to a blender, add the coconut milk, salt and pepper, pulse well, divide into bowls, sprinkle nutmeg, cayenne and parsley on top and serve.
Enjoy!
Nutrition: calories 210, fat 2, fiber 5, carbs 10, protein 7

74) Chicken Casserole

PREPARATION TIME: 10 minutes
COOKING TIME: 50 minutes
SERVINGS: 4
INGREDIENTS:
4 cups broccoli florets
1 yellow onion, chopped
2 tablespoons olive oil
Salt and black pepper to the taste
8 ounces mushrooms, sliced
3 cups chicken, cooked and shredded
1 cup chicken stock
½ teaspoon ground nutmeg
2 eggs
DIRECTIONS:
Heat up a pan with the oil over medium heat, add onions, mushrooms, salt and pepper, stir, cook for 10 minutes. Pour into a baking dish and top with the chicken and the broccoli. In a bowl, mix stock, eggs, nutmeg, salt and pepper. Stir well, spread over the chicken mix and cook at 350 degrees F for 40 minutes. Divide between plates and serve. Enjoy!
Nutrition: calories 318, fat 18, fiber 3, carbs 5, protein 33

75) Chicken Salad

PREPARATION TIME: 10 minutes
COOKING TIME: 10 minutes
SERVINGS: 4
INGREDIENTS:
2 sweet potatoes, baked
A drizzle of olive oil
1 yellow onion, chopped
12 ounces mushrooms, chopped
2 garlic cloves, minced
½ teaspoon dried thyme
3 cups chicken, already cooked and shredded
2 cups baby spinach
A pinch of salt and cayenne pepper
A splash of balsamic vinegar
DIRECTIONS:
Cut potatoes in half lengthwise, scoop out the flesh, chop it and put in a bowl. Heat up a pan with the oil over medium-high heat. Add onion, potato flesh, garlic, mushrooms, thyme, chicken, salt and cayenne pepper, toss, cook for 10 minutes, take off heat and transfer to the bowl with the sweet potato flesh. Add the spinach and the vinegar, toss and serve.
Enjoy!
Nutrition: calories 260, fat 2, fiber 8, carbs 17, protein 11

76) Italian Zucchini Mix

PREPARATION TIME: 10 minutes
COOKING TIME: 20 minutes
SERVINGS: 4
INGREDIENTS:
¼ cup olive oil
2 zucchinis, cut into small rounds
1 red bell pepper, cut into thin strips
1 yellow onion, cut into medium wedges

1 eggplant, cubed
A pinch of ground turmeric
A pinch of salt and black pepper
1 tablespoons capers
10 cherry tomatoes, halved
2 tablespoons pine nuts
1 tablespoons raisins
1 bunch basil , chopped

DIRECTIONS:

Heat up a pan with the oil over medium-high heat, add the onion, salt, pepper and turmeric, mix and cook for 5 minutes. Add the zucchini, bell pepper and eggplant, mix and cook for 5 minutes more. Add the capers, tomatoes, pine nuts and raisins, mix and cook for 10 minutes over medium heat. Add the basil, stir, cook for another minute more. Divide into bowls and serve for lunch.
Enjoy!
Nutrition: calories 162, fat 3, fiber 4, carbs 12, protein 7

77) <u>Cauliflower Stew</u>

PREPARATION TIME: 10 minutes
COOKING TIME: 35 minutes
SERVINGS: 2
INGREDIENTS:
½ teaspoon olive oil
1 small cauliflower head, florets separated
½ teaspoon cumin seeds
½ cup red onion, chopped
2 tomatoes, chopped
1 teaspoon fresh grated ginger
4 garlic cloves, minced
1 teaspoon ground coriander
½ teaspoon ground turmeric
A pinch of cayenne pepper
½ teaspoon garam masala
2 cups vegetable stock
A pinch of salt and black pepper
1 teaspoon lemon juice

DIRECTIONS:

In your blender, add the tomatoes with garlic, onions, ginger, salt, pepper, garam masala, cayenne, coriander and turmeric and pulse really well. Heat up a pot with the oil over medium heat, add the tomato mix, stir and sauté for 15 minutes. Add cauliflower, stock, salt, pepper, lemon juice and cumin, stir, cover and simmer over medium heat for 20 minutes. Divide into bowls and serve.
Enjoy!
Nutrition: calories 200, fat 6, fiber 7, carbs 10, protein 8

Sides

78) Lettuce Side Salad

PREPARATION TIME: 10 minutes
COOKING TIME: 0 minutes
SERVINGS: 4
INGREDIENTS:
½ cup olive oil
A pinch of salt and black pepper
2 tablespoons chopped shallot
¼ cup mustard
Juice of 2 lemons
½ cup chopped basil
Baby romaine lettuce heads, chopped
3 radicchio, sliced
3 endives, cut into medium pieces
DIRECTIONS:
In a salad bowl, mix romaine lettuce with the radicchio and endives and stir gently. In another bowl, whisk the oil with salt, pepper, shallot, mustard, lemon juice and basil. Drizzle this over your salad, toss to coat and serve as a side salad.
Enjoy!
Nutrition: calories 190, fat 2, fiber 6, carbs 11, protein 7
Radish and Tomatoes Salad
PREPARATION TIME: 10 minutes
COOKING TIME: 0 minutes
SERVINGS: 4
INGREDIENTS:
12 ounces tomatoes, chopped
1 cucumber, chopped
3 red onions, chopped
8 ounces red radishes, cut into wedges
3 tablespoons olive oil
1 teaspoon mustard
1 teaspoon mustard seeds
Juice of 2 limes
2 teaspoons agave nectar
3 tablespoons chopped mint
1 red chili pepper, chopped
DIRECTIONS:
In a salad bowl, mix tomatoes with cucumber, onions and radishes. In another bowl, whisk the mustard with mustard seeds, lime juice, agave nectar, chili pepper and mint. Pour the dressing over the salad, toss and serve as a side salad.
Enjoy!
Nutrition: calories 129, fat 3, fiber 2, carbs 8, protein 6

79) Cucumber and Radish Salad

PREPARATION TIME: 10 minutes
COOKING TIME: 0 minutes
SERVINGS: 4
INGREDIENTS:
1 cup sliced red onion
2 cups sliced radishes
1 garlic clove, minced
A pinch of salt and black pepper
2 tablespoons balsamic vinegar
1 cup sliced cucumber
1 teaspoon chopped dill
½ cup olive oil
DIRECTIONS:
In a salad bowl, mix onion with cucumber, radishes, garlic, salt, black pepper, oil, vinegar and dill. Toss to coat and serve.
Enjoy!
Nutrition: calories 110, fat 4, fiber 2, carbs 7, protein 7

80) Okra and Avocado Side Salad

PREPARATION TIME: 40 minutes
COOKING TIME: 0 minutes
SERVINGS: 4
INGREDIENTS:
1 pound okra, cut into medium pieces
A pinch of sea salt and black pepper
15 ounces canned black beans, drained
1 pound cherry tomatoes, halved
1 white onion, chopped
3 tablespoons olive oil
1 avocado, pitted, peeled and chopped
DIRECTIONS:
Put okra in a salad bowl, add beans, onion, tomatoes, avocado, salt, black pepper and

olive oil. Toss to coat and keep in the fridge for 30 minutes before serving as a side salad. Enjoy!
Nutrition: calories 120, fat 1, fiber 1, carbs 8, protein 7

81) **Tomato and Okra Salad**

PREPARATION TIME: 10 minutes
COOKING TIME: 0 minutes
SERVINGS: 4
INGREDIENTS:
3 cups chopped okra
1 big tomato, chopped
3 celery stalks, chopped
1 onion, chopped
3 cups chopped cauliflower florets
1 yellow bell pepper, chopped
A pinch of sea salt and black pepper
Juice of 1 lemon
½ teaspoon red pepper flakes
1 teaspoon garlic powder
DIRECTIONS:
In a salad bowl, mix okra with tomato, celery stalks, onion, cauliflower and bell pepper. Add the salt, black pepper, lemon juice, pepper flakes and garlic powder. Toss everything together and serve as a side dish. Enjoy!
Nutrition: calories 80, fat 3, fiber 1, carbs 8, protein 5

82) **Simple Corn Side Salad**

PREPARATION TIME: 10 minutes
COOKING TIME: 0 minutes
SERVINGS: 4
INGREDIENTS:
1 red bell pepper, thinly sliced
2 cups corn
Juice of 1 lemon
Zest of 1 lemon, grated
4 cups arugula
A pinch of sea salt and black pepper
DIRECTIONS:
In a salad bowl, mix arugula with the corn and bell pepper. Add the salt, pepper, lemon

zest and lemon juice. Toss to coat evenly and serve as a side dish.
Enjoy!
Nutrition: calories 90, fat 2, fiber 1, carbs 7, protein 5

83) **Bulgur with Corn Salad**

PREPARATION TIME: 30 minutes
COOKING TIME: 0 minutes
SERVINGS: 4
INGREDIENTS:
1 cup bulgur
2 cups hot water
A pinch of sea salt and black pepper
2 cups corn
1 cucumber, chopped
2 tablespoons lemon juice
2 tablespoons balsamic vinegar
¼ cup olive oil
DIRECTIONS:
In a bowl, mix bulgur with the water, cover and set aside for 25 minutes. Uncover the bulgur and fluff with a fork. Transfer the bulgur to a salad bowl, add the corn and cucumber and toss. In a separate small bowl, whisk the oil with lemon juice, vinegar, salt and pepper. Add the dressing to your salad, toss to coat well and serve as a side dish. Enjoy!
Nutrition: calories 253, fat 14, fiber 2, carbs 30, protein 4

84) **Asparagus Salad**

PREPARATION TIME: 15 minutes
COOKING TIME: 0 minutes
SERVINGS: 4
INGREDIENTS:
½ cup chopped walnuts
Salt and black pepper to the taste
1 teaspoon lemon zest
A pinch of chili flakes
¼ cup lemon juice
1 pound asparagus, trimmed and cut into medium pieces
¼ cup mint leaves
A drizzle of olive oil

DIRECTIONS:
In a bowl, mix together the walnuts, lemon zest, salt, pepper and chili flakes. Add the asparagus to the walnut mix and toss. Add the lemon juice, mint and oil as well then toss to coat and serve.
Enjoy!
Nutrition: calories 100, fat 1, fiber 6, carbs 8, protein 6

85) Cabbage Salad

PREPARATION TIME: 10 minutes
COOKING TIME: 0 minutes
SERVINGS: 4
INGREDIENTS:
½ cup red bell pepper, cut into thin strips
1 carrot, grated
4 cups napa cabbage, shredded
3 green onions, chopped
1 tablespoon sesame oil
2 teaspoons fresh grated ginger
½ teaspoon red pepper flakes, crushed
3 tablespoons balsamic vinegar
1 tablespoon coconut aminos
DIRECTIONS:
In a salad bowl, mix the bell pepper with carrot, cabbage, green onions, oil, ginger, pepper flakes, vinegar and aminos. Toss and serve as a side dish.
Enjoy!
Nutrition: calories 160, fat 10, fiber 3, carbs 10, protein 5

86) Almond with Cabbage Salad

PREPARATION TIME: 10 minutes
COOKING TIME: 0 minutes
SERVINGS: 4
INGREDIENTS:
1 Napa cabbage, shredded
1 cup chopped almonds
1 bunch green onions, chopped
¼ cup blueberries
¼ cup balsamic vinegar
2 tablespoons coconut aminos
½ cup olive oil

¼ teaspoon fresh grated ginger
A pinch of black pepper
DIRECTIONS:
In a salad bowl, mix the cabbage with the almonds, green onions, blueberries, vinegar, coconut aminos, oil, ginger and black pepper. Mix well and serve as a side dish.
Enjoy!
Nutrition: calories 140, fat 3, fiber 3, carbs 8, protein 6

87) Scallions with Cabbage Salad

PREPARATION TIME: 10 minutes
COOKING TIME: 0 minutes
SERVINGS: 4
INGREDIENTS:
3 scallions, chopped
1 green cabbage head, shredded
1 red bell pepper, halved and cut into thin strips
2 carrots, chopped
½ cup chopped cilantro
3 tablespoons sunflower seeds
2 tablespoons sesame seeds
¼ cup balsamic vinegar
3½ tablespoons olive oil
1 tablespoon maple syrup
DIRECTIONS:
In a salad bowl, mix the cabbage with the scallions, bell pepper, carrots, cilantro, vinegar, oil, maple syrup, sunflower and sesame seeds. Toss everything together well and serve as a side dish.
Enjoy!
Nutrition: calories 140, fat 4, fiber 3, carbs 5, protein 6

88) Raisin and Celery Salad

PREPARATION TIME: 10 minutes
COOKING TIME: 0 minutes
SERVINGS: 4
INGREDIENTS:
½ cup raisins
4 cups sliced celery
¼ cup chopped parsley

½ cup chopped walnuts
Juice of ½ lemon
2 tablespoons olive oil
Salt and black pepper to the taste
DIRECTIONS:
In a salad bowl, mix celery with raisins, walnuts and parsley and stir. Add lemon juice, oil, salt and pepper, toss to coat and serve as a side dish.
Enjoy!
Nutrition: calories 120, fat 1, fiber 2, carbs 3, protein 5

89) **Cumin Carrots**

PREPARATION TIME: 10 minutes
COOKING TIME: 40 minutes
SERVINGS: 4
INGREDIENTS:
8 carrots, peeled
1 teaspoon cumin, ground
A pinch of salt and black pepper
1 teaspoon dried thyme
3 tablespoons tahini
2½ tablespoons water
¼ tablespoon apple vinegar
1 tablespoon coconut aminos
1 teaspoon ground turmeric
DIRECTIONS:
Spread the carrots on a lined baking sheet, add cumin, salt, pepper, thyme and the oil. Toss well then bake in the oven at 360 degrees F for 40 minutes. In a small bowl, mix whisk the tahini with the water, apple vinegar, coconut aminos and turmeric. Divide the carrots between plates, spread the tahini mix all over and serve as a side dish.
Enjoy!
Nutrition: calories 181, fat 9, fiber 6, carbs 24, protein 7

90) **Baked Green Beans**

PREPARATION TIME: 10 minutes
COOKING TIME: 30 minutes
SERVINGS: 4
INGREDIENTS:
2 pounds green beans, trimmed

A drizzle of olive oil
2 garlic cloves, minced
2 teaspoons lemon zest
½ cup coconut cream
A pinch of red pepper flakes
A pinch of salt and black pepper
DIRECTIONS:
Grease a baking dish with the olive oil and add the green beans, lemon zest, coconut cream, pepper flakes, salt and pepper. Toss a bit then bake in the oven at 400 degrees F for 30 minutes. Divide between plates and serve.
Enjoy!
Nutrition: calories 200, fat 4, fiber 4, carbs 11, protein 7

91) **Green Bean Casserole**

PREPARATION TIME: 10 minutes
COOKING TIME: 30 minutes
SERVINGS: 6
INGREDIENTS:
28 ounces canned green beans, drained
¼ cup almond milk
A pinch of salt and black pepper
10 ounces coconut cream
DIRECTIONS:
In a baking dish, combine the green beans with the almond milk, salt, pepper and cream. Toss a bit and bake in the oven at 350 degrees F for 30 minutes. Divide between plates and serve as a side dish.
Enjoy!
Nutrition: calories 121, fat 3, fiber 4, carbs 10, protein 3

92) **Easy Roasted Cauliflower**

PREPARATION TIME: 10 minutes
COOKING TIME: 1 hour
SERVINGS: 6
INGREDIENTS:
1 cauliflower head, florets separated
1 red onion, cut into wedges
2 cups chopped tomatoes
½ pound green beans, trimmed
A pinch of salt and black pepper

3 tablespoons olive oil
1 cup balsamic vinegar
2 tablespoon chopped parsley
DIRECTIONS:
In a baking dish, mix the cauliflower with the onion, tomatoes, green beans, salt, pepper, oil and vinegar. Bake in the oven at 400 degrees F for 1 hour then divide between plates, sprinkle the parsley on top and serve. Enjoy!
Nutrition: calories 162, fat 4, fiber 9, carbs 11, protein 7

93)**Easy Roasted Vegetables**

PREPARATION TIME: 10 minutes
COOKING TIME: 25 minutes
SERVINGS: 4
INGREDIENTS:
¾ pound Brussel sprouts, halved
2 carrots, sliced
A drizzle of olive oil
1 teaspoon chopped rosemary
1 tablespoon balsamic vinegar
1 teaspoon chopped thyme
½ cup cranberries, dried
½ cup chopped walnuts
DIRECTIONS:
In a baking dish, mix the Brussel sprouts with the carrots, rosemary, oil, vinegar, thyme, cranberries and walnuts. Place in the oven and bake at 400 degrees F for 25 minutes. Divide between plates and serve as a side dish.
Enjoy!
Nutrition: calories 191, fat 5, fiber 8, carbs 13, protein 7

94) **Creamy Corn**

PREPARATION TIME: 10 minutes
COOKING TIME: 2 hours
SERVINGS: 4
INGREDIENTS:
40 ounces canned corn, drained
1 cup coconut milk, unsweetened
A pinch of salt and black pepper
2 tablespoons chopped green onions

DIRECTIONS:
In your slow cooker, mix the corn with the coconut milk, salt, pepper and green onions. Cover and cook on High for 2 hours then divide between plates and serve as a side dish. Enjoy!
Nutrition: calories 132, fat 4, fiber 4, carbs 6, protein 4

95)**Spinach and Squash**

PREPARATION TIME: 10 minutes
COOKING TIME: 25 minutes
SERVINGS: 4
INGREDIENTS:
1 butternut squash, peeled and cubed
1 tablespoon olive oil
A pinch of salt and black pepper
1 shallot, chopped
¼ cup red vinegar
7 cups baby spinach
½ cup chopped pecans, toasted
DIRECTIONS:
Arrange the squash cubes on a lined baking sheet, drizzle with half of the oil, add salt and pepper and toss a little bit. Bake in the oven at 425 degrees F for 25 minutes. Then, in a salad bowl, mix the cooked and cooled squash with shallot, vinegar, spinach, pecans and the rest of the oil and serve.
Enjoy!
Nutrition: calories 307, fat 6, fiber 4, carbs 9, protein 6

96) **Acorn Squash**

PREPARATION TIME: 10 minutes
COOKING TIME: 50 minutes
SERVINGS: 4
INGREDIENTS:
4 acorn squash, quartered
3 tablespoons ground cinnamon
¼ cup coconut oil, melted
DIRECTIONS:
Arrange the squash quarters on a lined baking sheet, drizzle with the coconut oil, sprinkle with the cinnamon and bake in the oven

at 360 degrees F for 50 minutes. Divide between plates and serve as a side dish.
Enjoy!
Nutrition: calories 305, fat 14, fiber 9, carbs 49, protein 4

97) **Tomato Chickpea Side Salad**

PREPARATION TIME: 10 minutes
COOKING TIME: 6 minutes
SERVINGS: 4
INGREDIENTS:
2 tablespoons olive oil
15 ounces canned chickpeas, drained and rinsed
2 pints cherry tomatoes, halved
2 teaspoons ground cumin
¼ cup chopped parsley
A pinch of salt and black pepper
For the vinaigrette:
2 tablespoons olive oil
1 teaspoon minced shallot
1 tablespoon sherry vinegar
DIRECTIONS:
Heat up a pan with 2 tablespoons oil over medium-high heat and add the chickpeas. Spread the chickpeas evenly in the pan and cook for 4 minutes. Add the cumin, salt and pepper and toss a bit then cook for 2 minutes more. Remove from heat and cool down then transfer to a bowl. Add the tomatoes and the parsley and toss. In another bowl, whisk together the 2 tablespoons oil with shallot and vinegar and pour over the salad. Toss well and serve as a side dish.
Enjoy!
Nutrition: calories 168, fat 9, fiber 3, carbs 8, protein 5

98) **Fresh Green Beans**

PREPARATION TIME: 10 minutes
COOKING TIME: 35 minutes
SERVINGS: 6
INGREDIENTS:
3 tablespoons olive oil
1 ½ cups chopped onion

1 tablespoon minced garlic
A pinch of salt and black pepper
2 teaspoons garam masala
2 teaspoons fresh grated ginger
½ teaspoon ground cinnamon
½ teaspoon ground coriander
2 cups chopped tomatoes
½ cup vegetable stock
½ teaspoon brown mustard seeds
1½ pounds green beans, trimmed
Juice of 1 lemon
DIRECTIONS:
Heat up a large pan with the oil over medium-high heat and add the onion and the garlic. Stir and cook for 5 minutes. Add salt, pepper, garam masala, ginger, cinnamon, coriander, tomatoes, stock, mustard seeds and green beans. Mix well then reduce heat to medium-low and cook everything for 30 minutes. Add lemon juice, toss, divide between plates and serve.
Enjoy!
Nutrition: calories 181, fat 3, fiber 6, carbs 12, protein 6

99) **Easy Tomato Salad**

PREPARATION TIME: 10 minutes
COOKING TIME: 0 minutes
SERVINGS: 4
INGREDIENTS:
4 mixed colored tomatoes, chopped
1 cucumber, sliced
A drizzle of olive oil
1 tablespoon chopped dill
1 red onion, chopped
A pinch of salt and black pepper
DIRECTIONS:
In a bowl, mix the tomatoes with the cucumber, onion, salt, pepper, dill and oil. Serve as a side dish.
Enjoy!
Nutrition: calories 171, fat 4, fiber 7, carbs 13, protein 6

100) Daikon Radish and Cabbage

PREPARATION TIME: 10 minutes
COOKING TIME: 0 minutes
SERVINGS: 6
INGREDIENTS:
1 pound Napa cabbage, chopped
1 carrot, julienned
A pinch of salt and black pepper
½ cup daikon radish
3 green onion stalks, chopped
3 tablespoons chili flakes
3 garlic cloves, minced
1 tablespoon sesame oil
½ inch fresh ginger, grated
DIRECTIONS:
In a bowl, mix the cabbage with the carrot, daikon radish, onion, chili flakes, garlic, salt, pepper, ginger and oil. Toss well and serve as a side salad.
Enjoy!
Nutrition: calories 60, fat 3, fiber 2, carbs 5, protein 1

101) Minty Snap Peas

PREPARATION TIME: 10 minutes
COOKING TIME: 5 minutes
SERVINGS: 4
INGREDIENTS:
¾ pound sugar snap peas, trimmed
Salt and black pepper to the taste
1 tablespoon chopped mint leaves
2 teaspoons olive oil
3 green onions, chopped
1 garlic clove, minced
DIRECTIONS:
Heat up a pan with the oil over medium-high heat and add snap peas, salt, pepper, green onions, garlic and mint. Toss the mix well and then cook for 5 minutes. Divide between plates and serve as a side dish.
Enjoy!
Nutrition: calories 120, fat 6, fiber 1, carbs 5, protein 6

102) Collard Greens Mix

PREPARATION TIME: 10 minutes
COOKING TIME: 10 minutes
SERVINGS: 4
INGREDIENTS:
5 bunches collard greens, chopped
Salt and black pepper to the taste
1 tablespoon crushed red pepper flakes
3 tablespoons chicken stock
2 tablespoons minced garlic
¼ cup olive oil
DIRECTIONS:
Heat up a pot with the oil over medium heat and add the garlic. Stir and cook for 2 minutes. Add the collard greens, pepper flakes, stock, salt and pepper. Mix well and cook for 8 minutes then divide between plates and serve as a side dish.
Enjoy!
Nutrition: calories 212, fat 16, fiber 10, carbs 7, protein 6

103) Fast Swiss Chard

PREPARATION TIME: 10 minutes
COOKING TIME: 10 minutes
SERVINGS: 4
INGREDIENTS:
2 tablespoons olive oil
2 bunches Swiss chard, roughly chopped
½ teaspoon garlic paste
3 tablespoons lemon juice
Salt and black pepper to the taste
DIRECTIONS:
Heat a pan with the olive oil over medium heat and add the garlic paste. Stir and cook for 1 minute. Add Swiss chard, lemon juice, salt and pepper. Toss and cook for 8-9 minutes then divide between plates and serve as a side dish.
Enjoy!
Nutrition: calories 69, fat 7, fiber 1, carbs 2, protein 1

104) Watercress and Endives Salad

PREPARATION TIME: 10 minutes
COOKING TIME: 0 minutes
SERVINGS: 4
INGREDIENTS:
4 medium endives, trimmed and thinly sliced
1 tablespoon lemon juice
1 shallot, finely chopped
1 tablespoon balsamic vinegar
2 tablespoons olive oil
6 tablespoons coconut cream
Salt and black pepper to the taste
4 ounces watercress, cut into medium springs
1 tablespoon chopped chervil
1 tablespoon chopped tarragon
1 tablespoon chopped chives
1/3 cup chopped almonds
1 tablespoon chopped parsley
DIRECTIONS:
In a small bowl, whisk together the lemon juice with vinegar, salt, pepper, oil and shallot then set aside for 10 minutes. In a separate salad bowl, mix the endives with watercress, chives, tarragon, parsley, chervil, cream and the lemon juice mix. Toss and serve as a side dish with almonds sprinkled on top.
Enjoy!
Nutrition: calories 142, fat 3, fiber 5, carbs 4, protein 7

105) Carrot and Zucchini Mix

PREPARATION TIME: 15 minutes
COOKING TIME: 0 minutes
SERVINGS: 6
INGREDIENTS:
3 carrots, grated
2 zucchinis, sliced
A bunch of radishes, sliced
½ red onion, chopped
6 mint leaves, roughly chopped
For the salad dressing:
1 teaspoon mustard
1 tablespoons balsamic vinegar
2 tablespoons olive oil
A pinch of salt and black pepper
DIRECTIONS:
In a bowl, mix the carrots with the radishes, zucchinis, onion and mint. In another bowl, whisk together the mustard with the vinegar, oil, salt and pepper. Add the dressing to the salad, toss and serve as a side dish.
Enjoy!
Nutrition: calories 117, fat 7, fiber 3, carbs 13, protein 1

106) Chili Eggplant Mix

PREPARATION TIME: 10 minutes
COOKING TIME: 15 minutes
SERVINGS: 4
INGREDIENTS:
1 big Asian eggplant, cubed
1 yellow onion, thinly sliced
2 tablespoon olive oil
2 teaspoons minced garlic
2 teaspoons chili paste
¼ cup coconut cream
4 green onions, chopped
DIRECTIONS:
Heat up a pan with the oil over medium-high heat then add the onion, stir and cook for 3-4 minutes. Add the garlic, chili paste, green onions and coconut cream and stir, cooking for 2-3 minutes more. Add the eggplant, toss and cook for 7-8 minutes more. Divide between plates and serve as a side dish.
Enjoy!
Nutrition: calories 142, fat 7, fiber 4, carbs 5, protein 3

107) Simple Spinach Mix

PREPARATION TIME: 10 minutes
COOKING TIME: 12 minutes
SERVINGS: 4
INGREDIENTS:
1 apple, cored and chopped
1 yellow onion, sliced
3 tablespoons olive oil
6 garlic cloves, chopped

¼ cup pine nuts, toasted
¼ cup balsamic vinegar
5 cups mixed spinach and Swiss chard
Salt and black pepper to the taste
A pinch of ground nutmeg
DIRECTIONS:
Heat up a pan with the oil over medium-high heat, add onion, stir and cook for 3 minutes. Add apple, garlic, vinegar and spinach chard mix. Stir and cook for 10 minutes over medium-low heat. Add nutmeg, salt and pepper and toss. Divide between plates and serve. Enjoy!
Nutrition: calories 120, fat 1, fiber 2, carbs 3, protein 6

Seafood

108) Chipotle Salmon Patties

PREPARATION TIME: 15 minutes
COOKING TIME: 10 minutes
SERVINGS: 6
INGREDIENTS:
1-pound salmon fillet
2 chipotle peppers
1 tablespoon coconut flour
½ teaspoon ground black pepper
1 egg, beaten
½ teaspoon ground coriander
2 tablespoons avocado oil
¾ cup almond flour
DIRECTIONS:
Mince the chipotle peppers and place them in the big mixing bowl.
Chop the salmon fillet and transfer it in the food processor. Process the fish until smooth.
Add the salmon in the chipotle pepper.
Then add coconut flour, ground black pepper, egg, ground coriander, and mix up the mixture.
Make the medium size patties from the mixture.
Pour avocado oil in the skillet and preheat it well.
Coat the patties in the almond flour and put in the skillet.
Roast the salmon patties for 2-3 minutes and then flip onto another side.
Cook the patties for 2 minutes more.
Dry the cooked meal with the help of the paper towel if needed.
Nutrition: calories 153, fat 8.1, fiber 1.7, carbs 3.9, protein 17.1

109) Creamy Halibut

PREPARATION TIME: 15 minutes
COOKING TIME: 25 minutes
SERVINGS: 6
INGREDIENTS:
6 halibut fillets
½ cup heavy cream
1 tablespoon butter
½ teaspoon onion powder
¾ teaspoon ground cinnamon
1 teaspoon dried oregano
½ teaspoon salt
1 tablespoon almond flour
1 tablespoon fresh parsley, chopped
DIRECTIONS:
Mix up together onion powder, ground cinnamon, dried oregano, salt, and almond flour.
Coat the fillets into the spice mixture carefully.
Spread the baking mold with butter.
Arrange the halibut fillets in the mold. Add remaining spice mixture.
After this, add chopped fresh parsley and heavy cream.
Cover the surface of the baking mold with foil. Secure the edges.
Place the fish in the preheated to 375F oven and cook for 25 minutes.
Serve the cooked fish with the creamy sauce from it.
Nutrition: calories 206, fat 9.4, fiber 0.4, carbs 1.1, protein 29.6

110) Fish Quesadillas

PREPARATION TIME: 15 minutes
COOKING TIME: 10 minutes
SERVINGS: 4
INGREDIENTS:
¾ cup almond flour
1 tablespoon butter
1 teaspoon Psyllium Husk
½ teaspoon salt
8 oz tuna, canned, chopped
1 teaspoon cream cheese
¼ teaspoon chili flakes
4 oz Cheddar cheese, shredded
DIRECTIONS:
In the mixing bowl, mix up together almond flour, butter, salt, and Psyllium Husk.
Knead the soft and non-sticky dough.
Cut the dough into 2 pieces.
Roll up every dough piece with the help of the rolling pin. Keto tortillas are prepared.

After this, preheat the non-sticky skillet well.
Place the first dough round in the skillet and cook it for 1 minute from each side.
Remove the first tortilla from the skillet.
Place the second tortilla in the skillet and cook it for 1 minute from one side.
Then flip it onto another side.
Mix up together chopped tuna, cream cheese, chili flakes, and shredded cheese.
Place the mixture over the tortilla (which one is in the skillet and cover with the second tortilla.
Cook the quesadillas for 2 minutes from each side over the medium heat.
Slice the cooked meal into the servings and transfer in the serving plates.
Nutrition: calories 285, fat 19.8, fiber 2.9, carbs 4.3, protein 23.3

111) **Mahi Mahi with Walnut Sauce**

PREPARATION TIME: 15 minutes
COOKING TIME: 20 minutes
SERVINGS: 4
INGREDIENTS:
1-pound mahi-mahi
3 tablespoons walnuts, chopped
¼ cup coconut cream
1 teaspoon psyllium husk
½ teaspoon ground black pepper
1 teaspoon butter
¾ jalapeno pepper, minced
½ white onion
DIRECTIONS:
Rub the fish with ground black pepper.
Peel and slice the onion.
Spread the baking form with butter from inside.
Place the mahi-mahi in the baking form.
Then in the mixing bowl, mix up together chopped walnuts, coconut cream, psyllium husk, and minced jalapeno.
Pour the mixture (sauce over the fish. Arrange the white pepper over the fish.
Preheat the oven to 365F.
Place the fish in the oven and bake it for 20 minutes.

When the time is over, transfer the fish in the serving plates and sprinkle with hot walnut sauce.
Nutrition: calories 377, fat 22, fiber 2.4, carbs 5.1, protein 40.2

112) **Cheese Fish Nuggets**

PREPARATION TIME: 10 minutes
COOKING TIME: 10 minutes
SERVINGS: 6
INGREDIENTS:
½ cup almond flour
4 oz Parmesan, grated
1-pound salmon fillet
½ teaspoon ground black pepper
1 teaspoon salt
1 tablespoon olive oil
DIRECTIONS:
In the mixing bowl, mix up together Parmesan, almond flour, ground black pepper, and salt.
Chop the salmon filet into the nuggets.
Pour olive oil in the skillet and preheat it well.
Coat every fish nugget in the almond flour mixture.
Then transfer the coated fish nuggets in the preheated skillet.
Cook them for 1 minute from each side or until they are light brown.
Nutrition: calories 195 fat 12.2, fiber 0.3, carbs 1.3, protein 21.3

113) **Fish Balls**

PREPARATION TIME: 15 minutes
COOKING TIME: 5 minutes
SERVINGS: 4
INGREDIENTS:
8 oz tuna, canned
3 tablespoons cream cheese
1 teaspoon dried dill
½ teaspoon turmeric
2 oz bacon, chopped
½ teaspoon minced garlic
¾ teaspoon ground nutmeg
DIRECTIONS:

Place the bacon in the skillet and roast it for 5 minutes over the medium-high heat. The cooked bacon has to be crunchy.

Meanwhile, shred the canned tuna and mix it up with the dried dill, turmeric, minced garlic, and ground nutmeg.

Add cream cheese and cooked crunchy bacon. Mix up the tuna mixture well.

Make the fish balls from the fish mixture with the help of 2 spoons.

Chill the fish balls little before serving.

Nutrition: calories 213, fat 13.3, fiber 0.2, carbs 1, protein 21

114) Fried Seabass Steak

PREPARATION TIME: 10 minutes
COOKING TIME: 10 minutes
SERVINGS: 4
INGREDIENTS:
4 seabass fillets
1 teaspoon salt
1 teaspoon ground coriander
½ teaspoon fresh thyme
1 tablespoon lemon juice
1 tablespoon butter
½ teaspoon canola oil
DIRECTIONS:
In the shallow bowl, mix up together salt, ground coriander, lemon juice, and canola oil.

Brush the seabass steaks with the spice mixture from each side well.

Toss butter in the skillet and preheat it. Add fresh thyme.

Place the seabass fillets in the skillet and cook them for 4 minutes from each side over the medium-high heat.

It is recommended to serve steaks hot.

Nutrition: calories 267, fat 17.6, fiber 1, carbs 0.2, protein 26.2

115) Ginger Tuna

PREPARATION TIME: 10 minutes
COOKING TIME: 10 minutes
SERVINGS: 4
INGREDIENTS:

4 servings tuna fillet
1 teaspoon minced gingerroot
½ teaspoon ground paprika
1 tablespoon apple cider vinegar
½ teaspoon salt
1 tablespoon avocado oil
¾ teaspoon cayenne pepper
DIRECTIONS:
Rub the tuna fillets with the gingerroot and ground paprika.

Then sprinkle the fish with salt and cayenne pepper.

Massage the fish gently with the help of the fingertips. Sprinkle the tuna with apple cider vinegar.

Pour avocado oil in the skillet.

Preheat it and add tuna fillets.

Cook the fish over the medium-high heat for 2 minutes from each side.

Nutrition: calories 372, fat 31.6, fiber 0.4, carbs 0.9, protein 21.2

116) Garlic Snapper

PREPARATION TIME: 10 minutes
COOKING TIME: 10 minutes
SERVINGS: 2
INGREDIENTS:
2 red snapper fillets
½ teaspoon garlic powder
½ teaspoon garlic, diced
2 teaspoons olive oil
½ teaspoon ground black pepper
1 teaspoon butter
½ teaspoon dried marjoram
DIRECTIONS:
Mix up together ground black pepper and garlic powder.

Rub the snapper fillets with spices.

Toss the butter in the skillet.

Add dried marjoram, olive oil, and diced garlic.

Bring the mixture to boil. Then remove the diced garlic from the skillet.

Add snapper fillets and roast them for 3 minutes from each side over the medium-low heat.

Dry the cooked fish with the help of the paper towel if needed and transfer on the serving plates.
Nutrition: calories 280, fat 9.5, fiber 0.3, carbs 1.5, protein 45

117) **Stuffed Fish Avocado**

PREPARATION TIME: 15 minutes
COOKING TIME: 4 minutes
SERVINGS: 2
INGREDIENTS:
1 avocado
½ teaspoon ground thyme
1 can mackerel, drained
¼ white onion, diced
1 tablespoon fresh parsley
1 tablespoon mayonnaise
½ teaspoon olive oil
1 egg, boiled
DIRECTIONS:
Preheat the olive oil in the skillet. Add diced onion.
Cook the onion for 3-4 minutes over the medium heat or until it is truculent.
Then peel the egg and chop it.
Cut the avocado into halves. Remove the pit.
Scoop ½ part of all avocado flesh and mash it.
Shred the mackerel and place it in the mixing bowl.
Add chopped egg, cooked onion, and ground thyme.
Chop the parsley and add it in the fishbowl.
Add mayonnaise and mix up the mixture.
When it is homogenous, transfer it into the avocado halves.
Store the stuffed avocado in the fridge up to 2 days.
Nutrition: calories 845, fat 48.2, fiber 7.2, carbs 12.1, protein 88.7

118) **Parmesan Tilapia**

PREPARATION TIME: 10 minutes
COOKING TIME: 8 minutes
SERVINGS: 4
INGREDIENTS:
4 tilapia fillets
1/3 cup almond flour
4 oz Parmesan, grated
½ teaspoon ground black pepper
1 tablespoon olive oil
½ teaspoon chili flakes
DIRECTIONS:
In the mixing bowl, mix up together almond flour, ground black pepper, and chili flakes.
Pour olive oil in the skillet and preheat it well.
Coat the tilapia fillets in the almond flour mixture and transfer in the hot skillet.
Cook the fish for 4 minutes over the medium-high heat.
When the fish is cooked, it will have little bit crunchy surface.
Nutrition: calories 228, fat 11.8, fiber 0.3, carbs 1.7, protein 30.7

119) **Crab Legs**

PREPARATION TIME: 5 minutes
COOKING TIME: 10 minutes
SERVINGS: 4
INGREDIENTS:
1-pound king crab legs
1 bay leaf
1 teaspoon salt
2 cups water, for cooking
DIRECTIONS:
Pour water in the saucepan.
Add bay leaf and salt.
Bring the water to boil.
Add king crab legs and close the lid.
Boil the crab legs for 4 minutes over the medium heat.
Then drain the water and transfer the crab legs on the serving plates.
Nutrition: calories 483, fat 4.4, fiber 0.1, carbs 2.7, protein 0

120) **Tuna Salad**

PREPARATION TIME: 10 minutes
SERVINGS: 3
INGREDIENTS:
5 oz celery stalk, chopped

1 white onion, diced
1 cayenne pepper, pickled
1 tablespoon mayonnaise
¼ teaspoon minced garlic
8 oz tuna, canned, drained
1 tablespoon fresh dill, chopped
DIRECTIONS:
Shred the canned tuna and place it in the salad bowl.
Add chopped dill, minced garlic, diced onion, and celery stalk.
Mince the pickled cayenne pepper and add it in the salad bowl.
Add mayonnaise and mix up the salad.
If you don't serve the salad immediately, store it in the fridge.
Nutrition: calories 185, fat 7.9, fiber 1.7, carbs 6.6, protein 21.1

121) **Fish Casserole**

PREPARATION TIME: 15 minutes
COOKING TIME: 35 minutes
SERVINGS: 4
INGREDIENTS:
1 cup broccoli florets
½ cup heavy cream
6 oz Cheddar cheese
10 oz cod fillet, chopped
1 oz green onion, chopped
¾ teaspoon chili flakes
1 teaspoon salt
1 tablespoon butter
1 teaspoon capers
DIRECTIONS:
Chop the broccoli florets roughly.
Shred Cheddar cheese.
Sprinkle the chopped cod fillet with the chili flakes and salt. Mix up well.
Spread the casserole dish with the butter. Place the chopped cod inside.
Then sprinkle the fish with capers and chopped broccoli florets.
Arrange the chopped green onion over the broccoli.
Then add shredded cheese and heavy cream.
Preheat the oven to 375F and place the casserole inside.
Cook it for 35 minutes.

Nutrition: calories 319, fat 23.3, fiber 0.8, carbs 3.1, protein 25.1

122) **Mexican Style Tilapia**

PREPARATION TIME: 20 minutes
COOKING TIME: 7 minutes
SERVINGS: 2
INGREDIENTS:
1 teaspoon Mexican chili spices
2 tilapia fillets
¾ teaspoon dried rosemary
1 tablespoon lime juice
1 tablespoon canola oil
1 teaspoon sour cream
DIRECTIONS:
Rub the tilapia fillets with Mexican chili spices and dried rosemary.
Then sprinkle the fish with lime juice and sour cream/
Massage it well with the help of the fingertips.
Brush the fish gently with the canola oil.
Let it marinate for 15 minutes.
Meanwhile, preheat the grill well.
Place the marinated fish in the grill and roast it for 3 minutes from each side or until it is light brown.
Nutrition: calories 161, fat 8.5, fiber 0.2, carbs 0.4, protein 21.1

123) **Rosemary Haddock**

PREPARATION TIME: 15 minutes
COOKING TIME: 20 minutes
SERVINGS: 4
INGREDIENTS:
1 teaspoon tarragon
1 teaspoon dried rosemary
1-pound haddock fillet
½ teaspoon onion powder
¾ teaspoon salt
2 tablespoons olive oil
1 oz Parmesan, grated
1 tablespoon butter
DIRECTIONS:
Mix up together tarragon, dried rosemary, onion powder, and salt.

Sprinkle the haddock fillet with the spice mixture.

Then cut it into 4 pieces.

Brush the baking dish with the olive oil.

Place the haddock fillets inside.

Sprinkle the fish with the grated cheese. Add butter.

Cook the haddock for 20 minutes in the preheated to the 365F oven.

Nutrition: calories 238, fat 12.5, fiber 0.2, carbs 0.8, protein 29.9

124) Oregano Tuna Patties

PREPARATION TIME: 15 minutes
COOKING TIME: 5 minutes
SERVINGS: 4
INGREDIENTS:
1 teaspoon dried oregano
1 egg, beaten
3 tablespoons almond flour
10 oz tuna, canned
1 teaspoon salt
1 tablespoon olive oil
1 teaspoon dried dill
½ teaspoon ground paprika
1 teaspoon chives, chopped
DIRECTIONS:
Place the canned tuna in the blender, add beaten egg, oregano, salt, dried dill, and paprika,

Blend the mixture until smooth and transfer in the mixing bowl.

Add almond flour and chives. Mix up the mixture.

Then pour olive oil in the skillet.

Make the small patties with the help of the spoon and place them in the preheated skillet.

Cook the patties for 2 minutes and then flip them onto another side.

The cooked tuna patties will have a golden brown color.

Nutrition: calories 300, fat 20.9, fiber 2.6, carbs 5.1, protein 24.8

125) Crab Cakes

PREPARATION TIME: 10 minutes
COOKING TIME: 6 minutes
SERVINGS: 7
INGREDIENTS:
12 oz crabmeat, chopped
1 tablespoon chives, chopped
½ teaspoon turmeric
½ teaspoon garlic, diced
3 tablespoons coconut flour
1/3 teaspoon salt
½ teaspoon ground black pepper
1 tablespoon olive oil
1 egg, beaten
DIRECTIONS:
In the mixing bowl, mix up together chopped crab meat, chives, turmeric, diced garlic, coconut flour, salt, ground black pepper, and beaten egg.

Mix up the crab mixture with the help of the spoon.

Put olive oil in the pan and bring it to boil.

Make the crab cakes with the help of 2 spoons and transfer them in the boiled oil.

Cook the crab cakes for 6 minutes (for 3 minutes from each side over the medium heat.

Chill the cooked crab cakes little before serving.

Nutrition: calories 87, fat 3.3, fiber 1.4, carbs 9.3, protein 5

126) Fish Fillets in Tomato Sauce

PREPARATION TIME: 10 minutes
COOKING TIME: 15 minutes
SERVINGS: 4
INGREDIENTS:
4 mackerel fillets
1 teaspoon tomato paste
¾ cup of coconut milk
½ teaspoon salt
¾ teaspoon white pepper
1 teaspoon butter
DIRECTIONS:
Toss the butter in the skillet.

Sprinkle the mackerel fillets with the salt and white pepper.

Place the fish fillets on the melted butter and cook them for 3 minutes from each side over the medium-high heat.

Meanwhile, pour the coconut milk in the saucepan and bring it to boil.

Add tomato paste and whisk it until smooth. Bring it to boil again.

Pour the coconut mixture (sauce over the fish and close the lid.

Saute the mackerel for 10 minutes over the low heat.

Nutrition: calories 345, fat 27.4, fiber 1.1, carbs 3, protein 22.1

127) Stuffed Mushroom Caps with Halibut

PREPARATION TIME: 15 minutes
COOKING TIME: 20 minutes
SERVINGS: 5
INGREDIENTS:
1 cup mushroom caps
½ teaspoon dried marjoram
10 oz halibut
½ onion, diced
¾ teaspoon chili flakes
½ teaspoon dried oregano
1 tablespoon butter
1 teaspoon olive oil
½ teaspoon garlic powder
DIRECTIONS:
Finely chop the halibut and mix it up with the diced onion, chili flakes, dried oregano, and garlic powder. Add dried marjoram.

Mix up the mixture and transfer it in the pan. Add olive oil.

Cook the fish mixture for 10 minutes over the medium heat.

Then fill the mushroom caps with the halibut mixture and transfer them in the baking tray.

Cover the tray with foil and secure the edges. Cook the mushroom caps for 10 minutes at 370F.

When the time is over, let the mushroom caps rest for 10 minutes in the switched off oven.

Then discard the foil and transfer the mushrooms in the serving plates.

Nutrition: calories 142, fat 5.5, fiber 0.5, carbs 1.8, protein 20.7

128) Keto Salmon Burger

PREPARATION TIME: 10 minutes
COOKING TIME: 10 minutes
SERVINGS: 4
INGREDIENTS:
1-pound salmon fillet
1 tablespoon almond flour
½ teaspoon ground black pepper
1 egg, beaten
¼ cup coconut flakes
1 tablespoon olive oil
1 tablespoon chives, chopped
1 teaspoon dried dill
1 teaspoon dried parsley
¼ teaspoon ground ginger
DIRECTIONS:
Chop the salmon fillet and transfer in the food processor.

Blend it for 1 minute or until it is smooth.

Then add almond flour, ground black pepper, egg, chives, dried dill, parsley, and ground ginger.

Pulse the mixture for 30 seconds.

After this, transfer the fish mixture in the mixing bowl.

Make the medium size burgers and coat them in the coconut flakes.

Preheat the olive oil over the medium heat.

Place the salmon burgers in the hot oil and cook them for 4 minutes from each side.

The salmon burgers are cooked when they are light brown color.

Nutrition: calories 255, fat 16.8, fiber 1.3, carbs 2.8, protein 25.2

129) Shrimp Scampi

PREPARATION TIME: 6 minutes
COOKING TIME: 10 minutes

SERVINGS: 7
INGREDIENTS:
12 oz shrimps, peeled
2 tablespoons butter
1 teaspoon garlic, diced
4 tablespoons lemon juice
1 teaspoon apple cider vinegar
2 tablespoons fresh parsley, chopped
1 tablespoon fresh dill, chopped
¼ teaspoon ground cardamom
1 teaspoon chili flakes
1 tablespoon avocado oil
½ teaspoon salt
DIRECTIONS:
Toss the butter in the pan and melt it.
Add diced garlic, chopped parsley, dill, ground cardamom, chili flakes, avocado oil, and salt. Mix up the mixture gently.
Add peeled shrimps and mix up with the help of the spatula.
Then sprinkle the shrimps with apple cider vinegar and lemon juice. Mix up them gently one more time.
Close the lid and cook scampi for 5 minutes over the medium heat.
Stir the cooked meal well before serving.
Nutrition: calories 94, fat 4.5, fiber 0.3, carbs 1.6, protein 11.4

130) Creamed Mussels

PREPARATION TIME: 15 minutes
COOKING TIME: 10 minutes
SERVINGS: 5
INGREDIENTS:
1-pound mussels
½ cup heavy cream
¾ cup of water
½ lemon, juiced
1 garlic clove, crushed
½ onion, chopped
1 teaspoon chili flakes
1 teaspoon thyme
½ teaspoon cumin seeds
1 tablespoon butter
½ teaspoon lime zest, grated
½ teaspoon white pepper
3 tablespoons fresh cilantro, chopped
DIRECTIONS:

Pour heavy cream and water in the saucepan.
Add crushed garlic, chopped onion, chili flakes, thyme, cumin seeds, butter, lime zest, white pepper, and chopped cilantro.
Bring the liquid to boil.
Then add mussels and stir the meal well.
Close the lid and cook it for 6 minutes over the medium-low heat.
When the mussels are cooked, let them rest for 10 minutes before serving.
Nutrition: calories 148, fat 8.9, fiber 0.5, carbs 5.4, protein 11.4

131) Garlic Clam Chowder

PREPARATION TIME: 10 minutes
COOKING TIME: 15 minutes
SERVINGS: 5
INGREDIENTS:
2 cups organic almond milk
1 cup of water
4 oz celery stalk, chopped
1 tablespoon celery root, grated
8 oz clams
1 garlic clove, diced
1 teaspoon ground cinnamon
1 chili pepper, chopped
½ teaspoon salt
1 teaspoon butter
½ carrot, chopped
DIRECTIONS:
Place the chopped carrot in the pan.
Add butter and start to preheat it over the medium heat.
Then add celery stalk, celery root, diced garlic, ground cinnamon, chili pepper, and salt.
Stir the mixture and add water.
Then add almond milk and bring the liquid to boil.
Add clams and close the lid.
Simmer the chowder for 10 minutes over the low heat.
Nutrition: calories 59, fat 1.9, fiber .9, carbs 9.7, protein 0.9

132) **Chili Oysters**

PREPARATION TIME: 10 minutes
COOKING TIME: 5 minutes
SERVINGS: 2
INGREDIENTS:
6 oysters
1 chili pepper, minced
3 oz bacon, chopped
½ teaspoon chili pepper
3 tablespoons lemon juice
DIRECTIONS:
Put the bacon in the skillet and roast it for 5 minutes.
Sprinkle the bacon with chili pepper and mix up.
Open the oysters and sprinkle them with lemon juice. Add cooked chili bacon and transfer on the serving plates.
Nutrition: calories 366, fat 22.3, fiber 0.3, carbs 8.3, protein 30.4

133) **Stuffed Calamari**

PREPARATION TIME: 15 minutes
COOKING TIME: 25 minutes
SERVINGS: 4
INGREDIENTS:
4 calamari tubes, trimmed
½ cup mushrooms, chopped
1 tablespoon butter
½ onion, diced
1 teaspoon ground black pepper
½ teaspoon chili flakes
½ teaspoon salt
¼ cup heavy cream
DIRECTIONS:
Place the butter in the skillet.
Add chopped mushrooms, diced onion, chili flakes, ground black pepper, and salt.
Saute the mushrooms for 10 minutes. Stir them from time to time.
Preheat the oven to 365F.
Fill the calamari tubes with the mushroom mixture and secure them with the tooth-picks.
Transfer the calamari in the baking dish.

Pour the heavy cream over the calamari and bake them for 15 minutes in the preheated oven.
Nutrition: calories 170, fat 7.8, fiber 0.5, carbs 5.1, protein 17.7

134) **Tender Crabs**

PREPARATION TIME: 6 minutes
COOKING TIME: 12 minutes
SERVINGS: 2
INGREDIENTS:
4 crabs (3 oz each, trimmed
1 teaspoon curry powder
2 tablespoons olive oil
1 teaspoon butter
2 garlic cloves, diced
1 teaspoon chili flakes
¾ cup of coconut milk
1 teaspoon salt
DIRECTIONS:
Por olive oil in the pan.
Add butter, chili flakes, coconut milk, and salt.
Then add curry powder and bring the mixture to boil.
Then add crabs and garlic cloves.
Cook the crab for 10 minutes. Flip them onto another side from time to time.
When the crabs are cooked, transfer them in the serving plates and sprinkle over with the remaining coconut mixture.
Nutrition: calories 525, fat 40.5, fiber 2.4, carbs 6.6, protein 36.8

135) **Creamy Dill Sauce with Salmon or Trout**

PREPARATION TIME: 10 minutes
COOKING TIME: 5 minutes
SERVINGS: 4 People
INGREDIENTS:
Dill Sauce:
☐   ¾ cup of sour cream (1
☐   2 teaspoons of Dijon or hot English mustard (2
☐   ½ teaspoon of garlic powder or 1 small garlic clove, minced

☐ 2½ tablespoons of fresh dill, finely chopped
☐ 1 teaspoon of lemon zest
☐ 1 to 2 tablespoon of lemon juice
☐ 2 tablespoons of milk (or olive oil, for richness
☐ ¼ to ½ teaspoon of salt
☐ ½ teaspoon of white sugar

Fish:
☐ ½ to 1 tablespoon of oil
☐ 4 salmon or trout fillets (125g / 4 ounces each
☐ Salt and pepper

DIRECTIONS:
Gather all the Dill Sauce ingredients together and mix well to loosen the sour cream. Set aside for 10 minutes. If using fresh garlic, set aside for 20 minutes.

Pat fish dry with paper towel. Sprinkle with salt and pepper. Over medium high heat, add oil to skillet and place the fish skin side down.

Cook for 2 minutes, then flip and cook the other side for 1½ or 2 minutes. Remove from skillet onto serving plates.

Serve with Dill Sauce on the side, garnished with fresh dill and lemon wedges if desired. Enjoy.

136) **Stew with Oyster Mushrooms**

SERVINGS: 4
PREPARATION TIME: 20 minutes
COOKING TIME: 8 hours
Total time: 8 hours 20 minutes
INGREDIENTS:
☐ 2 tablespoons of lard or coconut oil
☐ 1 medium onion, chopped
☐ 1 clove garlic, chopped
☐ 2 pounds of pork loin, cut into 1" cubes and patted dry
☐ ½ teaspoon of Himalayan salt
☐ ½ teaspoon of freshly cracked black pepper
☐ 2 tablespoons of dried oregano
☐ 2 tablespoons of dried mustard

☐ ½ teaspoon of freshly ground whole nutmeg
☐ 1½ cups bone broth
☐ 2 tablespoons of white wine vinegar
☐ 2 pounds of oyster mushrooms
☐ ¼ cup full fat coconut milk
☐ ¼ cup ghee
☐ 3 tablespoons capers

DIRECTIONS:
Over high heat, melt the lard or coconut oil in a heavy skillet.

Add the meat in a single layer, making sure that the pieces do not touch, and cook until brown on all sides.

Repeat in several batches if you have to so you don't overcrowd the pan. Remove the cooked pieces of meat to a bowl to collect the juices and set aside.

Turn the heat to medium, add a little fat to the pan if necessary, then throw in the onion and garlic and cook until the onion is fragrant.

Add oregano, mustard, ground nutmeg, stir to coat then add broth and white wine vinegar.

Then add meat and juices back into the pan, bring to a simmer then transfer to slow cooker and cook for 6 hours on low or high for 4 hours.

Add an extra cup of water and add mushrooms and continue cooking for 1 hour on high or 2 hours on low.

Ladle a little bit of the cooking liquid into a measuring cup. Whisk in coconut milk and ghee then return to slow cooker.

Lastly, add capers, mix one final time and serve. Enjoy.

137) **Salmon with avocado and basil**

PREPARATION TIME: 7 minutes
COOKING TIME: 8 minutes
SERVINGS: 4
INGREDIENTS:
☐ 2 teaspoons of coconut oil
☐ 1½ teaspoons of coarse kosher salt, divided

- ☐ 1 teaspoon of Italian seasonings
- ☐ ½ teaspoon of crushed red pepper
- ☐ ¼ teaspoon of ground black pepper
- ☐ 1½ pounds of boneless salmon filet, skin removed
- ☐ 1 avocado
- ☐ ¼ cup of chopped basil
- ☐ 1 tablespoon lime juice
- ☐ chopped scallions, for garnish

DIRECTIONS:

Over medium high heat, heat oil in a large cast-iron skillet.

Sprinkle ¾ teaspoon salt, Italian seasonings, crushed red pepper and black pepper all over the salmon.

Place the salmon filet skinned side up in the hot oil. Let cook, undisturbed until browned and crispy along the bottom edge.

Turn the salmon over and remove skillet from heat. Allow salmon to remain in hot skillet to allow the carry-over heat to continue cooking.

While waiting, peel pit and mash avocado with basil, lime juice and the remaining ¾ teaspoon salt.

Serve salmon topped with avocado mash sprinkled with scallions if desired.

- ☐

138) **Maple Walnut Crusted Salmon**

SERVINGS: 4
COOKING TIME: 3 hours
PREPARATION TIME: 20 minutes
Total time: 3 hours 20 minutes
INGREDIENTS:

- ☐ 2 tablespoons of ghee (or make your own for pan
- ☐ 4- 175g salmon fillets
- ☐ Sprinkle of salt and pepper
- ☐ Maple Walnut Crust
- ☐ ½ cup of finely chopped walnuts
- ☐ 1 teaspoon of smoked paprika
- ☐ ½ teaspoon of chipotle powder
- ☐ ½ teaspoon of onion powder
- ☐ ½ teaspoon of cracked black pepper
- ☐ 3 tablespoons of pure maple syrup

- ☐ 1 tablespoons of apple cider vinegar
- ☐ 1 teaspoon of coconut aminos

DIRECTIONS:

Mix all the ingredients listed under "Maple Walnut Crust" in a small mixing bowl and stir until well combined.

Lay your salmon fillets on a plate and spoon the mixture over each piece of fish. Place in the refrigerator, uncovered, for 2 to 3 hours. Preheat your oven to 425F. Melt the ghee in a large oven-safe skillet and set over high heat.

Add the pieces of fish and let them cook undisturbed for about 2 minutes, to sear the skin nice and good.

Transfer the pan to the oven and continue cooking the fish for about 5 to 8 minutes, depending on desired doneness and thickness of the fillets.

Drizzle with a little bit of melted ghee and additional maple syrup at the moment of serving, if desired. Enjoy.

139) **Sweet Chilli Salmon**

SERVINGS: 4
PREPARATION TIME: 5 minutes
COOKING TIME: 5 minutes
INGREDIENTS:

- ☐ 4 x fillets of salmon (approximately 125-150 grams each
- ☐ Oil for searing
- ☐ For the marinade
- ☐ ¼ cup of liquid aminos (can use soy sauce
- ☐ small handful of baby spinach, chopped very finely
- ☐ 1 tsp. black pepper
- ☐ 2 tsp. red pepper flakes (optional
- ☐ For the sweet chilli sauce topping
- ☐ ¼ cup of homemade chili sauce
- ☐ 2 tsp. sesame oil
- ☐ 1 tsp. liquid aminos (can use soy sauce

DIRECTIONS:

In a small bowl, make the marinade and mix well. In a separate bowl, make the sweet chilli sauce topping. Set aside.

Coat a large frying pan with oil and heat on medium. Once hot and nice, quickly coat the salmon fillets in the marinade before adding to the pan.

Sear on each side for 1 to 3 minutes. Remove from the pan and cover in aluminium foil for 3 minutes to rest.

Evenly divide the sweet chilli sauce topping amongst the four salmon fillets.

Serve and enjoy.

140) **Buttered Cod in Skillet**

PREPARATION TIME: 5 minutes
COOKING TIME: 5 minutes
SERVINGS: 4
INGREDIENTS:
Cod:
- [ ] 1½ pounds of cod fillets
- [ ] 6 tablespoons of unsalted butter, sliced

Seasoning:
- [ ] ¼ teaspoon of garlic powder
- [ ] ½ teaspoon of table salt
- [ ] ¼ teaspoon of ground pepper
- [ ] ¾ teaspoon of ground paprika
- [ ] Few lemon slices
- [ ] Herbs, parsley or cilantro

DIRECTIONS:
Make Buttered Cod in Skillet; Stir together the ingredients for seasoning in a small bowl.

Then cut cod into smaller pieces, if desired. Season all sides of the cod with the seasoning.

Over medium-high heat, heat 2 tablespoons of butter in a large skillet. Once butter melts, add cod to skillet and cook for 2 minutes.

Set heat down to medium. Turn cod over, top with remaining butter and cook another 3 to 4 minutes.

Butter will completely melt and the fish will cook. (Don't overcook the cod, it will become mushy and completely fall apart.

Drizzle cod with fresh lemon juice. Top with fresh herbs, if desired.

Serve immediately. Enjoy, friends.

141) **Baked Butter Garlic Shrimp**

PREPARATION TIME: 10 minutes
COOKING TIME: 20 minutes
SERVINGS: 5 to 6 people
INGREDIENTS:
- [ ] 1 pound of raw shrimp, peeled and cleaned
- [ ] 5 tablespoons softened butter
- [ ] 3 to 4 large cloves garlic, crushed
- [ ] salt and fresh ground pepper
- [ ] fresh or dried parsley for garnish
- [ ] Lemon wedges, for serving, if desired

DIRECTIONS:
First heat oven to 425 degrees. Smear butter evenly over the bottom of the baking dish.

Add the crushed garlic over the butter, sprinkle evenly. Add the shrimp, trying not to overlap if possible

Sprinkle everything with salt and pepper. Bake for 7 minutes and then stir the shrimp and bake for 7 to 10 more minutes, or until shrimp is done.

Garnish with parsley, if desired, and squeeze a lemon wedge over it, if desired.

Serve as a side with steak, or toss the cooked shrimp and butter sauce with pasta. Enjoy.

142) **Baked Lobster Tails with Garlic Butter**

PREPARATION TIME: 10 minutes
COOKING TIME: 15 minutes
SERVINGS: 4
INGREDIENTS:
- [ ] 4 lobster tails
- [ ] 5 cloves garlic, minced
- [ ] ¼ cup grated Parmesan, plus more for serving
- [ ] Juice of 1 lemon
- [ ] 1 teaspoon of Italian seasoning
- [ ] 4 tablespoons of melted butter

DIRECTIONS:
Preheat oven to 350 degrees F. Mix together garlic, Parmesan, Italian seasoning, and melted butter and season with salt in a bowl.

Using sharp scissors or knife, cut the clear skin off the lobster and rub the lobster tails with the garlic butter seasoning.

Line a baking sheet with parchment and place the lobster tails. Bake the lobster tails for 15 minutes.

The lobster meat inside will be firm and opaque. Internal temperature should read 140 to 145 degrees.

Serve immediately friend. Enjoy.

☐

143) **Salmon and Summer Veggies in Foil**

SERVINGS: 4
PREPARATION TIME: 15 minutes
COOKING TIME: 30 minutes
INGREDIENTS:
☐ 4 (5 to 6 ounces skinless salmon fillets
☐ 2 small zucchinis (13 ounces sliced into half moons
☐ 2 small yellow squash (13 ounces sliced into half moons
☐ 2 shallots, 1 thinly sliced and 1 chopped (there are usually two in a whole shallot
☐ 1 clove garlic, minced
☐ 2½ tablespoons of olive oil, divided
☐ Salt and freshly ground black pepper
☐ 1½ tablespoons of fresh lemon juice
☐ 2 large Roma tomatoes, diced
☐ 1 tablespoon of chopped fresh thyme (or 1 teaspoon dried
☐ ¾ teaspoon of dried oregano
☐ ½ teaspoon of dried marjoram
DIRECTIONS:
First heat oven to about 400 degrees. Then cut 4 sheets of aluminium foil into 17-inch lengths.

Toss zucchini, squash, sliced shallot and garlic together with 1 tablespoon of olive oil.

Add salt and pepper to taste and divide among 4 sheets of foil, placing veggies in centre of foil.

Rub salmon fillets with 1 tablespoon of the olive oil and season bottom side with salt and pepper then place one fillet over each layer of veggies on foil.

Drizzle lemon juice over salmon and season top with salt and pepper. Mix together tomatoes, remaining diced shallot, thyme, oregano and marjoram with remaining 1½ teaspoon of olive oil and season lightly with salt and pepper.

Divide the tomato mixture over salmon fillets. Wrap sides of foil inward then fold up ends to seal.

Place on a rimmed baking sheet and bake in preheated oven until salmon has cooked through, about 25 to 30 minutes.

Carefully open foil packets and serve warm. Enjoy.

144) **Fish Curry with Coconut and Spinach**

PREPARATION TIME: 5 minutes
COOKING TIME: 20 minutes
SERVINGS: 5 to 6
INGREDIENTS:
☐ Metric - Cups/Ounces
☐ 1 kg firm white fish cut into cubes
☐ 2 to 4 tablespoons of curry paste of choice
☐ 400 ml coconut cream
☐ 400 ml water
☐ 500 g spinach washed and sliced
DIRECTIONS:
Heat the oil in a large saucepan, add the curry paste and sauté on a moderate heat for 2 to 3 minutes to activate the spices.

Add the coconut cream and water, and bring to the boil. Then carefully add the fish pieces and reduce the heat. Cook for 10 to 15 minutes.

Add the prepared spinach and cook for another 3 to 4 minutes.

Serve in large bowls. Enjoy.

145) **Buttered Cod**

PREPARATION TIME: 5 minutes
COOKING TIME: 5 minutes
SERVINGS: 4

INGREDIENTS:
Cod;
- ☐ 1½ pounds of cod fillets
- ☐ 6 tablespoons of unsalted butter, sliced

Seasoning;
- ☐ ¼ teaspoon of garlic powder
- ☐ ½ teaspoon of table salt
- ☐ ¼ teaspoon of ground pepper
- ☐ ¾ teaspoon of ground paprika
- ☐ Few lemon slices
- ☐ Herbs, parsley or cilantro

DIRECTIONS:
Make Buttered Cod in Skillet; Stir together ingredients for seasoning in a small bowl.

Cut cod into smaller pieces, if desired. Season all sides of the cod with the seasoning.

At medium-high heat, heat 2 tablespoons of butter in a large skillet. Once butter melts, add cod to skillet. Cook for 2 minutes.

Set heat down to medium. Turn cod over, top with remaining butter and cook another 3 to 4 minutes.

Butter will completely melt and the fish will cook. (Don't overcook the cod, it will become mushy and completely fall apart.

Drizzle cod with fresh lemon juice. Top with fresh herbs, if desired.

Serve immediately. Enjoy, friends.

146) **Garlic Shrimp Asparagus Skillet**

SERVINGS: 4 people
PREPARATION TIME: 10 Minutes
COOKING TIME: 15 Minutes
INGREDIENTS:
- ☐ 1 pound of uncooked extra-large shrimp — peeled, 454g
- ☐ Kosher salt and freshly ground black pepper to taste
- ☐ A pinch of crushed red pepper or red pepper flakes
- ☐ 1 teaspoon of onion powder
- ☐ 2 tablespoons of grass-fed ghee butter or extra virgin olive oil
- ☐ 1 tablespoon of extra virgin olive oil
- ☐ 3 cloves garlic — minced

- ☐ 2 cups of mushrooms — sliced
- ☐ 1 bunch of asparagus — ends trimmed and cut in half
- ☐ 1 tablespoon fresh parsley — chopped

DIRECTIONS:
Mix the shrimp, salt, pepper, red pepper flakes, and onion powder in mixing bowl. Mix everything well.

In a cast iron skillet, add 2 tablespoons of olive oil or grass-fed ghee butter over medium heat.

Add the garlic, and sauté for 30 seconds. Then add the shrimp, and sauté for about 4 minutes or until the shrimp are cooked through and done. Set aside.

In the same skillet, add 1 tablespoon of olive oil and the mushrooms. Sauté for 5 minutes. Then, add the asparagus, and cook until it's soft. Stir occasionally.

Add the shrimp back to the skillet and mix everything well to combine.

Garnish with fresh parsley. Enjoy!

147) **Grilled Salmon with Creamy Pesto Sauce**

SERVINGS: 4
PREPARATION TIME: 15 minutes
COOKING TIME: 10 minutes
INGREDIENTS:
- ☐ 4 to 6 (6 ounces skin on or skinless salmon fillets
- ☐ Olive oil, for brushing salmon and grill
- ☐ Salt and freshly ground black pepper
- ☐ 4 ounces of cream cheese, diced into small cubes
- ☐ ¼ cup of milk
- ☐ 3 tablespoons of homemade or store-bought pesto, plus more for serving* (I used homemade

DIRECTIONS:
Preheat a grill over medium-high heat to about 425 degrees.

Rub both sides of salmon with olive oil (about 1 tablespoon total and season both sides with salt and pepper.

Brush grill grates with oil and grill salmon. Do this for about 3 minutes per side or to desired doneness (if using skin-on salmon grill skin side up first.

While waiting for the salmon is, heat cream cheese with milk in a saucepan set over medium heat, stirring constantly until melted. Remove from heat and stir in pesto.

Serve salmon warm with creamy pesto sauce.

Spoon about 1 teaspoon of pesto over creamy pesto sauce for added flavor.

□

148) **Lobster Bisque**

PREPARATION TIME: 10 minutes
COOKING TIME: 40 minutes
SERVINGS: 6 people
INGREDIENTS:
□   4 lobster tails frozen in shells (or fresh
□   2 tablespoons of olive oil extra virgin
□   ½ cup of onion chopped
□   1½ teaspoons of garlic minced
□   1 cup of dry white wine
□   2 teaspoons of Worcestershire sauce
□   1 teaspoon of celery salt
□   1 teaspoon of dried thyme
□   ½ teaspoon of paprika
□   ½ teaspoon of ground cayenne pepper
□   ¼ teaspoon of ground black pepper
□   1 tablespoon of tomato paste increase to 2 tablespoons for more tomato flavour
□   2 cups of lobster stock
□   2 cups of heavy cream
□   4 tablespoons of butter
DIRECTIONS:
Boil lobster tails until shells are bright red. Remove tails to cool and reserve water to use as lobster stock.

Remove meat from shells then return the shell to water and boil for another 10 minutes. Using fine mesh strainer, strain lobster stock and reserve 2 cups.

Chop lobster meat into bite sized pieces. Set aside. Heat a sauce pan over medium high

heat and add olive oil. Sauté onion and garlic, cook for 5 minutes.

Slowly add the wine, then stir in the Worcestershire, celery salt, thyme, paprika, cayenne pepper, and black pepper. Stir gently.

Stir in the tomato paste and reserved lobster stock. Cook for 10 minutes. Puree mixture in blender or use a stick blender in the pot until smooth.

Pour mixture back to the pot, if needed, and add in the heavy cream and butter. Add additional salt if needed.

Add lobster meat and continue to simmer for another 5 to 10 minutes. Serve and enjoy.

149) **Lobster roll salad**

SERVINGS: 4 people
INGREDIENTS:
For the lobster salad:
□   2 cups of cooked lobster meat, chopped into bite sized pieces
□   1½ cups of cauliflower florets, cooked until tender and chilled
□   ½ cup of sugar free mayonnaise
□   1 teaspoon of fresh tarragon leaves, chopped
To serve:
□   8 fresh romaine lettuce leaves
□   ½ cup of chopped tomatoes
□   ½ cup of cooked bacon, chopped
DIRECTIONS:
Gather and mix the cooked lobster, cooked cauliflower, mayonnaise and tarragon in a medium bowl. Stir until well mixed and creamy.

Lay the lettuce leaves on a platter. Divide the lobster salad mixture between the 8 leaves. Sprinkle with chopped tomatoes and chopped bacon.

Serve cold or at room temperature. Enjoy.

150) **Lemon garlic steamed clams**

PREPARATION TIME: 25 minutes
COOKING TIME: 5 minutes
SERVINGS: 2

INGREDIENTS:
- ☐ 2 pounds of fresh clams
- ☐ 1 cup chicken stock
- ☐ 3 cloves garlic, minced
- ☐ 1 small onion, diced
- ☐ 2 tablespoons of grass-fed butter or ghee
- ☐ 2 tablespoons of chopped fresh flat-leaf parsley
- ☐ ½ lemon, juiced
- ☐ ½ teaspoon of dried thyme (I use this brand
- ☐ ½ teaspoon of sea salt
- ☐ ½ teaspoon of crushed red pepper flakes

DIRECTIONS:

Before cooking, add salt to a bowl of water and soak the clams for 20 minutes. The salt will help draw the sand out of the clams.

Mix the clams, chicken stock, garlic, onions, butter, a tablespoon of the parsley, lemon juice, thyme, sea salt, and red pepper flakes in a large pot.

Boil over medium-high heat, cover and cook until the clams have opened. About 3 to 5 minutes.

Pour clams and broth into large bowl and garnish with the remaining parsley and any extra lemon.

Serve and enjoy friends.

151) **Spicy Mussels in Tomato Chorizo Broth**

SERVINGS: 6
PREPARATION TIME: 5 minutes
COOKING TIME: 20 minutes
INGREDIENTS:
- ☐ 1 pound of chorizo or other spicy sausage casings removed
- ☐ 3 garlic cloves minced
- ☐ ¼ teaspoon of red pepper flakes
- ☐ 1 14- oz. can diced tomatoes
- ☐ 1 cup Apothic White Winemaker's Blend
- ☐ ¼ teaspoon of dried thyme

- ☐ 2 pounds of mussels cleaned (discard any that have cracked shells or are open and won't close when tapped gently on counter
- ☐ Salt and pepper to taste

DIRECTIONS:

Set a large pot or Dutch oven over medium heat, brown sausage until cooked through, and break up any chunks with the back of a wooden spoon.

Remove sausage to a paper towel-lined plate to drain (use a slotted spoon, leaving drippings in pan.

Add garlic and red pepper flakes to pot and cook until fragrant, about 1 minute.

Add tomatoes, wine, and dried thyme and turn heat to medium high. Bring to a boil and add mussels.

Cover and cook for 3 minutes. Remove lid, stir gently and re-cover. Cook another 3 to 4 minutes, or until most mussels have opened. Remove mussels from pot with a slotted spoon or skimmer. Return sausage to pot.

Season broth with salt and pepper and bring back to a boil for a few minutes until it thickens.

Place mussels in large bowls and spooning sauce over. Enjoy.

152) **Garlic Lemon Butter Crab Legs Recipe**

PREPARATION TIME: 10 minutes
COOKING TIME: 5 minutes
Servings 2 people
INGREDIENTS:
- ☐ 1 pound of king crab legs
- ☐ ½ stick salted butter, melted (4 tablespoons
- ☐ 3 cloves garlic, minced
- ☐ 1 tablespoon of chopped parsley
- ☐ ½ tablespoon of lemon juice
- ☐ lemon slices

DIRECTIONS:

Preheat oven to 375F.

Thaw the crab legs if they are frozen. Cut or slice the crab legs into halves to expose the flesh. Arrange them evenly on a baking sheet or tray.

Melt the butter in a microwave, for about 30 seconds. Add the garlic, parsley and lemon juice to the melted butter. Give a good stir. Drizzle and spread the butter mixture on the crab. Save some for dipping. Bake the crab legs in the oven for about 5 minutes.

Serve immediately with the remaining garlic lemon butter and lemon slices. Squeeze some lemon juice on the crab before eating. Enjoy friends.

☐

153) **Crab Rangoon Fat Bombs**

PREPARATION TIME: 5 minutes
COOKING TIME: 15 minutes
INGREDIENTS:
☐   1 Pkg. 80 ounces Cream Cheese
☐   1 can crab 170 g
☐   ¾ cup of Shredded Mozzarella Cheese
☐   ½ teaspoon of Finely Minced Garlic
☐   ½ teaspoon of Garlic Powder
☐   ½ teaspoon of Onion Powder
☐   Dash of Salt and Pepper
☐   10 Slices Bacon
DIRECTIONS:
Soften the Cream Cheese.

Then in a large bowl combine it with the strained canned crab, the shredded mozzarella cheese, the garlic and onion powder and the salt and pepper.

Mix until well combined. Place the bowl in the fridge for ½ hour. Cook the bacon until it is Crispy. Then set aside to cool. Then chop into small pieces.

Scoop 1 tablespoon size balls of the cream cheese and crab mixture, then use your fingers to make them ball shaped.

Roll the balls in the chopped up bacon. (I washed my hands between each ball. Store in the fridge until ready to serve.

Makes 24 Bacon Crab Rangoon Fat Bombs. Serve and enjoy.

154) **Ginger Sesame Glazed Salmon**

COOKING TIME: 25 minutes
PREPARATION TIME: 15 minutes
INGREDIENTS:
☐   10 oz. Salmon Filet
☐   2 tablespoons of Soy Sauce (or coconut aminos
☐   2 teaspoons of Sesame Oil
☐   1 tablespoon of Rice Vinegar
☐   1 teaspoon of Minced Ginger
☐   2 teaspoons of Minced Garlic
☐   1 tablespoon of Red Boat Fish Sauce
☐   1 tablespoon of Sugar Free Ketchup
☐   2 tablespoons of White Wine
Cooking Instruction:
Combine all of the ingredients except for sesame oil, ketchup and white wine in a small Tupperware container.

Marinade ingredients in the liquids for about 10 to 15 minutes. Then add sesame oil to a high heated pan.

Add fish skin when you see the first wisp of smoke. Let fish cook and skin crisp, then flip and cook on the other side (about 3-4 minutes per side.

Add all marinate liquids to the pan and let it boil with the fish when you flip it. Bring out the fish from the pan and set aside.

Add ketchup, and white wine to marinate liquids. Cook for 5 minutes to reduce. Serve on the side. Enjoy.

155) **Cucumber Dill Salmon**

COOKING TIME: 20 minutes
PREPARATION TIME: 10 minutes
INGREDIENTS:
☐   Olive oil
☐   3 to 4 salmon filets
☐   Salt and pepper
☐   1 lemon cut in 6 wedges
☐   1/3 cup English cucumber cut in pea size cubes
☐   4 ounces of light or Greek yogurt cream cheese
☐   2 tablespoons of fresh dill minced

☐   ¼ cup + an additional 2 to 3 table-spoons of skim milk

DIRECTIONS:

Pre-heat the oven to 400 degrees.

Drizzle olive oil into pan and warm over medium heat. Pat moisture from salmon using a paper towel and season with salt and pepper.

Sear the salmon on both sides then squeeze the juice from one lemon wedge over the top of the salmon pieces.

Bake the salmon 6 to 8 minutes. Remove the salmon from the pan onto a serving platter and on top of the stove over low-medium heat.

Add the milk and cream cheese to the same skillet then season with salt and pepper.

Combine ¼ cup of the skim milk and cream cheese using an 'S' motion (if the mixture is too thick, add more milk one tablespoon at a time.

Switch off the heat and add the diced cucumber and 1 tablespoon of the fresh dill (stir well. Spoon the creamy dill sauce over the salmon filets.

Garnish with the additional dill and serve with a lemon wedge. Enjoy.

Poultry

156) Chicken with Mushrooms Soup

PREPARATION TIME: 10 minutes
COOKING TIME: 15 minutes
SERVINGS: 4
INGREDIENTS:
2 tablespoons olive oil
3 garlic cloves, minced
8 ounces baby Bella mushrooms, sliced
3 carrots, sliced
1 yellow onion, chopped
2 celery stalks, chopped
¼ cup coconut cream
1 tablespoon chopped thyme
4 cups chicken stock
1 cup coconut milk
1 cup brown rice
2 chicken breasts, skinless, boneless and cubed
DIRECTIONS:
Heat up a pot with the oil over medium heat then add carrots, mushrooms, onion and celery, stir and cook for 6 minutes. Add the chicken, toss and cook for 5 minutes more. Add thyme, garlic, salt, pepper, stock and milk. Stir well and cook for 2-3 minutes. Add the rice, stir, bring to a simmer over medium heat and cook for 10 more minutes until the rice is done. Divide the soup into bowls and serve.
Enjoy!
Nutrition: calories 300, fat 6, fiber 7, carbs 15, protein 16

157) Chicken and Plum Sauce

PREPARATION TIME: 10 minutes
COOKING TIME: 1 hour and 40 minutes
SERVINGS: 6
INGREDIENTS:
1 whole chicken
A pinch of salt and black pepper
1 red onion, chopped

3 tablespoons olive oil
1 teaspoon grated fresh ginger
4 garlic cloves, minced
21-ounces plums, stones removed and chopped
6 tablespoons coconut aminos
1 tablespoon balsamic vinegar
4 tablespoons sriracha
DIRECTIONS:
Arrange the chicken in a roasting pan and season with salt and pepper. Drizzle half of the oil over the chicken and rub the seasonings and oil into the chicken. Place in the oven at 400 degrees F and roast for 1 hour and 10 minutes. Heat up a pan with the rest of the oil over medium heat then add onion, stir and cook for 5 minutes. Add the garlic, ginger, plums, coconut aminos, sriracha and vinegar. Stir, bring to a simmer and cook for 20 minutes. Transfer this mix to your blender, pulse a few times and then brush the cooked chicken with this mix. Cook the chicken for 10 minutes more in the oven then carve and serve with the sauce from the pan drizzled all over.
Enjoy!
Nutrition: calories 280, fat 8, fiber 4, carbs 12, protein 17

158) Adobo Lime Chicken Mix

PREPARATION TIME: 10 minutes
COOKING TIME: 40 minutes
SERVINGS: 6
INGREDIENTS:
6 chicken thighs
Salt and black pepper to the taste
1 tablespoon olive oil
Zest of 1 lime
1½ teaspoons chipotle peppers in adobo sauce
1 cup sliced peach
1 tablespoon lime juice
DIRECTIONS:
Heat up a pan with the oil over medium-high heat and add the chicken thighs. Season with salt and pepper then brown for 4 minutes on each side and bake in the oven at 375 degrees F for 20 minutes. In your food processor,

mix the peaches with the chipotle, lime zest and lime juice then blend and pour over the chicken. Bake for 10 minutes more, divide everything between plates and serve. Enjoy!

Nutrition: calories 309, fat 6, fiber 4, carbs 16, protein 15

159) Chicken and Cauliflower Rice with Mango

PREPARATION TIME: 10 minutes
COOKING TIME: 25 minutes
SERVINGS: 2
INGREDIENTS:
2 tablespoons coconut oil
8 ounces chicken breast, cubed
3 tablespoons almond flour
Salt and black pepper to the taste
For the cauliflower rice:
3 cups chopped cauliflower
2 tablespoons coconut flakes
2 teaspoons coconut oil
1 mango, cored and cubed
1 tablespoon chopped cilantro
1 tablespoon chopped green onions
1 tablespoon sesame seeds, toasted
DIRECTIONS:
In a bowl, mix the almond flour with the chicken, salt and pepper and toss to coat. Heat up a pan with 2 tablespoons coconut oil over medium-high heat then add chicken, stir, cook for 5 minutes on each side and divide between plates. In your food processor, mix cauliflower with salt and pepper and blend well to turn the cauliflower into "rice". Heat up a pan with 2 teaspoons coconut oil over medium-high heat. Add cauliflower and coconut flakes, stir and cook for 3 minutes. Reduce heat and add mango, cilantro, green onions and sesame seeds. Stir, cover the pan, cook for 5 minutes more. Divide between two plates and serve next to the chicken. Enjoy!

Nutrition: calories 260, fat 22, fiber 6, carbs 13, protein 19

160) Chicken and Berry Sauce

PREPARATION TIME: 10 minutes
COOKING TIME: 25 minutes
SERVINGS: 2
INGREDIENTS:
1 shallot, chopped
2 chicken breasts, skinless and boneless
2 garlic cloves, minced
1/3 cup balsamic vinegar
1 cup chicken stock
2 tablespoons coconut oil
2 cups raspberries
Salt and black pepper to the taste
DIRECTIONS:
Heat up a pan with half of the coconut oil over medium-high heat. Add the chicken, season with salt and pepper and cook for 5 minutes. Place the chicken in the oven, roast for 10 minutes at 325 degrees F then divide between plates. Meanwhile, heat up the pan with the rest of the oil over medium-high heat and add shallot and garlic, stir and cook for 3 minutes. Add vinegar, stock, raspberries, salt and pepper. Stir, cook for 5 minutes more, drizzle over the chicken and serve. Enjoy!

Nutrition: calories 280, fat 6, fiber 3, carbs 15, protein 16

161) Chicken Curry

PREPARATION TIME: 10 minutes
COOKING TIME: 5 hours
SERVINGS: 4
INGREDIENTS:
2 sweet potatoes, cubed
3 chicken breasts, boneless, skinless and chopped
1 red bell pepper, chopped
1 small yellow onion, chopped
2 cups coconut milk
2 cups chicken stock
1 teaspoon ground cumin
3 tablespoons curry powder
2 tablespoons chopped cilantro
Salt and cayenne pepper to the taste
DIRECTIONS:

In your slow cooker, mix the chicken the sweet potatoes, bell pepper, onion, stock, milk, cumin, curry powder, salt and cayenne. Cover and cook on Low for 5 hours then divide into bowls, sprinkle the cilantro on top and serve.

Enjoy!

Nutrition: calories 280, fat 13, fiber 7, carbs 8, protein 15

162) **Cumin Chicken Mix**

PREPARATION TIME: 2 hours
COOKING TIME: 25 minutes
SERVINGS: 4
INGREDIENTS:
4 garlic cloves, minced
2 pounds chicken thighs, skinless and boneless
4 tablespoons extra-virgin olive oil
4 tablespoons chopped cilantro
2 tablespoons lime juice
A pinch of salt and black pepper
2 tablespoons olive oil
1 teaspoon cumin, ground
1 teaspoon red chili flakes
Lime wedges for serving
DIRECTIONS:
In a bowl, whisk the olive oil with salt, pepper, cilantro, garlic, lime juice, cumin and chili flakes. Add the chicken, toss, cover and leave aside for 2 hours. Heat up a pan with the oil over medium-high heat, add chicken, cook for 3 minutes on each side and transfer to a baking dish. Cook in the oven at 375 degrees F for 20 minutes then divide between plates and serve with lime wedges on the side.

Enjoy!

Nutrition: calories 200, fat 10, fiber 1, carbs 12, protein 24

163) **Herbed Chicken Thighs**

PREPARATION TIME: 10 minutes
COOKING TIME: 40 minutes
SERVINGS: 2
INGREDIENTS:

14 ounces chicken thighs, bone-in
1 tablespoon lemon juice
1 teaspoon chili powder
A pinch of salt and black pepper
1 tablespoon fresh minced ginger
1 tablespoon olive oil
4 onions, chopped
2 rosemary springs, chopped
DIRECTIONS:
In a bowl, mix chili powder with lemon juice and ginger. Add the chicken, rub it with this mix and then let sit for 10 minutes. Heat up a pan with the oil over medium-high heat, add the marinated chicken pieces and cook for 3 minutes on each side. Add rosemary, onions, salt and pepper. Reduce heat to medium, cover pan, cook for 25 minutes. Divide between plates and serve.

Enjoy!

Nutrition: calories 210, fat 8, fiber 9, carbs 12, protein 17

164) **Turkey with Tomatoes Stew**

PREPARATION TIME: 10 minutes
COOKING TIME: 1 hour and 20 minutes
SERVINGS: 6
INGREDIENTS:
3 teaspoons olive oil
1 green bell pepper, chopped
1 pound ground turkey meat
1 tablespoons garlic, minced
1 yellow onion, chopped
1 teaspoon ground ancho chilies
1 tablespoon chili powder
2 teaspoons ground cumin
8 ounces canned green chilies and juice, chopped
8 ounces tomato paste
15 ounces canned tomatoes, chopped
2 cups veggie stock
A pinch of salt and black pepper
DIRECTIONS:
Heat up a pan with 2 teaspoons oil over medium heat, add turkey, stir, brown well on all sides and transfer to a pot. Heat up the pan with the rest of the oil over medium heat and

add onion and green bell pepper. Stir and cook for 3 minutes. Add garlic, chili powder, ancho chili powder, salt, pepper and cumin, stir and cook for 2 more minutes. Transfer this to the pot with the turkey meat, add chilies and juice, tomato sauce, chopped tomatoes, stock, salt and pepper. Stir, bring to a boil, cover the pot and cook for 1 hour. Divide into bowls and serve.
Enjoy!
Nutrition: calories 327, fat 8, fiber 13, carbs 24, protein 27

Chicken and Mushroom Salad
PREPARATION TIME: 10 minutes
COOKING TIME: 0 minutes
SERVINGS: 4
INGREDIENTS:
1 yellow onion, chopped
12 ounces canned mushrooms, drained and chopped
2 garlic cloves, minced
2 teaspoons chopped rosemary
3 cups chicken, already cooked and shredded
2 cups baby spinach
Salt and black pepper to the tastes
A splash of balsamic vinegar
A drizzle of olive oil
DIRECTIONS:
In a bowl, mix the mushrooms with the chicken, onion, garlic, rosemary, spinach, salt, pepper, vinegar and oil, toss and serve.
Enjoy!
Nutrition: calories 210, fat 5, fiber 8, carbs 15, protein 11

165) **Rosemary Chicken Roast**

PREPARATION TIME: 10 minutes
COOKING TIME: 1 hour and 10 minutes
SERVINGS: 4
INGREDIENTS:
1 whole chicken
A pinch of salt and black pepper
2 tablespoons olive oil
2 green onions, chopped
1 cup chicken stock
2 teaspoons lemon juice
2 teaspoons chopped rosemary

DIRECTIONS:
Place chicken in a roasting pan, add salt, pepper, oil, green onions, stock, lemon juice and rosemary. Toss the ingredients together, place in the oven and bake at 450 degrees F for 1 hour. Slice the meat, divide it between plates and serve with cooking juices drizzled on top.
Enjoy!
Nutrition: calories 495, fat 8, fiber 4, carbs 10, protein 27

166) **Ginger Chicken Thighs**

PREPARATION TIME: 12 hours
COOKING TIME: 1 hour
SERVINGS: 4
INGREDIENTS:
8 chicken thighs, bone in and skin on
A pinch of sea salt and black pepper
1 tablespoon apple cider vinegar
3 tablespoons chopped onion
1 tablespoon fresh grated ginger
½ teaspoon dried thyme
¾ cup apple juice
½ cup maple syrup
DIRECTIONS:
In a bowl, combine chicken thighs with salt, pepper, vinegar, onion, ginger, thyme, apple juice and maple syrup. Cover and keep in the fridge for 12 hours to marinate. Transfer this whole mix to a baking dish, cover dish, bake in the oven at 400 degrees F for 1 hour. Divide the meat and sauce between plates and serve.
Enjoy!
Nutrition: calories 274, fat 6, fiber 8, carbs 14, protein 12

167) **Spicy Chicken Thighs**

PREPARATION TIME: 10 minutes
COOKING TIME: 6 hours and 10 minutes
SERVINGS: 6
INGREDIENTS:
4 pounds chicken thighs, skin-on and bone-in
1 bunch green onions, chopped

½ cup Thai sweet chili sauce
DIRECTIONS:
Heat up a pan over medium-high heat, add chicken thighs and brown them for 5 minutes on each side. Transfer the chicken to your slow cooker, add green onions and chili sauce, cover and cook on Low for 6 hours. Divide between plates and serve.
Enjoy!
Nutrition: calories 260, fat 4, fiber 2, carbs 12, protein 14

168) Chicken with Parsley Sauce

PREPARATION TIME: 30 minutes
COOKING TIME: 40 minutes
SERVINGS: 6
INGREDIENTS:
1 cup chopped parsley
1 teaspoon dried oregano
½ cup olive oil
¼ cup vegetable stock
4 garlic cloves
A pinch of salt and black pepper
12 chicken thighs
DIRECTIONS:
In your food processor, mix parsley with oregano, garlic, salt, oil and the stock. Pulse well until smooth. In a bowl, mix the chicken with the parsley sauce and toss, cover and keep in the fridge for 30 minutes. Heat up your kitchen grill over medium heat and place the chicken pieces on the grill. Close the lid and cook for 20 minutes. Flip the chicken and cook for 20 minutes more. Divide between plates and serve with the parsley sauce on top.
Enjoy!
Nutrition: calories 254, fat 3, fiber 3, carbs 7, protein 12

169) Simple Chicken and Veggie Casserole

PREPARATION TIME: 10 minutes
COOKING TIME: 1 hour and 40 minutes
SERVINGS: 8

INGREDIENTS:
1½ cups green lentils
3 cups clean chicken stock
2 pound chicken breasts, skinless, boneless and cubed
A pinch of sea salt and cayenne pepper
3 teaspoons ground cumin
Cooking spray
5 garlic cloves, minced
1 yellow onion, chopped
2 red bell peppers, chopped
14 ounces canned tomatoes, chopped
2 cups corn
2 tablespoons chopped jalapeno pepper
1 tablespoon garlic powder
1 cup chopped parsley
DIRECTIONS:
Put the stock in a pot, add a pinch of salt and the lentils. Stir, bring to a boil over medium heat, cover and simmer for 35 minutes. Heat up a pan with some cooking spray over medium-high heat and add the chicken, season with salt, cayenne pepper and 1 teaspoon cumin. Cook for 5 minutes on each side then transfer to a bowl. Heat up the pan again over medium heat, add bell peppers, garlic, onion, tomatoes, salt, cayenne and 1 teaspoon cumin. Stir, cook for 7 minutes and transfer to the bowl with the chicken. Drain the lentils, add them to the bowl with the meat and then add jalapeno pepper, garlic powder, the rest of the cumin, corn and parsley. Toss, transfer the whole mix to a baking dish and place in the oven at 350 degrees F and bake for 50 minutes. Divide between plates and serve.
Enjoy!
Nutrition: calories 244, fat 11, fiber 4, carbs 10, protein 13

170) Chicken Breasts and Mushrooms

PREPARATION TIME: 10 minutes
COOKING TIME: 30 minutes
SERVINGS: 6
INGREDIENTS:

3 pounds chicken breasts, skinless and boneless
1 yellow onion, chopped
1 garlic clove, minced
A pinch of salt and black pepper
10 mushrooms, chopped
1 tablespoon olive oil
2 red bell peppers, chopped

DIRECTIONS:

Put chicken in a baking dish, add onion, garlic, salt, pepper, mushrooms, oil and bell peppers. Mix briefly and bake in the oven at 425 degrees F for 30 minutes. Divide between plates and serve.

Enjoy!

Nutrition: calories 285, fat 12, fiber 1, carbs 13, protein 16

171) Spicy Chicken and Cauliflower

PREPARATION TIME: 10 minutes
COOKING TIME: 25 minutes
SERVINGS: 4
INGREDIENTS:

2 pounds chicken breasts, skinless, boneless and cubed
1 tablespoon rice vinegar
4 tablespoons raw honey
6 tablespoons coconut aminos
2 garlic cloves, minced
2 pounds cauliflower, florets separated
½ cup water
1 tablespoon whole wheat flour
2 tablespoons olive oil
3 green onions, chopped
2 tablespoons sesame seeds

DIRECTIONS:

In a bowl, mix 3 tablespoons honey with 3 tablespoons coconut aminos, garlic, vinegar and the chicken. Heat up a pan with half of the oil over medium heat, add cauliflower and stir then cook for 5 minutes and transfer to a bowl. Heat up the pan with the rest of the oil over medium heat, Drain the chicken, reserving the marinade, then add it to the pan. Toss and cook for 6 minutes. In a separate bowl, whisk together the rest of the aminos with the remaining honey, water, whole wheat flour and the reserved marinade. Add over the chicken, cover the pan and cook on low heat for 10 minutes, take off the heat, add the cauliflower and toss. Divide between plates, sprinkle green onions and sesame seeds on top and serve.

Enjoy!

Nutrition: calories 250, fat 4, fiber 5, carbs 10, protein 12

172) Chicken and Corn Soup

PREPARATION TIME: 10 minutes
COOKING TIME: 8 hours
SERVINGS: 6
INGREDIENTS:

8 cups chicken stock
2 teaspoons garlic powder
A pinch of salt and black pepper
14 ounces coconut milk
1½ cups green lentils
2 pounds chicken breasts, skinless, boneless and cubed
1/3 cup chopped parsley
3 cups corn
3 handfuls spinach
3 green onions, chopped

DIRECTIONS:

In your slow cooker, mix the stock with salt, pepper, chicken, lentils, garlic powder and corn. Cover and cook on Low for 7 hours and 30 minutes. Add the coconut milk, spinach and green onions the recover and cook on Low for 30 minutes more. Add the parsley, stir, divide into bowls and serve.

Enjoy!

Nutrition: calories 265, fat 8, fiber 10, carbs 10, protein 24

173) Chicken with Artichokes

PREPARATION TIME: 10 minutes
COOKING TIME: 1 hour
SERVINGS: 8
INGREDIENTS:

2 yellow onions, chopped
2 pounds chicken thighs, skinless, boneless and chopped
5 garlic cloves, minced
2 tablespoons olive oil
16 ounces canned artichoke hearts, drained and chopped
1 tablespoon maple syrup
2 cups vegetable stock
A pinch of sea salt and black pepper
2 tablespoons chopped cilantro
DIRECTIONS:
Heat up a pot with half of the oil over medium heat, add chicken, cook for 4 minutes on each side and transfer to a bowl. Heat up the pot again with the rest of the oil over medium-high heat, add garlic and onion then stir and cook for 1 minute. Add the stock, maple syrup, artichokes, salt and pepper. Stir well, bring to a simmer and cook for 3-4 minutes. Return chicken to the pot, stir, cover, reduce heat to low and cook for 45 minutes. Add the cilantro, toss, divide into bowls and serve.
Enjoy!
Nutrition: calories 200, fat 4, fiber 4, carbs 10, protein 16

174) **Chicken with Green Beans**

PREPARATION TIME: 10 minutes
COOKING TIME: 30 minutes
SERVINGS: 4
INGREDIENTS:
1½ pounds chicken breasts, cubed
2 tablespoons olive oil
2 pounds green beans, trimmed
25 ounces canned tomato sauce
2 tablespoons chopped parsley
6 ounces canned tomato paste
A pinch of salt and black pepper
DIRECTIONS:
Heat up a pan with half of the oil over medium heat, add chicken, stir, cook for 5 minutes on each side and transfer to a bowl. Set the cooked chicken aside. Heat up the pan with the rest of the oil over medium

heat, add green beans, stir and cook for 10 minutes. Return chicken to the pan, add salt, pepper, tomato sauce, tomato paste and parsley. Stir and cook for 5 minutes more then divide between plates and serve.
Enjoy!
Nutrition: calories 250, fat 4, fiber 2, carbs 6, protein 12

175) **Chicken and Pumpkin Soup**

PREPARATION TIME: 10 minutes
COOKING TIME: 20 minutes
SERVINGS: 4
INGREDIENTS:
2 chicken breasts, skinless, boneless and cubed
1 yellow onion, chopped
2 tablespoons olive oil
1 garlic clove, chopped
20 ounces pumpkin , peeled, seedless and cubed
2 carrots, chopped
½ teaspoon fresh grated ginger
½ teaspoon ground cumin
1 teaspoon ground turmeric
A pinch of salt and black pepper
12 ounces coconut milk
16 ounces chicken stock
DIRECTIONS:
Heat up a pot with the oil over medium-high heat then add garlic and onion. Stir and cook for 2 minutes. Add carrots, pumpkin, ginger, cumin, turmeric, stock, coconut milk and chicken, Stir, bring to a boil, reduce heat to medium and simmer for 15 minutes. Add salt and pepper, blend slightly using an immersion blender then divide into bowls and serve.
Enjoy!
Nutrition: calories 220, fat 3, fiber 9, carbs 7, protein 11

176) **Chicken and Kale Soup**

PREPARATION TIME: 10 minutes
COOKING TIME: 15 minutes

SERVINGS: 2
INGREDIENTS:
1 red bell pepper, chopped
1 yellow onion, chopped
¼ cup chopped pickled jalapeno peppers
2 garlic cloves, minced
1 tablespoon olive oil
1 teaspoon ground cumin
1 teaspoon ground coriander
1 teaspoon dried oregano
1 ½ cups chicken breast, cooked and shredded
2 ½ cups chicken stock
2 cups kale, torn
Zest of 1 lime, grated
Juice of 1 lime
A pinch of salt and black pepper
15 ounces canned tomatoes, chopped
2 tablespoons chopped spring onions
1 avocado, peeled, pitted and sliced
1 teaspoon sweet paprika
3 tablespoons chopped coriander
DIRECTIONS:
Heat up a pot with the oil over medium heat, add onion, stir and cook for 2 minutes. Add red bell peppers, garlic, jalapenos, oregano, cumin, coriander, tomatoes, kale, chicken, lime zest, stock, lime juice, salt and pepper. Stir the mix, bring to a boil, cook for 10 minutes and take off heat. Ladle soup into bowls, top with green onion, paprika, chopped coriander and avocado and serve. Enjoy!
Nutrition: calories 170, fat 3, fiber 3, carbs 12, protein 11

177) **Chicken and Sweet Potatoes Stew**

PREPARATION TIME: 10 minutes
COOKING TIME: 8 hours
SERVINGS: 4
INGREDIENTS:
2 carrots, chopped
5 garlic cloves, minced
2 celery sticks, chopped
2 onions, chopped
2 sweet potatoes, cubed

14 ounces tomato juice
1-quart chicken stock
2 cups chicken meat, skinless, boneless and cubed
A pinch of salt and black pepper
¼ teaspoon cayenne pepper
½ pound baby spinach
DIRECTIONS:
In your slow cooker, combine the carrots with the garlic, celery, onions, sweet potatoes, tomato juice, stock, chicken, salt, pepper and cayenne. Mix and cover then cook on Low for 7 hours and 40 minutes. Add the spinach, cover and cook on Low for 20 minutes more. Divide into bowls and serve. Enjoy!
Nutrition: calories 250, fat 3, fiber 3, carbs 14, protein 7

178) **Chicken and Carrot Stew**

PREPARATION TIME: 10 minutes
COOKING TIME: 7 hours
SERVINGS: 4
INGREDIENTS:
2 tablespoons olive oil
8 carrots, chopped
1 ½ pounds chicken breasts, skinless, boneless and cubed
½ teaspoon black peppercorns
1 yellow onion, chopped
¼ cup tapioca flour
1 tablespoon chopped thyme
4 cups chicken stock
A pinch of salt and black pepper
DIRECTIONS:
Heat up a pan with the oil over medium-high heat, add the chicken and stir. Brown for 4 minutes on all sides and transfer to your slow cooker. Add the carrots, peppercorns, onion, tapioca, thyme, stock, salt and pepper to the slow cooker as well. Stir, cover and cook on Low for 7 hours. Divide into bowls and serve.
Enjoy!
Nutrition: calories 260, fat 8, fiber 5, carbs 14, protein 11

179) Squash Soup with Turkey

PREPARATION TIME: 10 minutes
COOKING TIME: 35 minutes
SERVINGS: 4
INGREDIENTS:
3 celery stalks, chopped
1 yellow onion, chopped
1 tablespoon olive oil
6 cups chicken stock
Salt and black pepper to the taste
¼ cup chopped parsley
3 cups baked spaghetti squash, chopped
3 cups turkey, cooked and shredded
DIRECTIONS:
Heat up a pot with the oil over medium-high heat, add celery and onion then stir and cook for 5 minutes. Add parsley, stock, turkey meat, salt and pepper. Stir and cook for 20 minutes. Add spaghetti squash, stir, cook for 10 minutes more, divide into bowls and serve.
Enjoy!
Nutrition: calories 180, fat 4, fiber 8, carbs 11, protein 10

180) Turkey Casserole with Coconut Cream

PREPARATION TIME: 10 minutes
COOKING TIME: 45 minutes
SERVINGS: 8
INGREDIENTS:
4 cups spiralzed zucchinis
1 egg, whisked
3 cups shredded cabbage
3 cups turkey meat, cooked and shredded
½ cup chicken stock
½ cup coconut cream
Salt and black pepper to the taste
¼ teaspoon garlic powder
DIRECTIONS:
Heat up a pan with the stock over medium-low heat, add the egg, cream, salt, pepper and garlic powder. Stir and bring to a simmer then add the cabbage and the turkey. Stir and take off the heat. Arrange the zucchini noodles in a baking dish and pour turkey mix on top as well. Spread the mix across the pan then cover the dish and bake in the oven at 400 degrees F for 35 minutes. Divide between plates and serve.
Enjoy!
Nutrition: calories 240, fat 15, fiber 1, carbs 9, protein 15

181) Coconut Chicken Dish

PREPARATION TIME: 10 minutes
COOKING TIME: 50 minutes
SERVINGS: 4
INGREDIENTS:
3 pounds chicken breasts, boneless and skinless
Cooking spray
4 ounces coconut cream
1 zucchini, shredded
1 carrot, shredded
Salt and black pepper to the taste
1 teaspoon minced garlic
DIRECTIONS:
In a bowl, mix the cream with the zucchini, carrot, garlic, salt and pepper. Arrange the chicken in a baking dish greased with cooking spray then add the cream mixture and spread evenly into the pan. Place in the oven at 400 degrees F, bake for 45 minutes, divide between plates and serve.
Enjoy!
Nutrition: calories 425, fat 5, fiber 1, carbs 8, protein 20

182) Thyme Chicken and Veggies

PREPARATION TIME: 10 minutes
COOKING TIME: 40 minutes
SERVINGS: 6
INGREDIENTS:
2 cups coconut cream
40 ounces rotisserie chicken pieces, boneless, skinless and shredded
3 tablespoons coconut oil, melted
½ cup chopped yellow onion
¾ cup chopped red peppers

29 ounces chicken stock
Salt and black pepper to the taste
8 ounces mushrooms, chopped
1 cup green beans
17 ounces asparagus, trimmed
3 teaspoons chopped thyme
DIRECTIONS:
Heat up a pan with the cream over medium heat, bring to a simmer and cook for 6-7 minutes. Heat up a pan with the oil over medium heat, add onion and peppers, stir and cook for 3 minutes. Add stock, salt and pepper and then bring to a boil and cook for 10 minutes. Add asparagus, Green Beans with Mushroomss, stir and cook for 7 minutes. Add chicken pieces, cream, thyme, salt and pepper. Stir and cook for 3-4 minutes more then divide between plates and serve.
Enjoy!
Nutrition: calories 430, fat 27, fiber 3, carbs 4, protein 47

183) Chicken and Avocado Salad

PREPARATION TIME: 10 minutes
COOKING TIME: 0 minutes
SERVINGS: 2
INGREDIENTS:
1 avocado, pitted, peeled and sliced
Salt and black pepper to the taste
3 tablespoons coconut cream
1 chicken breast, grilled and shredded
DIRECTIONS:
In a salad bowl, mix the avocado with the chicken, salt, pepper and coconut cream. Toss well and serve right away
Enjoy!
Nutrition: calories 218, fat 14, fiber 5, carbs 10, protein 15

184) Chicken and Egg Salad

PREPARATION TIME: 10 minutes
COOKING TIME: 0 minutes
SERVINGS: 3
INGREDIENTS:
1 green onion, chopped

1 celery rib, chopped
2 eggs, hard-boiled, peeled and chopped
5 ounces chicken breast, roasted and chopped
2 tablespoons chopped parsley
½ tablespoons dill relish
Salt and black pepper to the taste
1/3 cup mayonnaise
DIRECTIONS:
In a salad bowl, mix the chicken with the eggs, celery, onion, parsley, dill, salt, pepper and mayo and serve.
Enjoy!
Nutrition: calories 253, fat 7, fiber 5, carbs 8, protein 12

185) Balsamic Chicken and Salad

PREPARATION TIME: 10 minutes
COOKING TIME: 40 minutes
SERVINGS: 4
INGREDIENTS:
1½ pound chicken breasts, skinless and boneless
3 tablespoons olive oil
Salt and black pepper to the taste
¼ cup balsamic vinegar
6 ounces sweet onion, chopped
1 lettuce head, chopped
2 garlic cloves, minced
4 ounces mushrooms, sliced
1 avocado, pitted, peeled and sliced
3 ounces sun-dried tomatoes, chopped
1 orange bell pepper, sliced
1 teaspoon Italian seasoning
1 teaspoon red pepper flakes
1 teaspoon onion powder
DIRECTIONS:
In a bowl, mix the chicken with salt, pepper, Italian seasoning, pepper flakes, onion powder and balsamic vinegar and toss. Heat up your grill over medium-high heat then add the chicken, cook for 6-7 minutes on each side and divide between plates. Heat up another pan with the oil over medium-low heat, add mushrooms, garlic, salt, pepper and onion. Stir and cook for 20 minutes. In

a bowl, mix lettuce leaves with the bell pepper, sun-dried tomatoes, avocado and the mushrooms mix and add this salad next to the chicken and serve.
Enjoy!
Nutrition: calories 235, fat 13, fiber 7, carbs 15, protein 15

Meat

186) Lemony Pork Chops

PREPARATION TIME: 10 minutes
COOKING TIME: 20 minutes
SERVINGS: 4
INGREDIENTS:
4 pork chops
1 cup pork rinds
1 egg
½ cup coconut cream
2 tablespoons olive oil
½ cup chicken stock
3 tablespoons lemon juice
A pinch of salt and black pepper
2 tablespoons chopped chives
DIRECTIONS:
In a bowl, whisk the egg with salt and pepper. Put the pork rinds in another bowl. Dip pork chops in egg and then in pork rinds. Heat up a pan with the oil over medium-high heat and add the coated pork chops. Cook them for 4 minutes on one side, flip the place in the oven and cook at 400 degrees F for 10 minutes. Meanwhile, heat up a pan with the stock over medium heat, add the cream, lemon juice, salt, pepper and chives. Toss and cook for 5-6 minutes and take off the heat. Divide the pork chops between plates and drizzle the lemon sauce over the meat then serve.
Enjoy!
Nutrition: calories 299, fat 7, fiber 5, carbs 13, protein 17

187) Pork Chops with Berry Sauce

PREPARATION TIME: 10 minutes
COOKING TIME: 15 minutes
SERVINGS: 4
INGREDIENTS:
2 pounds pork chops
1 teaspoon ground cinnamon
A pinch of salt and black pepper
12 ounces blackberries
½ teaspoon dried thyme
2 tablespoons water
½ cup balsamic vinegar
A pinch of salt and black pepper
DIRECTIONS:
Season pork chops with salt and pepper and sprinkle the cinnamon and thyme all over as well. Heat up a small pot with the blackberries over medium heat. Add the vinegar, water, salt and pepper then stir, bring to a simmer and cook for 3-5 minutes. Take off the heat and brush the pork chops with half of this mix. Place the pork on the preheated grill and cook over medium heat for 6 minutes on each side. Divide the pork chops between plates, drizzle the rest of the blackberry sauce all over and serve.
Enjoy!
Nutrition: calories 261, fat 7, fiber 8, carbs 15, protein 16

188) Sweet Paprika Grilled Pork Chops

PREPARATION TIME: 10 minutes
COOKING TIME: 25 minutes
SERVINGS: 4
INGREDIENTS:
4 pork chops
A drizzle of olive oil
A pinch of salt and black pepper
½ teaspoon ground cinnamon
½ teaspoon sweet paprika
DIRECTIONS:
In a bowl, rub the pork chops with salt, pepper, oil, cinnamon and paprika. Heat up a grill over medium-high heat, add the pork chops and cook them for 2 minutes on each side. Close the grill lid and continue to cook for 20 minutes more. Divide between plates and serve with a side salad.
Enjoy!
Nutrition: calories 251, fat 6, fiber 8, carbs 14, protein 16

189) Rosemary Pork Chops

PREPARATION TIME: 1 hour and 10 minutes
COOKING TIME: 10 minutes
SERVINGS: 4
INGREDIENTS:
4 pork chops
¼ cup olive oil
2 rosemary springs
Juice of 2 lemons
Zest of 2 lemons
2 garlic cloves
1 teaspoon crushed red pepper
A pinch of salt and black pepper
DIRECTIONS:
In your blender, mix the oil with the rosemary, lemon juice, lemon zest, garlic and red pepper and pulse well. In a bowl, mix the pork chops with the rosemary mix, salt and pepper. Toss well and keep in the fridge for 1 hour. Place the pork chops on your preheated grill, cook for 5 minutes on each side, divide between plates and serve.
Enjoy!
Nutrition: calories 211, fat 4, fiber 4, carbs 15, protein 17

190) Basil Pork Chops

PREPARATION TIME: 10 minutes
COOKING TIME: 10 minutes
SERVINGS: 4
INGREDIENTS:
4 pork chops, bone-in
Zest of 1 lemon
3 tablespoons olive oil
Juice of 1 lemon
3 garlic cloves, minced
1 tablespoon chopped thyme
1 tablespoon chopped basil
½ tablespoon ground black pepper
DIRECTIONS:
In a bowl, mix the pork chops with lemon zest, lemon juice, oil, garlic, thyme, basil and black pepper. Mix and set aside for 10 minutes to marinate. Heat up your kitchen grill over medium-high heat, add the pork

chops and cook them for 5 minutes on each side. Divide between plates and serve.
Enjoy!
Nutrition: calories 251, fat 5, fiber 9, carbs 15, protein 7

191) Crusted Pork Chops with Garlic

PREPARATION TIME: 10 minutes
COOKING TIME: 14 minutes
SERVINGS: 4
INGREDIENTS:
4 pork chops, bone-in
2 garlic cloves, minced
3 tablespoons olive oil
A pinch of salt and black pepper
½ cup mustard
DIRECTIONS:
In a bowl, mix the garlic with the oil, salt, pepper and mustard and whisk well. Brush the pork chops with this mix and set them aside for 10 minutes. Heat up your grill over medium-high heat, add the pork chops and cook them for 6-7 minutes on each side. Divide between plates and serve.
Enjoy!
Nutrition: calories 194, fat 15, fiber 0, carbs 0, protein 15

192) Basil Pork Chops

PREPARATION TIME: 10 minutes
COOKING TIME: 12 minutes
SERVINGS: 4
INGREDIENTS:
4 pork chops
2 tablespoons minced garlic
2 tablespoons olive oil
1 cup minced basil
2 tablespoons lemon juice
A pinch of salt and black pepper
DIRECTIONS:
In a bowl, whisk the garlic with oil, basil, lemon juice, salt and pepper. Add pork chops and toss them well. Place the chops on the preheated grill over medium-high heat and

cook for 6 minutes on each side. Divide between plates and serve.
Enjoy!
Nutrition: calories 261, fat 6, fiber 7, carbs 15, protein 16

193) **Baked Pork Chops with Cashew**

PREPARATION TIME: 10 minutes
COOKING TIME: 25 minutes
SERVINGS: 4
INGREDIENTS:
4 pork chops
2 eggs, whisked
½ cup cashew meal
1/3 cup sunflower seeds, minced
2 teaspoons garlic powder
A pinch of salt and black pepper
1½ teaspoon smoked paprika
1 teaspoon chipotle chili powder
DIRECTIONS:
In a bowl, mix the cashew meal with sunflower seeds, garlic powder, salt, pepper, paprika and chili powder. Dip the pork chops in whisked eggs, then in cashew mix and place them on a lined baking sheet and bake at 400 degrees F for 25 minutes. Divide between plates and serve.
Enjoy!
Nutrition: calories 251, fat 12, fiber 4, carbs 7, protein 16

194) **Roasted Pork Chops with Garlic**

PREPARATION TIME: 10 minutes
COOKING TIME: 15 minutes
SERVINGS: 4
INGREDIENTS:
4 pork chops, bone-in
A pinch of salt and black pepper
1 tablespoon olive oil
6 garlic cloves, minced
DIRECTIONS:
Heat up a pan with the oil over medium-high heat and add the pork chops. Season with salt and pepper and cook for 3 minutes. Flip

the pork chops, add the garlic and place in the oven to roast at 400 degrees F for 4 minutes. Divide between plates and serve.
Enjoy!
Nutrition: calories 282, fat 12, fiber 1, carbs 6, protein 17

195) **Skillet Pork Chops with Rosemary**

PREPARATION TIME: 10 minutes
COOKING TIME: 25 minutes
SERVINGS: 6
INGREDIENTS:
6 pork chops, bone-in
3 tablespoons olive oil
A pinch of salt and black pepper
¼ teaspoon ground cumin
¼ teaspoon dried rosemary
DIRECTIONS:
Heat up a pan with the oil over medium-high heat, add pork chops, season with salt, pepper, cumin and rosemary and cook for 5 minutes on each side. Place the pan in the oven and roast at 350 degrees F for 15 minutes. Divide between plates and serve.
Enjoy!
Nutrition: calories 261, fat 6, fiber 5, carbs 11, protein 18

196) **Cranberry Pork**

PREPARATION TIME: 10 minutes
COOKING TIME: 8 hours
SERVINGS: 4
INGREDIENTS:
1 ½ pounds pork roast
½ teaspoon fresh grated ginger
1 tablespoon coconut flour
A pinch of mustard powder
A pinch of salt and black pepper
½ cup cranberries
¼ cup water
Juice of ½ lemon
2 garlic cloves, minced
DIRECTIONS:
In your slow cooker, mix the roast with the ginger, flour, mustard, salt, pepper,

cranberries, water, lemon juice and garlic. Cover and cook on Low for 8 hours. Slice and divide everything between plates and serve. Enjoy!

Nutrition: calories 261, fat 4, fiber 8, carbs 9, protein 17

197) Spicy Pork with Veggies

PREPARATION TIME: 10 minutes
COOKING TIME: 12 hours
SERVINGS: 6
INGREDIENTS:
6 pork chops
3 chipotle peppers, chopped
¼ cup lime juice
1 small yellow onion, chopped
¼ cup tomato paste
4 garlic cloves, minced
1 ½ tablespoons apple cider vinegar
1 teaspoon dried oregano
2 teaspoons ground cumin
1 cup chicken stock
1 teaspoon cloves
3 bay leaves
DIRECTIONS:
In your slow cooker, combine the pork chops with chipotle peppers, lime juice, onion, tomato paste, garlic, vinegar, oregano, cumin, stock, cloves and bay leaves. Mix together then cover and cook on Low for 12 hours. Discard bay leaves and cloves then divide the pork mix between plates and serve. Enjoy!

Nutrition: calories 271, fat 3, fiber 5, carbs 9, protein 16

198) Pork Chops and Brussel Sprouts

PREPARATION TIME: 10 minutes
COOKING TIME: 20 minutes
SERVINGS: 4
INGREDIENTS:
1 pound pork chops, boneless
A pinch of salt and black pepper
1½ tablespoons olive oil
2/3 cup chicken stock

1 teaspoon mustard
½ tablespoon balsamic vinegar
¼ cup onion, chopped
¼ cup applesauce, unsweetened
2 garlic cloves, minced
1¼ cup Brussel sprouts, halved
1 tablespoon chopped rosemary
1 tablespoon chopped sage
DIRECTIONS:
Heat up a pan with half of the oil over medium-high heat and add pork chops. Season with salt and pepper, cook for 6 minutes on each side and transfer to a plate. Heat up the pan again with the rest of the oil over medium heat, add stock, mustard, vinegar, onion, applesauce, garlic, rosemary and sage. Whisk well, bring to a simmer and cook for 5-6 minutes. Add brussel sprouts, toss and cook for 4-5 minutes more. Add the pork chops, toss, cook the whole mixture for a few minutes then divide everything between plates and serve. Enjoy!

Nutrition: calories 251, fat 6, fiber 8, carbs 12, protein 17

199) Herbs de Provence Pork Chops

PREPARATION TIME: 10 minutes
COOKING TIME: 1 hour
SERVINGS: 4
INGREDIENTS:
2 tablespoons olive oil
4 pork chops
A pinch of salt and black pepper
2 garlic cloves, minced
1 yellow onion, chopped
28 ounces canned tomatoes, chopped
¼ cup chicken stock
1 cup tomato sauce
¼ cup balsamic vinegar
1 tablespoon herbs de Provence
2 tablespoons chopped parsley
1 tablespoon chopped basil
DIRECTIONS:
Heat up a pan with the oil over medium heat and add the pork chops. Season with salt and

pepper, cook for 3 minutes on each side and transfer to a plate. Heat up the pan again over medium heat, add the garlic and onion, stir and cook for 10 minutes. Add tomatoes, stock, tomato sauce, vinegar, herbs and parsley, stir and cook for 10 minutes. Return the pork, also add the basil, stir, cook for 5 minutes more, divide between plates and serve.

Enjoy!

Nutrition: calories 251, fat 11, fiber 6, carbs 9, protein 16

200) Pork Chops and Vinegar Sauce

PREPARATION TIME: 10 minutes
COOKING TIME: 30 minutes
SERVINGS: 2
INGREDIENTS:
2 pork chops, boneless
½ cup apple cider vinegar
2 tablespoons olive oil
1 yellow onion, chopped
1 teaspoon fresh grated ginger
½ teaspoon ground cinnamon
A pinch of salt and black pepper
DIRECTIONS:
Heat up a pan with the oil over medium-high heat, add the pork chops and season with salt and pepper. Cook for 3-4 minutes on each side. Add vinegar, onion, ginger and cinnamon. Mix everything together and place in the oven to bake at 400 degrees F for 20 minutes. Divide pork chops and sauce between plates and serve.

Enjoy!

Nutrition: calories 271, fat 5, fiber 8, carbs 10, protein 17

201) Simple Pork Stew

PREPARATION TIME: 10 minutes
COOKING TIME: 1 hour and 40 minutes
SERVINGS: 4
INGREDIENTS:
3 tablespoons olive oil
3 pounds pork shoulder, cubed

2 cups almond flour
A pinch of salt and black pepper
2 yellow onions, chopped
2 tablespoons minced garlic
1 teaspoon chili pepper flakes, dried
4 tablespoons chopped sage
3 cups chicken stock
¼ cup tomato paste
½ teaspoon allspice
DIRECTIONS:
In a bowl, mix the flour with salt and pepper and dredge the pork in this mix. Heat up a pot with the oil over medium-high heat, add the pork, brown for a few minutes on each side and transfer to a bowl. Add the garlic, onion, sage and pepper flakes to the pan and cook for 8 minutes. Return the pork to the pan and also add stock, allspice and tomato paste. Stir and cook everything for 1 hour and 30 minutes. Divide the stew into bowls and serve.

Enjoy!

Nutrition: calories 290, fat 8, fiber 7, carbs 12, protein 18

202) Easy Pork Chili

PREPARATION TIME: 10 minutes
COOKING TIME: 5 hours
SERVINGS: 6
INGREDIENTS:
1 green bell pepper, chopped
1 pound pork, cubed
1 yellow onion, chopped
4 carrots, chopped
Salt and black pepper to the taste
26 ounces canned tomatoes, chopped
1 teaspoon onion powder
1 tablespoon chopped parsley
4 teaspoons chili powder
1 teaspoon garlic powder
1 teaspoon sweet paprika
DIRECTIONS:
Heat up a pan over medium-high heat, add meat and brown for a few minutes then transfer to your slow cooker. Add bell pepper, carrots, onions, tomatoes, salt, pepper, onion powder, parsley, chili powder, paprika

and garlic powder. Stir, cover, cook on High for 5 hours then divide into bowls and serve. Enjoy!
Nutrition: calories 274, fat 6, fiber 3, carbs 11, protein 24

203) **Cinnamon Simple Pork Stew**

PREPARATION TIME: 10 minutes
COOKING TIME: 1 hour and 40 minutes
SERVINGS: 4
INGREDIENTS:
2 pounds sweet potatoes, chopped
A drizzle of olive oil
1 yellow onion, chopped
1 pound ground pork
1 tablespoon chili powder
Salt and black pepper to the taste
1 teaspoon ground cumin
½ teaspoon garlic powder
½ teaspoon chopped oregano
½ teaspoon ground cinnamon
A pinch of cayenne pepper
1 bunch kale, chopped
1 cup water
2 avocados, pitted, peeled and chopped
½ cup chopped parsley
DIRECTIONS:
Heat up a pan with the oil over medium-high heat then add sweet potatoes and onion. Stir and cook for 15 minutes then transfer to a bowl. Heat up the pan again over medium-high heat, add pork, stir and brown for a few minutes. Add salt, pepper, cumin, garlic powder, oregano, cinnamon, cayenne, water, cooked sweet potatoes, and onion. Stir and cook for 1 hour. Add kale and stir then cook for 15 minutes more. Divide into bowls and serve with avocado and parsley on top. Enjoy!
Nutrition: calories 300, fat 7, fiber 6, carbs 19, protein 15

204) **Pork and Peach Salad**

PREPARATION TIME: 10 minutes
COOKING TIME: 12 minutes

SERVINGS: 2
INGREDIENTS:
2 peaches, chopped
3 handfuls kale, chopped
8 ounces pork, cut into thin strips
1 tablespoon olive oil
A splash of balsamic vinegar
Salt and black pepper to the taste
DIRECTIONS:
Heat up a pan with the oil over medium-high heat, add the pork and peaches, toss and cook for 12 minutes. Transfer to a bowl, add kale, vinegar, salt and pepper, toss and serve.
Enjoy!
Nutrition: calories 260, fat 5, fiber 4, carbs 12, protein 14

205) **Balsamic Pork Roast with Garlic**

PREPARATION TIME: 10 minutes
COOKING TIME: 8 hours
SERVINGS: 6
INGREDIENTS:
4 pound pork roast
6 garlic cloves, minced
1 yellow onion, chopped
½ cup balsamic vinegar
1 cup chicken stock
2 tablespoons coconut aminos
Salt and black pepper to the taste
A pinch of red chili pepper flakes
DIRECTIONS:
In your slow cooker, mix the roast with the garlic, onion, vinegar, stock, aminos, salt, pepper and chili flakes. Mix, cover and cook on Low for 8 hours. Slice the roast, divide it between plates and serve with the cooking juices.
Enjoy!
Nutrition: calories 255, fat 7, fiber 1, carbs 12, protein 17

206) **Pork Tenderloin with Date Gravy and Mustard**

PREPARATION TIME: 10 minutes

COOKING TIME: 40 minutes
SERVINGS: 6
INGREDIENTS:
1 ½ pounds pork tenderloin
2 tablespoons veggie stock
1/3 cup dates, pitted
¼ teaspoon onion powder
¼ teaspoon smoked paprika
2 tablespoons mustard
¼ cup coconut aminos
Salt and black pepper to the taste
DIRECTIONS:
In your food processor, mix dates with the stock, coconut aminos, mustard, paprika, salt, pepper and onion powder and blend well. Put pork tenderloin in a baking dish, drizzle the date sauce all over, toss and bake in the oven at 400 degrees F for 40 minutes. Divide between plates and serve.
Enjoy!
Nutrition: calories 270, fat 8, fiber 5, carbs 13, protein 24

207) Thyme Pork with Apples

PREPARATION TIME: 10 minutes
COOKING TIME: 1 hour
SERVINGS: 4
INGREDIENTS:
1½ cups chicken stock
Salt and black pepper to the taste
1 teaspoon coconut aminos
4 pork chops
1 yellow onion, chopped
1 tablespoon chopped thyme
2 garlic cloves, minced
2 apples, cored and sliced
DIRECTIONS:
Arrange the pork chops in a roasting pan, add stock, salt, pepper, aminos, onion, thyme, garlic and apples. Mix and place in the oven and bake at 400 degrees F for 1 hour. Divide everything between plates and serve.
Enjoy!
Nutrition: calories 260, fat 12, fiber 9, carbs 14, protein 18

208) Smoked Paprika Pork

PREPARATION TIME: 10 minutes
COOKING TIME: 10 hours
SERVINGS: 4
INGREDIENTS:
5 pounds pork butt, boneless
1½ cups apple cider vinegar
1 sweet onion, chopped
Salt and black pepper to the taste
2 teaspoons smoked paprika
½ teaspoon ground ginger
½ teaspoon chili powder
DIRECTIONS:
In your slow cooker, mix the pork with the cider vinegar, onion, salt, pepper, paprika, ginger and chili powder. Cover and cook on Low for 10 hours. Divide everything between plates and serve.
Enjoy!
Nutrition: calories 280, fat 7, fiber 8, carbs 12, protein 8

209) Pork and Pineapple Mix

PREPARATION TIME: 10 minutes
COOKING TIME: 40 minutes
SERVINGS: 4
INGREDIENTS:
8 ounces canned pineapple, crushed
1 tablespoon olive oil
1 pound ground pork
1 teaspoon chili powder
1 teaspoon garlic powder
1 teaspoon cumin
Salt and black pepper to the taste
1 mango, chopped
Juice of 1 lime
2 avocados, pitted, peeled and chopped
¼ cup chopped cilantro
DIRECTIONS:
Heat up a pan with the oil over medium heat, add the pork, stir and brown for 3 minutes. Add garlic, cumin, chili powder, salt and pepper and stir then cook for 8 minutes. Add pineapple, mango, avocados, lime juice, cilantro, salt and pepper and stir. Cook for 5-

6 minutes more then divide between plates and serve.
Enjoy!
Nutrition: calories 200, fat 6, fiber 7, carbs 12, protein 16

210) **Basil Pork Steaks and Pesto**

PREPARATION TIME: 4 hours
COOKING TIME: 15 minutes
SERVINGS: 4
INGREDIENTS:
¼ cup balsamic vinegar
1 pound pork steaks
¼ cup chopped basil
1 tablespoons minced garlic
2 tablespoons olive oil
Salt and black pepper to the taste
1 teaspoon onion powder
For the pesto:
½ cup bell peppers, roasted
½ cup chopped basil
¼ cup olive oil
¼ cup pine nuts
1 garlic clove
Salt and black pepper to the taste
DIRECTIONS:
In a bowl, mix steaks with vinegar, 2 tablespoons oil, basil, garlic, onion, salt and pepper. Toss to coat and keep in the fridge for 4 hours. Heat up a grill over medium-high heat and add the steaks, cooking for 4 minutes. Flip the steaks and cook for another 4 minutes. In your food processor, mix the basil with the roasted peppers, pine nuts, ¼ cup olive oil, garlic, salt and pepper. Pulse well and serve your steaks with the pesto on top.
Enjoy!
Nutrition: calories 270, fat 6, fiber 5, carbs 13, protein 18

211) **Pork egg roll in a bowl**

PREPARATION TIME: 5 minutes
COOKING TIME: 25 minutes
SERVINGS: 4 people

INGREDIENTS:
☐ 2 tablespoons of sesame oil
☐ 3 cloves of garlic, minced
☐ ½ cup of onion, diced
☐ 5 green onions, sliced on a bias (white and green parts
☐ 1 pound of ground pork
☐ ½ teaspoon ground ginger
☐ sea salt and black pepper, to taste
☐ 1 tablespoon of Sriracha or garlic chili sauce, more to taste (omit or use a compliant brand for Whole30
☐ 14 ounces' bag coleslaw mix
☐ 3 tablespoons Coconut Aminos or gluten free soy sauce
☐ 1 tablespoon of rice vinegar
☐ 2 tablespoons toasted sesame seeds
DIRECTIONS:
First, heat sesame oil in a large skillet over medium high heat and add the garlic, onion, and white part of the green onions.
Sauté until the onions are translucent and the garlic is fragrant. Then add the ground pork, ground ginger, sea salt, black pepper and Sriracha.
Cook until the pork is cooked through. Add the coleslaw mix, coconut aminos, and rice wine vinegar.
Cook until the coleslaw is soft. Top with green onions and sesame seeds. Serve and enjoy.

212) **Apple dijon pork chops**

PREPARATION TIME: 5 minutes
COOKING TIME: 10 minutes
SERVINGS: 2 people
INGREDIENTS:
☐ 2 pork chops (320 g
☐ 4 tablespoons of ghee (60 ml
☐ 2 tablespoons of applesauce (30 ml
☐ 2 tablespoons of ghee (30 ml
☐ 2 tablespoons of Dijon mustard (30 ml
☐ Salt and pepper, to taste
DIRECTIONS:
Melt the 4 tablespoons of ghee in a large pan. Then add in the pork chops. Position the

pork chops on its side so that the fat cooks in the ghee first.

Cook for 3-4 minutes on each side. Check the internal temperature of the pork using a meat thermometer. It should be at about 145 F (63 C.

When you cut into the pork chops, you'll find it has a medium rare pink inside. If you prefer your pork chops more cooked, then just leave it in there for longer.

While waiting, mix the applesauce, melted ghee, and mustard together well.

Serve the pork chops with the sauce and season with salt and pepper to taste.

213) **Bacon Covered Meatloaf**

PREPARATION TIME: 15 minutes
COOKING TIME: 50 minutes
INGREDIENTS:
- [ ] Metric - Cups/Ounces
- [ ] 1 spring onion sliced
- [ ] 2 cloves garlic crushed
- [ ] 750 g mince/ground beef
- [ ] 750 g mince/ground pork
- [ ] 2 eggs - medium lightly beaten
- [ ] handful fresh parsley chopped
- [ ] handful fresh basil chopped
- [ ] 2 slices bacon diced
- [ ] 2 tablespoons of sun-dried tomatoes chopped
- [ ] 2 teaspoons of dried oregano
- [ ] salt and pepper to taste
- [ ] vegetables of choice diced/grated/shredded
- [ ] 6 slices bacon to cover the meatloaf
- [ ] Optional - if not paleo you can add 100g / 3.5 grated cheese of choice to the meatloaf mixture

DIRECTIONS:
Start with oiling and lining a baking tray. Then mix all the ingredients in a large mixing bowl. Mix with your hand thoroughly.

Form a large meatloaf shape on the lined baking tray and cover with the bacon slices and sprinkle on parmesan cheese (optional.

Bake at 180C/350F for 50 minutes or until thoroughly cooked in the centre.

Serve and enjoy.

214) **Italian parmesan breaded pork cutlets**

PREPARATION TIME: 5 minutes
COOKING TIME: 15 minutes
SERVINGS: 6 people
INGREDIENTS:
- [ ] 6 pork cutlets
- [ ] ½ cup of Italian dressing
- [ ] ½ cup of grated parmesan
- [ ] 1 tablespoon of pork seasoning
- [ ] 1 to 2 tablespoons of Golden Ghee

DIRECTIONS:
Preheat a medium-sized frying pan to medium heat. Melt your ghee (or butter.

Then set up two bowls, one for your Italian dressing, and one for your seasoning and grated parmesan.

Coat each cutlet by dipping it in the Italian dressing and then your seasoning/parmesan. Do in a bowl. Set aside on some plates.

Depending on the size of your pan, you may need to cook them in batches because it's important not to crowd the pan.

Then add 1 tablespoon of ghee or butter and let melt. Add your cutlets to the pan and cook for about 3 to 5 minutes on each side

Do this for all until they're all done, and garnish with more parmesan and fresh herbs (optional.

Serve and enjoy.

215) **Pork Chops & Cabbage Recipe**

PREPARATION TIME: 5 minutes
COOKING TIME: 15 minutes
Total time 20 minutes
SERVINGS: 2
INGREDIENTS:
- [ ] The Pork Chops
- [ ] 2 boneless pork chops
- [ ] 1/8 teaspoon of coriander ground
- [ ] 1/8 teaspoon of garlic powder
- [ ] 1/8 teaspoon of sea salt
- [ ] 1 teaspoon of ghee
- [ ] The Cabbage
- [ ] 6 ounces of cabbage sliced into strips

- ☐ 1 tablespoon of apple cider vinegar
- ☐ ¼ cup of chicken broth
- ☐ 1/8 teaspoon of red chili flakes
- ☐ sea salt to taste

DIRECTIONS:

Season pork chops with coriander, garlic powder, and sea salt. Season each side.

Melt ghee in a cast-iron skillet over medium heat and cook pork chops for 4 to 5 minutes on each side. Set aside to rest 5 minutes prior to slicing.

Add cabbage, vinegar, broth, and sea salt in a medium skillet and boil over high heat.

Cook until the liquid has cooked off and the edges of the cabbage begin to brown (stir occasionally.

Serve pork chops sliced with cabbage on the side. Enjoy.

216) **Italian Pork Rollatini**

PREPARATION TIME: 10 minutes
COOKING TIME: 30 minutes
SERVINGS: 6
INGREDIENTS:
- ☐ 1 pound of boneless pork cutlets thin cutlets
- ☐ 6 slices prosciutto
- ☐ ⅓ cup of ricotta cheese whole ricotta
- ☐ 2 tablespoon of flat leaf Italian parsley
- ☐ 2 tablespoons of parmesan
- ☐ 3 cloves garlic minced
- ☐ ¼ cup of onions minced
- ☐ 1 tablespoon of olive oil
- ☐ ⅓ cup of chicken broth
- ☐ 14.5 oz. diced tomatoes
- ☐ ½ teaspoon of sea salt
- ☐ ½ teaspoon of Italian seasonings
- ☐ 1 ½ tablespoon of extra parmesan cheese *optional

DIRECTIONS:

Place a pork cutlet between 2 sheets of plastic wrap and flatten the pork cutlet with a kitchen mallet or pounder until very thin (about ¼ inch.

Remove the back top of plastic wrap and place a slice of prosciutto on the flattened pork.

Place about a tablespoon of ricotta on top and sprinkle with a little parsley and parmesan.

Roll pork cutlet up around filling, and use a toothpick to close. Pinch the side ends closed. Repeat with other cutlets.

Add olive oil in a large fry pan over medium high heat and place pork rolls toothpick side down in pan. Fry until it gets brown. Do for both side.

Remove pork rolls from pan, set aside on a plate, and leave it to cool. Remove toothpicks from pork rolls and set aside (they will return to the pan later.

In the same fry pan add onions and minced garlic. Sauté over medium heat until onions are translucent.

Add chicken broth to the fry pan and loosen garlic and onions from pan and stir together. Then add pork rolls back to the frying pan and cover with the diced tomatoes and liquid. Sprinkle with sea salt and Italian seasonings.

10. Heat to a boil, then turn heat to low, cover and simmer for 30 minutes.

11. Serve and enjoy.

☐

217) **Cajun pork sauté recipe with peppers and tomatoes**

PREPARATION TIME: 5 minutes
COOKING TIME: 20 minutes
SERVINGS: 2
INGREDIENTS:
- ☐ 1-pound of Cajun shredded pork, cooked
- ☐ 2 bell peppers, sliced
- ☐ 1 onion, sliced (optional
- ☐ 1 14 ounces (400g can of diced tomatoes (or use 2 to 3 fresh tomatoes
- ☐ 4 cloves garlic, minced
- ☐ salt to taste
- ☐ coconut oil to cook with

DIRECTIONS:
Cook the bell peppers and onions in 1 tablespoon of coconut oil.

Add the shredded pork followed by the tomatoes. Simmer for 5 more minutes, then add in the minced garlic and season with salt to taste.

Cook for 2 more minutes and serve. Enjoy.

218) **Dry Rub Pork Spare Ribs**

SERVINGS: 4
PREPARATION TIME: 15 minutes
COOKING TIME: 3 hours 30 minutes
Total time: 3 hours 45 minutes
INGREDIENTS:
- ☐ 2 tablespoons of Cacao
- ☐ 1 tablespoon of coriander
- ☐ ½ teaspoon of cumin
- ☐ ½ teaspoon of cinnamon
- ☐ ½ teaspoon of chili powder
- ☐ ½ teaspoon of black pepper
- ☐ ½ to 1 tablespoon of sea salt
- ☐ 2 racks ribs

DIRECTIONS:
Preheat your oven to 350 degrees. Add all the ingredients into a bowl and mix with a spoon thoroughly.

Lightly apply this rub to both sides of your rack until it is well coated. Next take two sheets of aluminium foil and sandwich the ribs.

Place them in your oven to bake for 3 to 3.25 hours. The meat should be falling off the bone by the time they are done.

Serve and enjoy.
- ☐

219) **Meatballs**

SERVINGS: 4 people
PREPARATION TIME: 20 minutes
COOKING TIME: 30 minutes
INGREDIENTS:
For the meatballs:
- ☐ 1 pound of ground beef
- ☐ 1 clove garlic, minced
- ☐ ½ cup of shredded mozzarella
- ☐ ¼ cup freshly grated Parmesan, plus more for serving
- ☐ 2 tablespoons of freshly chopped parsley
- ☐ 1 large egg, beaten
- ☐ 1 tsp. kosher salt
- ☐ ½ tsp. freshly ground black pepper
- ☐ 2 tbsp. extra-virgin olive oil

For the sauce:
- ☐ 1 medium onion, chopped
- ☐ 2 cloves garlic, minced
- ☐ 1 (28 ounces can crushed tomatoes
- ☐ 1 tsp. dried oregano
- ☐ Kosher salt
- ☐ Freshly ground black pepper

DIRECTIONS:
Combine the beef, garlic, mozzarella, Parmesan, parsley, egg, salt and pepper in a large bowl and form 16 meatballs.

Heat oil in a large skillet over medium heat. Add meatballs and cook. Turn occasionally, until golden on all sides, about 10 minutes. Remove from skillet and set aside on a paper towel-lined plate. To the same skillet, add onion and cook until soft, 5 minutes.

Add garlic and cook until fragrant, 1 minute more. Add tomatoes and oregano and season with salt and pepper.

Then add meatballs back to skillet, cover and simmer until sauce has thickened, 15 minutes.

Garnish with Parmesan before serving. Enjoy.

220) **Meatloaf**

SERVINGS: 6
PREPARATION TIME: 15 minutes
Gross time: 1 hour 15 minutes
INGREDIENTS:
- ☐ Cooking spray
- ☐ 1 tablespoon of extra-virgin olive oil
- ☐ 1 medium onion, chopped
- ☐ 1 stalk celery, chopped
- ☐ 3 cloves garlic, minced
- ☐ 1 teaspoon of dried oregano
- ☐ 1 teaspoon of chili powder
- ☐ 2 pound of ground beef
- ☐ 1 cup shredded cheddar

- ☐ ½ cup of almond flour
- ☐ ¼ cup of grated Parmesan
- ☐ 2 eggs
- ☐ 1 tablespoon of low-sodium soy sauce
- ☐ Kosher salt
- ☐ Freshly ground black pepper
- ☐ 6 thin strips bacon

DIRECTIONS:

Start by heating the oven to 400°. Grease a medium baking dish with cooking spray.

In a medium skillet over medium heat, heat oil. Then add onion and celery and cook until tender. Cook for 5 minutes.

Add in garlic, oregano, and chili powder and cook until fragrant, 1 minute (stir gently. Let mixture cool slightly.

Combine your ground beef, vegetable mixture, cheese, almond flour, Parmesan, eggs, soy sauce in a large bowl and season with salt and pepper.

Shape into a large loaf in baking dish, then lay bacon slices on top and cook until bacon is crispy and beef is cooked through, about 1 hour.

Cover dish with foil if the bacon is cooking too quickly.

Serve and enjoy.

221) **Burger Fat Bombs**

PREPARATION TIME: 15 minutes
COOKING TIME: 15 minutes
INGREDIENTS:
- ☐ Cooking spray, for muffin tin
- ☐ 1 pound of ground beef
- ☐ ½ teaspoon of garlic powder
- ☐ Kosher salt
- ☐ Freshly ground black pepper
- ☐ 2 tablespoons of cold butter, cut into 20 pieces
- ☐ ¼ (8 ounces block cheddar cheese, cut into 20 pieces
- ☐ Lettuce leaves, for serving
- ☐ Thinly sliced tomatoes, for serving
- ☐ Mustard, for serving

DIRECTIONS:

Heat oven to 375°. Grease a mini muffin tin with cooking spray. Season beef with garlic powder, salt, and pepper in a medium bowl.

Insert about 1 tablespoon of beef into the bottom of each muffin tin cup, completely covering the bottom.

Place a piece of butter on top then press about 1 tablespoon of beef over butter to completely cover.

Add a piece of cheese on top of meat in each cup then press remaining beef over cheese to completely cover.

Allow it to bake until meat is cooked through, about 15 minutes. Let cool slightly. Release each burger from the tin with a metal offset spatula. Do it gently.

Serve with lettuce leaves, tomatoes, and mustard. Enjoy.

222) **Taco Stuffed Avocados**

SERVINGS: 4 to 6 People
PREPARATION TIME: 10 minutes
COOKING TIME: 15 minutes
INGREDIENTS:
- ☐ 4 ripe avocados
- ☐ Juice of 1 lime
- ☐ 1 tablespoon of extra-virgin olive oil
- ☐ 1 medium onion, chopped
- ☐ 1 pound of ground beef
- ☐ 1 packet taco seasoning
- ☐ Kosher salt
- ☐ Freshly ground black pepper
- ☐ 2/3 cup shredded Mexican cheese
- ☐ ½ cup shredded lettuce
- ☐ ½ cup quartered grape tomatoes
- ☐ Sour cream, for topping

DIRECTIONS:

Halve and pit avocados. Use spoon to create a large well by scooping out a bit of the avocado.

Dice removed avocado and set aside to use later. Squeeze lime juice over all avocados (to prevent browning!.

Heat oil in a medium skillet over medium heat. Add onion and cook until it softens, about 5 minutes.

Then add ground beef and taco seasoning, breaking up the meat with a wooden spoon. Season with salt and pepper, and cook until the beef is no longer pink, about 6 minutes. Remove from heat and drain fat.

Fill each avocado half with beef, then top with reserved avocado, cheese, lettuce, tomato, and a dollop sour cream.
Serve and enjoy.

223) Taco Casserole

SERVINGS: 6 People
PREPARATION TIME: 15 minutes
COOKING TIME: 45 minutes
Total time: 1 hour
INGREDIENTS:
- [ ] 1 tablespoon of extra-virgin olive oil
- [ ] ½ yellow onion, diced
- [ ] 2 pounds ground beef
- [ ] 2 tablespoons of kosher salt
- [ ] Freshly ground black pepper
- [ ] 2 tablespoons of keto taco seasoning mix
- [ ] 1 jalapeño, seeded and minced, plus more sliced for garnish
- [ ] 6 large eggs, lightly beaten
- [ ] 2 cups of shredded Mexican cheese
- [ ] 2 tablespoons of freshly chopped parsley leaves
- [ ] 1 cup of sour cream, for serving (optional

DIRECTIONS:
Preheat oven to 350°. Heat oil in a large skillet over medium heat. Add onion and cook until tender (2 minutes.
Add ground beef and season with salt and pepper. Then cook, and break up meat with a wooden spoon, until it is no longer pink (6 minutes.
Sprinkle in taco seasoning and jalapeño and cook, stirring, until spices are lightly toasted (1 minute. Drain and let cool slightly.
Whisk eggs in a large mixing bowl, then add in meat mixture and spread mixture into an even layer in the bottom of a 2-quart baking dish.
Sprinkle with cheese and bake until set, about 25 minutes. Then sprinkle parsley and top each slice with a dollop of sour cream and jalapeno.
Serve and enjoy.

224) Ice burgers

SERVINGS: 4 people
COOKING TIME: 20 minutes
PREPARATION TIME: 10 minutes
INGREDIENTS:
- [ ] 1 large head iceberg lettuce
- [ ] 4 slices bacon
- [ ] 1 red onion, sliced
- [ ] 1 pound of ground beef
- [ ] Kosher salt
- [ ] Freshly ground black pepper
- [ ] 4 slices cheddar
- [ ] 1 tomato, sliced
- [ ] Ranch dressing, for serving

DIRECTIONS:
Start with slicing 8 large rounds from the edges of the head of iceberg to create buns.
Cook bacon in a large skillet over medium heat until it is crispy. Remove and place on a paper towel-lined plate to drain, reserving bacon fat in pan.
Add onion slices and cook until it softens (about 3 minutes per side. Set aside red onions and wipe skillet clean.
Return skillet over medium-high heat and shape ground beef into 4 large burger patties.
Season both sides of patties with salt and pepper and add to skillet. Cook until seared on both sides and cooked to your liking (4 minutes per side for medium.
Top each burger with a slice of cheese, then cover skillet with a lid and cook until cheese has melted, about 1 minute more.
Top one iceberg round with the cooked cheeseburger, a slice of bacon, and a tomato slice, then sprinkle with ranch. Top with second iceberg round.
Repeat with remaining ingredients and serve. Enjoy.

225) Cheese Taco Shells

SERVINGS: 4 people
PREPARATION TIME: 20 minutes
COOKING TIME: 10 minutes
INGREDIENTS:

- ☐ 2 cups of shredded Cheddar
- ☐ Freshly ground black pepper
- ☐ 1 tablespoon of vegetable oil
- ☐ 1 white onion, chopped
- ☐ 1 pound of ground beef
- ☐ 1 tablespoon of Taco Seasoning
- ☐ shredded lettuce, for serving
- ☐ Chopped tomatoes, for serving
- ☐ Hot sauce, for serving

DIRECTIONS:

First heat the oven to 375⁰. Prepare a baking sheet with parchment paper and spray with cooking spray.

Add ½ cup mounds of cheddar on baking sheet and season with pepper. Bake for 5 to 7 minutes. Blot grease with a paper towel.

Set up 4 stations of two upside-down glasses and a wooden spoon as a bridge. Transfer cheese mounds to wooden spoons to form shell (use a spatula for this.

In a large skillet over medium heat, heat oil. Add onions and cook for 5 minutes until tender.

Then add ground beef and cook until no longer pink, 6 minutes more. Drain the fat and season with taco seasoning.

Assemble tacos: Place beef in shells and top with lettuce, tomatoes, and hot sauce.

Serve and enjoy.

226) **Cream Cheese Stuffed Meatballs**

PREPARATION TIME: 15 minutes
COOKING TIME: 15 minutes
INGREDIENTS:

Meatballs:
- ☐ 1 spring onion finely sliced
- ☐ 1 clove garlic crushed
- ☐ 750 g ground/mincemeat. I used pork
- ☐ salt and pepper to taste
- ☐ 1 egg slightly beaten
- ☐ 2 slices bacon finely chopped
- ☐ 3 tablespoons of sun-dried tomatoes finely diced
- ☐ 2 tablespoons of favourite herbs - I use rosemary, thyme, oregano and sage

Filling:
- ☐ 110 g cream cheese diced into squares

DIRECTIONS:

Add all your meatball ingredients on a large mixing bowl. Mix thoroughly with your hands.

Scoop up a golf ball size of meatball mixture (use a desert spoon.

Squeeze the mixture into a ball then flatten into a circle.

Place a cube of cream cheese in the centre of the meatball circle then enclose the meatball mixture around the cream cheese.

On a greased baking tray, place the cream cheese stuffed meatball. Repeat until all the mixture has been used.

Spray them all with olive oil spray so they will crisp and brown beautifully.

Bake at 180C/350F for 15-20minutes depending on your oven.

Serve and enjoy.

227) **Taco Seasoning**

PREPARATION TIME: 5 minutes
COOKING TIME: 10 minutes
INGREDIENTS:
- ☐ 1 tablespoon of ground chili powder
- ☐ 1½ teaspoons of ground cumin
- ☐ 1 teaspoon of paprika
- ☐ ½ teaspoon of granulated garlic
- ☐ ½ teaspoon of granulated onion
- ☐ ½ teaspoon of dried oregano, rubbed
- ☐ ½ teaspoon of salt
- ☐ ¼ teaspoon of pepper

Optional:
- ☐ 1 teaspoon of Sukrin :1 (Swerve Granulated or sugar if not low carb

DIRECTIONS:

Measure and gather all of the ingredients into a small bowl and whisk with a fork. Keep them in an airtight container.

6-12 people depending on your taste. 1-carb per 2 teaspoons of seasoning or ½ carb per 1 teaspoon of seasoning.

Brown 1 pound of ground beef in a pan. Add 2 to 4 tablespoons (half of the recipe or the whole thing to the ground beef along with 2 tablespoons of tomato paste and ½ cup beef broth.

Cook gently until most of the sauce evaporates. Adjust seasoning with salt and pepper. Carb counts will depend on how much seasoning you use.

228) **Spicy Beef Ramen**

PREPARATION TIME: 10 minutes
COOKING TIME: 20minutes
SERVINGS: 4
INGREDIENTS:
☐ 1-pound 80/20 ground beef, browned and crumbled
☐ ½ small onion, diced
☐ 2 cloves minced garlic
☐ ¼ to ½ teaspoon ground ginger
☐ 2 tablespoons vegetable oil
☐ 1 teaspoon of sesame oil
☐ 2 cups of beef broth
☐ 2 tablespoons soy sauce
☐ 2 packages Miracle angel hair noodles
☐ ½ cup of green onions, chopped
☐ garnish: red pepper flakes
☐ Optional: Sriracha sauce for more heat. This is not factored in to the nutrition count. You would add 1.3-carbs per teaspoon added.
DIRECTIONS:
Prepare the ground beef and set aside. In the same pan, fry the onion, garlic, ginger, vegetable, and sesame oil. Sauté over medium for several minutes.

Then add the beef broth and soy sauce and cook for a few minutes. Turn heat to low to keep warm. Meanwhile, prepare noodles.

Empty and drain the packages of the noodles. Rinse with cold water for 20 seconds and drain in a colander.

Add noodles to a pot of boiling water and boil for 1 minute. Drain and pat dry with a paper towel.

Add the noodles to the warm broth mixture. Add in the ground beef, raising the temperature until everything is warmed through.

Garnish with chopped green onions and red pepper flakes.

Serve and enjoy.

229) **Lamb chops with fragrant curry sauce**

PREPARATION TIME: 15 minutes
COOKING TIME: 30 minutes
SERVINGS: 4
INGREDIENTS:
☐ 2 racks of lamb, Frenched (2 lbs each
☐ 1 teaspoon melted ghee or olive oil
☐ salt and pepper
☐ 1– 2 teaspoons garam masala
Indian Curry Sauce:
☐ 1 tablespoon ghee (or coconut oil
☐ 1 shallot- chopped
☐ 3 fat garlic cloves- rough chopped
☐ 1 tablespoon ginger- finely chopped
☐ ½ teaspoon turmeric
☐ ½ teaspoon fennel seed
☐ ½ teaspoon mustard seed
☐ 1½ cups diced tomatoes (about 2 medium tomatoes
☐ 1 can 13 ounce can coconut milk
☐ 1 teaspoon dry fenugreek leaves – optional, but delicious!
☐ 1 teaspoon salt
☐ 1 teaspoon brown sugar or honey
☐ Garnish- cilantro, toasted fennel seeds, Aleppo chili flakes
DIRECTIONS:
Heat oven to 425F. Remove any excess fat, and pat lamb dry. Brush with melted ghee or olive oil.

Sprinkle all sides with salt, pepper and garam masala spice blend (or use Indian curry powder and place on a baking sheet and set aside.

In a medium pot or large fry pan, heat ghee over medium heat. Add shallot, garlic and ginger and stir until golden (3 to 4 minutes.

Then add turmeric, fennel seed and mustard seeds and continue cooking for one more minute (stir occasionally.

Add diced tomato and their juices. Continue cooking and stirring about 5 more minutes. Add coconut milk, fenugreek leaves, salt, and sugar.

Give a good stir, taste, adjust salt. Bring to a simmer, switch heat to low and let simmer while you bake the lamb.

Place lamb in the hot oven, roast 10 minutes, flip, cook 10 more minutes, then flip once more and broil for a couple minutes if you like a crispy crust.

Remove lamb from oven and set aside for 5-10 minutes, then slice and plate or platter over top the fenugreek sauce.

Sprinkle with fresh cilantro, toasted fennel seeds (optional and chili flakes (Aleppo chili is nice if you like.

10. Serve immediately and enjoy!

230) Grilled lamb chops with charmoula

PREPARATION TIME: 10 minutes
COOKING TIME: 5 minutes
SERVINGS: 4
INGREDIENTS:
- [ ] 8 lamb loin chops
- [ ] 1 teaspoon of olive oil
- [ ] 2 tablespoons of Ras el Hanout
- [ ] salt

For the Charmoula:
- [ ] 2 tablespoons of fresh mint, roughly chopped
- [ ] ¼ cup of fresh parsley, roughly chopped
- [ ] 2 tablespoons of lemon zest
- [ ] 3 cloves garlic, roughly chopped
- [ ] ½ teaspoon of smoked paprika (use regular if you don't have smoked
- [ ] 1 teaspoon of red pepper flakes
- [ ] ¼ cup of olive oil
- [ ] 2 tablespoons of lemon juice
- [ ] salt and pepper to taste

DIRECTIONS:
Coat the lamb with olive oil, ras el hanout and salt. (If not using the ras el hanout, season generously with salt, pepper, and a little cumin.

Preheat your grill, then grill about 2 minutes per side for medium rare. Set aside. Let the meat rest a few minutes before serving.

Gather all of the Charmoula ingredients in a food processor or magic bullet and pulse until a pesto-like consistency. Don't over blend. It shouldn't be completely liquefied.

Serve the lamb chops with a generous helping of Charmoula and some fresh lemon zest. Perfect with grilled asparagus and cauliflower puree on the side.

231) Greek Lamb Chops with Tzatziki Sauce

PREPARATION TIME: 10 minutes
COOKING TIME: 10 minutes
SERVINGS: 4
INGREDIENTS:
- [ ] 8 lamb chops
- [ ] ¼ cup of lemon juice
- [ ] 2 tablespoons olive oil
- [ ] 1 clove garlic grated
- [ ] 1½ teaspoons kosher salt
- [ ] ½ teaspoon pepper

Tzatziki Sauce:
- [ ] 2 cups plain Greek yogurt
- [ ] 2 cups diced cucumber or shredded
- [ ] ½ cup fresh dill minced
- [ ] ¼ cup lemon juice
- [ ] 2 cloves garlic grated
- [ ] ½ teaspoon of salt
- [ ] ¼ teaspoon of pepper

DIRECTIONS:
Position the lamb chops on a large platter and pat dry with paper towel.

Combine the lemon juice, olive oil, garlic, salt and pepper in a glass dish. Add chops to the bag and seal.

Move bag around to make sure lamb chops are well coated with marinade. Marinate meat for 30 minutes or up to overnight.

Grill the lamb, let meat sit out at room temperature for 20-30 minutes and pre-heat grill to medium-high heat.

Grill 4-5 minutes per side or until meat thermometer reads 155 degrees. Remove from heat and set aside. Let rest 10 minutes before serving.

While lamb is resting, combine the ingredient for Tzatziki Sauce in a medium bowl.

Check for seasoning and adjust according to your taste.

Serve lamb chops with Tzatziki Sauce on the side. Enjoy

232) Grilled Lamb Chops with Dijon-Basil Butter

INGREDIENTS:
- ☐ 4 to 6 centre-cut lamb chops – depending on size
- ☐ 1 tablespoon of olive oil
- ☐ ½ teaspoon of garlic powder
- ☐ 1 tablespoon of chopped fresh basil
- ☐ 1 clove garlic, minced
- ☐ 1 teaspoon of Dijon-style mustard
- ☐ 2 tablespoons of soft butter
- ☐ Grilled Lamb Chops

DIRECTIONS:
Sprinkle chops with garlic powder, drizzle with oil and allow to sit until ready to cook.

Over medium-high, cook on barbecue grill for 2 to 5 minutes per side. When you think they might be close take one off, cut into center and peak.

When done to your liking remove from heat, divide basil butter to top each chop and serve.

Put garlic and basil into a small bowl, add mustard and butter and mix well. Can be made ahead, shaped into a log, chilled and sliced.

Serve and enjoy.

233) Lamb Kebabs with Coconut Curry Dipping Sauce

PREPARATION TIME: 10 minutes
COOKING TIME: 15 minutes
INGREDIENTS:
- ☐ Metric - Cups/Ounces
- ☐ Lamb Kebabs
- ☐ 800 g ground/minced lamb
- ☐ 1 spring onion finely sliced
- ☐ 1 teaspoon of dried cumin
- ☐ 1 teaspoon of dried coriander/cilantro
- ☐ 1 teaspoon of turmeric powder
- ☐ Coconut Curry Dipping Sauce
- ☐ 250 ml coconut cream
- ☐ 2 tablespoons of curry paste/powder to taste
- ☐ 12 bamboo or metal skewers

DIRECTIONS:
Combine and mix all the ingredients together with your hands and form into 12 long kebab shapes.

Gently push the skewer into the kebab and press firmly. Bake in the oven for 10 to 15 minutes.

You can also adopt the method of shallow frying. Mix the curry paste/powder with the coconut cream.

Serve on the side or drizzled across the lamb kebabs. Serve with cauliflower rice. Enjoy.

234) Kofta

PREPARATION TIME: 15 minutes
COOKING TIME: 15 minutes
SERVINGS: 3 to 4
INGREDIENTS:
- ☐ 14 wooden skewers
- ☐ 2 tablespoons finely minced garlic
- ☐ ¼ cup of red onion shredded on large holes of box grater and squeezed of all liquid
- ☐ ¼ cup of fresh parsley minced
- ☐ ¼ cup of fresh mint minced
- ☐ 1 tablespoon of fresh ginger grated
- ☐ ½ teaspoon of kosher salt
- ☐ 2 tablespoons of Garam Masala
- ☐ 1 pound of ground lamb
- ☐ Greek flat bread (sold in bread section of supermarkets or see our Gluten Free Flat Bread recipe here
- ☐ Shredded lettuce
- ☐ Diced tomato
- ☐ Tzatziki sauce

DIRECTIONS:
Soak skewers in water for two hours or longer. If using an outdoor grill, heat to medium heat. Or use a ribbed grill pan on your stove.

Mix all ingredients except lamb until combined in a medium bowl. Then add lamb and mix just enough to combine without over working the meat.

Form into seven oval shaped patties. Place two skewers side by side into each (two makes it easy to flip on grill.

Gill over medium heat flipping halfway through to a nicely seared exterior and cooked to your liking on the inside.

Place one or two patties on open flat bread and top with shredded lettuce, chopped tomato and a generous drizzle of Tzatziki. Enjoy.

235) **Ground Pork Tacos**

SERVINGS: 1 serving = about 5 wraps
PREPARATION TIME: 10 minutes
COOKING TIME: 15 minutes
INGREDIENTS:
- [ ] 400 grams of ground pork (about 13 ounces.
- [ ] ½ teaspoon of garlic powder
- [ ] ½ teaspoon of onion powder
- [ ] ½ teaspoon of sea salt
- [ ] 1/8 teaspoon of cumin
- [ ] 1/8 teaspoon of ground pepper
- [ ] 5 tablespoons of salsa
- [ ] 5 or more lettuce leaves (I used Boston Red Leaf Lettuce
- [ ] Taco toppings like diced green peppers/red peppers/avocado/onions etc.

DIRECTIONS:
Mix the ground pork and all the seasonings except the salsa in a small bowl. Mix with your hands.

Place the meat in a frying pan and turn the heat to medium. Constantly stir the meat making sure to breakup any large pieces.

Once the meat is cooked drain the fat from the pan. Then add the salsa and mix.

Place the meat on the lettuce wraps and top with your favourite taco toppings.

Serve and enjoy.

236) **Paleo Pork Dumplings**

PREPARATION TIME: 10 minutes
COOKING TIME: 15 minutes
SERVINGS: 6
INGREDIENTS:
- [ ] 1 pound of ground Pork
- [ ] 3 Green Onions
- [ ] ½ head Napa Cabbage
- [ ] 4 Garlic cloves
- [ ] 1 teaspoon of fresh Ginger
- [ ] 2 Bird's Eye Chili Peppers
- [ ] 2 tablespoons of Coconut Aminos
- [ ] 2 tablespoons of Sesame Oil
- [ ] Coconut Oil
- [ ] Paleo Thai Dipping Sauce

DIRECTIONS:
Carefully chop the green parts of the green onions and cabbage and mix together.

Mince the garlic, ginger, and chili peppers (sans stems and add them to the scallions and mix well.

Pour in the coconut aminos and sesame oil while stirring, then add in the pork and mix thoroughly. Or you can use a food processor and do this all at once.

Form about a 1" oval, dumpling shapes with the meat mixture and set aside. Pre-heat 1 tablespoon coconut oil over medium-high (~6 heat.

Cook dumplings in a single layer for 2 to 3 minutes on each side, or until the pork is cooked through and no longer pink.

Drain on a paper towel and serve hot. Repeat until all of the pork dumplings are cooked.

Serve with Paleo Sweet Chili Sauce or Paleo Thai Dipping Sauce for dipping!

237) **Pork and cashew stir-fry recipe**

PREPARATION TIME: 5 minutes
COOKING TIME: 10 minutes
SERVINGS: 2
INGREDIENTS:
- [ ] ½ pound of (225 g pork tenderloin, sliced thin
- [ ] 1 egg, whisked
- [ ] 1 bell pepper, diced
- [ ] 1 green onion, diced
- [ ] 1/3 cup (40 g of cashews
- [ ] 1 tablespoon (5 g of fresh ginger, grated
- [ ] 3 cloves of garlic, minced

☐ 1 teaspoon (5 ml of Chinese chili oil (optional

☐ 1 tablespoon (15 ml of sesame oil (optional

☐ 2 tablespoons (30 ml of gluten-free tamari sauce or coconut aminos

☐ Salt to taste

☐ Avocado oil to cook with

DIRECTIONS:

Add avocado oil into a frying pan and cook the whisked egg. Remove and set it aside on a plate.

Add additional avocado oil into the frying pan and cook the pork. Then add in the pepper, onion, and cashews.

Sauté until the pork is fully cooked, then add the cooked egg. Then add in the ginger, garlic, chili oil, sesame oil, tamari sauce, and salt to taste.

Serve immediately. Enjoy.

238) Pork tenderloin

PREPARATION TIME: 10 minutes
COOKING TIME: 20 minutes
SERVINGS: 2 people
INGREDIENTS:

☐ 1 pound of pork tenderloin

☐ salt and pepper to taste

☐ 1 tablespoon coconut oil

DIRECTIONS:

First cut the 1-pound pork tenderloin in half. Add coconut oil into a frying pan on a medium heat.

After the coconut oil melts, place the 2 pork tenderloin pieces into the pan. Leave the pork to cook on its side.

Once that side is cooked, turn using tongs to cook the other sides. Repeat until the pork looks cooked on all sides.

Cook all sides of the pork until the meat thermometer shows an internal temperature of just below 145F (63C.

Let the pork sit for a few minutes and then slice into 1-inch thick slices with a sharp knife.

Serve and enjoy.

239) Kalua Pork

SERVINGS: 5 to 6
PREPARATION TIME: 5 minutes
COOKING TIME: 6 hours
Total time: 6 hours 5 minutes
INGREDIENTS:

☐ 2 pounds of Pork tenderloin

☐ 10 ounces of Bacon

☐ ½ teaspoon black lava sea salt

DIRECTIONS:

Set your slow cooker on low for 6 hours. Add bacon on the bottom of the slow cooker and then set the pork tenderloin on top and cover with black see lava salt.

Pull the pork with a fork in the slow cooker and mix until well combined.

Serve and enjoy.

240) Andouille Sausage & Rice Stuffed Pork Tenderloin

PREPARATION TIME: 20 minutes
COOKING TIME: 30 minutes
SERVINGS: 3 to 4 people
INGREDIENTS:

☐ 4 tablespoons butter, ghee or coconut oil, divided

☐ 2 garlic cloves, minced

☐ 1 yellow onion, minced

☐ 1 red bell pepper, finely chopped

☐ 2 chicken Andouille sausages, chopped

☐ 1 small cauliflower, riced*

☐ 1 cup of chicken broth

☐ 1 teaspoon of fine sea salt

☐ ½ teaspoon of smoked paprika

☐ ½ teaspoon of chili powder

☐ ½ teaspoon of red pepper flakes

☐ 1 6 ounces can of tomato paste

☐ 1 to 1½ pound pork tenderloin

DIRECTIONS:

First, heat oven to 375 degrees.

Over medium heat, place 2 tablespoons of butter in a large fry pan. Add minced garlic and onion and sauté until onions are translucent.

Then add red pepper and sausage to the pan and cook for 3 to 4 minutes then add rice cauliflower and 1 cup of broth.

Then add all spices and salt. Mix and cook for about 10 minutes, until cauliflower cooks and becomes tender.

Lastly, add tomato paste and cook for a couple minutes until it is warm. Cut pork tenderloin open lengthwise.

Use about 1 cup of rice mixture and spread out lengthwise down the middle of the tenderloin.

Wrap tenderloin around the rice then tie multiple ties around the tenderloin to keep it secure.

Add 2 more tablespoons of butter to another large sauté pan over medium-high. Once hot, sear pork tenderloin on all side for about 2 minutes per side.

Place on a baking sheet, uncovered for 30 minutes, until meat thermometer reads 160 degrees.

10. Remove and let stand for 10 minutes before removing string and slicing it.

11. Serve with reheated Andouille rice. Enjoy.

Vegetables

241) **Cauliflower Pizza Crust**

PREPARATION TIME: 15 minutes
COOKING TIME: 20 minutes
SERVINGS: 6
INGREDIENTS:
2 cups cauliflower, chopped
1 egg, whisked
1 teaspoon butter
1 teaspoon dried basil
1 teaspoon salt
6 oz Cheddar cheese, shredded
1 tablespoon heavy cream
DIRECTIONS:
Place the cauliflower in the food processor and blend until you get cauliflower rice.
Then squeeze the juice from the cauliflower rice.
Line the baking tray with the parchment and then spread parchment with the butter.
Place the cauliflower rice in the tray in the shape of the pizza crust.
Bake the cauliflower pizza crust for 10 minutes at 365F.
Meanwhile, mix up together salt, shredded Cheddar cheese, heavy cream, and egg.
When the cauliflower crust is cooked, spread it with cheese mixture and flatten gently it.
Bake the meal for 10 minutes more at 375F.
When the pizza crust is cooked, cut it into 6 servings.
Nutrition: calories 147, fat 11.7, fiber 0.8, carbs 2.3, protein 8.7

242) **Zucchini Ravioli**

PREPARATION TIME: 20 minutes
COOKING TIME: 15 minutes
SERVINGS: 4
INGREDIENTS:
1 zucchini, trimmed
2 tablespoons ricotta cheese
½ cup spinach, chopped
1 teaspoon olive oil
½ teaspoon salt
1/3 cup marinara sauce
4 oz Parmesan, grated
DIRECTIONS:
Slice the zucchini with the help of the peeler to get long slices.
Then take 4 zucchini slices and make the cross from them.
Repeat the same steps with all remaining zucchini slices.
After this, place chopped spinach in the skillet.
Add salt and olive oil. Mix up spinach and cook it for 5 minutes. Stir it from time to time.
After this, mix up spinach with ricotta and stir well.
Pour marinara sauce in the casserole dish.
Place the ricotta mixture in the center of every zucchini cross and fold up them.
Transfer zucchini balls (ravioli in the casserole to dish on the marinara sauce.
Sprinkle the zucchini ravioli over with grated Parmesan and transfer the casserole dish in the preheated to the 395F oven. Cook the meal for 15 minutes.
Nutrition: calories 141, fat 8.9, fiber 1.2, carbs 5.9, protein 11.1

243) **Vegetable Crackers**

PREPARATION TIME: 20 minutes
COOKING TIME: 20 minutes
SERVINGS: 4
INGREDIENTS:
1 cup cauliflower
1 tablespoon flax meal
1 teaspoon chia seeds
1 teaspoon ground cumin
1 teaspoon salt
½ teaspoon ground paprika
1 tablespoon rice flour
1 teaspoon nutritional yeast
1 cup water, for the steamer
DIRECTIONS:
Chop the cauliflower roughly.
Pour water in the steamer and insert steamer rack. Place the cauliflower in the rack and close the lid.

Preheat the steamer and steam cauliflower for 5 minutes.

After this, place the vegetables in the food processor and blend well.

Transfer the blended cauliflower in the cheesecloth and squeeze the liquid from it.

Then transfer the cauliflower in the bowl.

Add all ingredients from the list above and mix up well.

Line the baking tray with the parchment and place cauliflower mixture over it.

Cover it with the second parchment sheet.

Roll up the cauliflower mixture into the rectangular.

Remove the upper parchment sheet and cut the cauliflower mixture into the crackers.

Transfer the tray in the preheated to the 365F oven.

Cook crackers for 15 minutes.

Chill the crackers well remove from the baking tray.

Nutrition: calories 35, fat 1.3, fiber 2.1, carbs 5.2, protein 1.8

244) Crunchy Okra Bites

PREPARATION TIME: 10 minutes
COOKING TIME: 12 minutes
SERVINGS: 2
INGREDIENTS:
1 cup okra, roughly sliced
¼ cup almond flour
1 tablespoon coconut flakes
1 teaspoon chili powder
½ teaspoon salt
3 eggs, whisked
DIRECTIONS:
In the mixing bowl, mix up together almond flour, coconut flakes, chili powder, and salt.

Place the sliced okra into the whisked egg and mix up well.

Then coat every okra bite into the almond flour mixture.

Line the tray with the parchment.

Place the okra bites into the tray to make the okra layer.

Preheat the oven to 375F.

Place the tray with okra bites in the oven and cook for 12 minutes.

Chill the hot okra bites little before serving.
Nutrition: calories 147, fat 9.5, fiber 2.7, carbs 6.1, protein 10.3

245) Arugula-Tomato Salad

PREPARATION TIME: 15 minutes
SERVINGS: 6
INGREDIENTS:
2 cups arugula, chopped
1 cup lettuce, chopped
½ cup cherry tomatoes
¼ cup fresh basil
1 tablespoon olive oil
½ teaspoon chili flakes
5 oz Mozzarella cheese balls, cherry size
DIRECTIONS:
Make the salad dressing: blend the fresh basil until smooth and add olive oil and chili flakes. Pulse the mixture for 5 seconds.

After this, place arugula and lettuce into the salad bowl.

Cut the cherry tomatoes into the halves and add in the salad bowl.

Then add Mozzarella cheese balls and shake the salad well.

Pour the salad dressing over the salad.
Nutrition: calories 93, fat 8.3, fiber 0.4, carbs 1.1, protein 4.5

246) Basil Bake

PREPARATION TIME: 15 minutes
COOKING TIME: 25 minutes
SERVINGS: 4
INGREDIENTS:
½ cup fresh basil
4 tablespoons coconut oil
1 zucchini, sliced
2 oz Parmesan, grated
1 tablespoon walnuts, chopped
½ teaspoon salt
2 tomatoes, sliced
DIRECTIONS:
Melt coconut oil and transfer it in the blender.

Add fresh basil, walnuts, and salt. Blend the mixture until smooth. Add grated Parmesan and stir it. The pesto sauce is cooked.

Place the sliced zucchini and tomatoes into the casserole dish one-by-one.

Then top it with pesto sauce.

Cover the casserole dish with the foil and transfer in the oven.

Bake the meal for 25 minutes at 375F.

Then discard the foil and remove the basil bake from the oven.

Nutrition: calories 194, fat 18, fiber 1.5, carbs 4.8, protein 6.2

247) **Roasted Bok Choy with Chili Sauce**

PREPARATION TIME: 10 minutes
COOKING TIME: 10 minutes
SERVINGS: 2
INGREDIENTS:
8 oz bok choy
4 tablespoons chili sauce
2 tablespoons almond butter
1 teaspoon dried dill
DIRECTIONS:
Slice bok choy into halves and place in the big bowl.

Add chili sauce and dried dill and mix up well.

Place the almond butter in the skillet and melt it.

Add the chili bok choy and roast it for 5 minutes from each side over the medium-low heat.

Gently transfer the cooked bok choy into the serving plates.

Nutrition: calories 117, fat 9.4, fiber 2.9, carbs 6.3, protein 5.4

248) **Vegan Moussaka**

PREPARATION TIME: 15 minutes
COOKING TIME: 35 minutes
SERVINGS: 88
INGREDIENTS:
2 eggplants, trimmed
1 white onion, chopped

1 garlic clove, diced
¼ cup tomatoes, crushed
½ teaspoon ground cinnamon
1 teaspoon salt
1 teaspoon ground black pepper
1 teaspoon ground paprika
2 tablespoons coconut oil
2 tablespoons ricotta cheese
1 oz Cheddar cheese, shredded
1 tablespoon heavy cream
DIRECTIONS:
Place the coconut oil in the saucepan and melt it.

Meanwhile, chop the eggplants.

Place the eggplants and onion in the hot coconut oil. Add diced garlic.

Mix up the vegetables and cook them for 10 minutes or until they start to be soft.

Meanwhile, mix up together heavy cream, ricotta cheese, and shredded Cheddar cheese.

Transfer the roasted vegetables in the blender and blend for 3 minutes or until they are smooth.

After this, add all spices and crushed tomatoes, Blend the mixture 1 minute more.

Transfer the eggplant mixture in the casserole dish and flatten it well with the help of the spatula.

Place ricotta mixture over the eggplant mixture.

Bake moussaka for 20 minutes at the preheated to the 360F oven.

Chill the cooked meal for 10 minutes before serving.

Nutrition: calories 99, fat 5.9, fiber 5.5, carbs 10.4, protein 3

249) **Cumin Fennel**

PREPARATION TIME: 10 minutes
COOKING TIME: 15 minutes
SERVINGS: 6
INGREDIENTS:
1-pound fennel bulb
2 tablespoons butter, softened
1 tablespoon ground cumin
1 teaspoon salt
¼ teaspoon garlic powder
DIRECTIONS:

Slice fennel bulb into the medium slices.
Line the baking tray with the baking paper.
Churn butter with the ground cumin, salt, and garlic powder.
Arrange the sliced fennel on the tray and spread it with the churned butter mixture.
Bake the fennel for 15 minutes at 360F.
When the fennel is cooked, it has a tender taste.
Nutrition: calories 62, fat 4.2, fiber 2.5, carbs 6, protein 1.2

250) Mushroom Tart

PREPARATION TIME: 15 minutes
COOKING TIME: 40 minutes
SERVINGS: 8
INGREDIENTS:
1 teaspoon baking powder
½ teaspoon salt
1 small egg, beaten
1 tablespoon coconut oil
½ cup almond flour
1 cup mushroom caps
1 tablespoon fresh dill, chopped
1 tablespoon butter
1 teaspoon ground turmeric
1 teaspoon ground paprika
2 oz Parmesan, grated
¼ cup heavy cream
DIRECTIONS:
Make the tart dough: mix up together salt, egg baking powder, coconut oil, and almond flour. Knead the dough and roll it up into the pie crust.
Place the dough into the pie form.
Then arrange the mushrooms caps inside the pie form.
Sprinkle them with chopped dill, ground turmeric, paprika, and butter.
Then add Parmesan and pour it over with the heavy cream.
Transfer the tart in the oven.
Cook the mushroom tart for 40 minutes at 360F.
Chill the cooked tart till them room temperature and after this cut it into the servings.
Nutrition: calories 85, fat 7.5, fiber 0.5, carbs 1.9, protein 3.8

251) Zucchini Pasta with Spices

PREPARATION TIME: 10 minutes
COOKING TIME: 5 minutes
SERVINGS: 4
INGREDIENTS:
2 zucchini, sliced
1 oz Parmesan, grated
1 teaspoon butter
¼ teaspoon ground nutmeg
¾ teaspoon ground cinnamon
½ teaspoon salt
½ teaspoon chili powder
½ teaspoon ground paprika
½ teaspoon dried oregano
¼ teaspoon dried cilantro
¼ teaspoon ground black pepper
¼ cup of coconut milk
DIRECTIONS:
Mix up together all spices.
Then make the noodles from zucchini with the help spiralizer.
Combine together zucchini noodles and spices.
Place butter in the skillet and melt it.
Add coconut milk and bring the liquid to boil.
After this, add zucchini noodles and carefully mix with the help of the spoon.
Close the lid and simmer zucchini pasta for 5 minutes over the medium-low heat.
Sprinkle the cooked meal with grated Parmesan.
Nutrition: calories 86, fat 6.4, fiber 2, carbs 5.3, protein 4

252) Cauliflower Cheese

PREPARATION TIME: 10 minutes
COOKING TIME: 25 minutes
SERVINGS: 5
INGREDIENTS:
2 cups cauliflower florets
1 cup organic almond milk
½ cup heavy cream
2 tablespoons coconut flour
1 teaspoon salt

6 oz Cheddar cheese, shredded
2 cups of water
DIRECTIONS:
Bring water to boil, add cauliflower florets and boil them for 10 minutes.
Then drain water and transfer cauliflower florets in the baking dish.
Pour almond milk and heavy cream in the saucepan. Bring the liquid to boil.
Add salt and coconut flour.
Whisk the liquid very fast for 1 minute.
Then switch off the heat and add shredded cheese.
Leave the liquid until cheese is melted. Mix it up.
Pour cheese over the cauliflower florets.
Bake the cauliflower cheese for 15 minutes at 375F or until it starts bubbling.
Nutrition: calories 225, fat 17.1, fiber 3, carbs 7.7, protein 10.5

253) **Spinach&Kale Salad**

PREPARATION TIME: 10 minutes
SERVINGS: 4
INGREDIENTS:
2 cups fresh spinach
1 cucumber, chopped
1 cup kale
¼ teaspoon salt
½ teaspoon ground black pepper
1 teaspoon flax seeds
1 bell pepper
2 tablespoons sesame oil
2 tablespoons lemon juice
½ cup lettuce
DIRECTIONS:
Remove stems from kale.
Roughly chop kale, spinach, and lettuce and transfer greens in the salad bowl.
Slice bell pepper.
Add sliced bell pepper and chopped cucumber in the salad bowl too.
Then sprinkle the meal with salt, ground black pepper, lemon juice, and sesame oil.
Mix up a salad with the help of 2 forks.
Nutrition: calories 99, fat 7.3, fiber 1.7, carbs 8, protein 2

254) **Cauliflower Anti Pasto**

PREPARATION TIME: 10 minutes
COOKING TIME: 20 minutes
SERVINGS: 4
INGREDIENTS:
1 cup mushrooms, marinated, chopped
1 cup cauliflower
2 oz Swiss cheese, chopped
1 bell pepper, chopped
1 teaspoon dried oregano
1 tablespoon lemon juice
1 tablespoon olive oil
½ teaspoon dried cilantro
1 cup water, for the steamer
DIRECTIONS:
Pour water in the steamer and insert trivet.
Place the cauliflower in the trivet and close the lid.
Steam the vegetable for 10 minutes totally (including preheating.
Preheat oven to 375F.
Place bell peppers in the tray and transfer in the oven.
Bake it for 5 minutes from each side.
Remove the cooked bell pepper from the oven, chill little and peel.
Then chop it roughly and put in the big bowl.
Remove the cauliflower from the steamer and cut it into the small florets.
Transfer the cauliflower in the zip log bag.
Add dried oregano, lemon juice, olive oil, and dried cilantro.
Shake the mixture well.
Remove the cauliflower from the zip log into the bowl with the bell pepper.
Add chopped Swiss cheese and marinated mushrooms.
Mix up antipasto well.
Nutrition: calories 105, fat 7.7, fiber 1.4, carbs 5.2, protein 5.2

255) **Sour Sweet Bok Choy**

PREPARATION TIME: 7 minutes
COOKING TIME: 12 minutes
SERVINGS: 1
INGREDIENTS:

6 oz bok choy, sliced
1 teaspoon Erythritol
1 teaspoon lime juice
¼ teaspoon ground paprika
1 tablespoon water
1 teaspoon apple cider vinegar
1 tablespoon almond butter
DIRECTIONS:
Put almond butter in the skillet and melt it.
Add sliced bok choy and roast it for 3 minutes from each side.
Meanwhile, whisk together Erythritol, lime juice, ground paprika, water, and apple cider vinegar.
When the bok choy is roasted from both sides sprinkle it with Erythritol mixture and mix up with the help of a spatula.
Bring to boil the meal and switch off the heat.
Let bok choy rest for 5 minutes.
Nutrition: calories 124, fat 9.4, fiber 3.5, carbs 7.4, protein 6

256) **Celery Rosti**

PREPARATION TIME: 10 minutes
COOKING TIME: 10 minutes
SERVINGS: 4
INGREDIENTS:
8 oz celery root, peeled
1/3 onion, diced
1 teaspoon olive oil
½ teaspoon ground black pepper
2 oz Parmesan, grated
¼ teaspoon ground turmeric
DIRECTIONS:
Put the diced onion in the skillet. Add olive oil and cook it until translucent.
Meanwhile, grated celery root and mix it up with ground black pepper, ground turmeric, and Parmesan.
When the mixture is homogenous, add it in the skillet.
Mix up well.
Then press the celery root mixture with the help of the spatula to get the shape of the pancake.
Close the lid and cook celery rosti for 6 minutes or until it is light brown.

Nutrition: calories 84, fat 4.4, fiber 1.3, carbs 6.9, protein 5.5

257) **Garlic Snap Peas**

PREPARATION TIME: 5 minutes
COOKING TIME: 10 minutes
SERVINGS: 3
INGREDIENTS:
1 cup snap peas
1 teaspoon Erythritol
1 teaspoon avocado oil
¼ teaspoon cayenne pepper
½ teaspoon garlic powder
¾ teaspoon garlic, diced
DIRECTIONS:
Pour avocado oil in the skillet.
Add diced garlic and cook it for 1 minute over the medium heat.
Sprinkle it with garlic powder, cayenne pepper, and Erythritol.
Then add snap peas and mix up well.
Cook the snap peas for 9 minutes. Stir it all the time.
The cooked snap peas should be tender and crispy.
Nutrition: calories 44, fat 0.4, fiber 2.6, carbs 7.7, protein 2.8

258) **Sheet Pan Rosemary Mushrooms**

PREPARATION TIME: 10 minutes
COOKING TIME: 15 minutes
SERVINGS: 2
INGREDIENTS:
1 cup mushrooms
1 teaspoon minced rosemary
½ teaspoon of sea salt
1 tablespoon sesame oil
DIRECTIONS:
Line the baking tray with baking paper.
Slice the mushrooms roughly and put them in the baking tray.
Sprinkle mushrooms with minced rosemary, sea salt, and sesame oil.
Mix up the vegetables well with the help of the hand palms.

Preheat the oven to 360F.
Cook mushrooms for 15 minutes.
Nutrition: calories 70, fat 7, fiber 0.6, carbs 1.5, protein 1.1

259) Buttered Sprouts

PREPARATION TIME: 7 minutes
COOKING TIME: 20 minutes
SERVINGS: 4
INGREDIENTS:
10 oz Brussel sprouts
2 oz prosciutto
3 teaspoons butter
1 cup of water
1 teaspoon salt
DIRECTIONS:
Chop prosciutto and place in the saucepan.
Roast it until it starts to be crispy.
Then add water and Brussel sprouts.
Bring the mixture to boil and close the lid.
Boil the vegetables for 15 minutes.
After this, drain ½ part of all liquid and add butter.
Mix it up until the butter is melted and bring the meal to boil one more time in the butter liquid.
Serve buttered sprouts with the butter liquid.
Nutrition: calories 76, fat 3.9, fiber 2.7, carbs 6.7, protein 5.4

260) Bacon Cabbage Slices

PREPARATION TIME: 10 minutes
COOKING TIME: 15 minutes
SERVINGS: 4
INGREDIENTS:
10 oz white cabbage
4 oz bacon, sliced
½ teaspoon ground black pepper
1 teaspoon butter
½ teaspoon salt
DIRECTIONS:
Slice the cabbage into medium slices and rub with butter.
Sprinkle the bacon slices with ground black pepper and salt.

Wrap every cabbage slice into the bacon and transfer in the tray.
Cook the cabbage slices in the oven at 370F for 15 minutes. You can flip the cabbage slices onto another side during cooking.
Nutrition: calories 180, fat 12.9, fiber 1.8, carbs 4.7, protein 11.5

261) Lemon Onion Mash

PREPARATION TIME: 15 minutes
COOKING TIME: 15 minutes
SERVINGS: 4
INGREDIENTS:
2 white onions
4 oz cauliflower
¼ cup heavy cream
4 oz Cheddar cheese, shredded
½ teaspoon Pink salt
1 teaspoon white pepper
½ teaspoon lemon zest
1 teaspoon lemon juice
1 teaspoon butter
DIRECTIONS:
Peel the onion and grind it.
Put grinded onion and butter in the saucepan.
Blend cauliflower until you get cauliflower rice.
Add cauliflower rice in the saucepan too.
Add Pink salt, white pepper, lemon zest, and lemon juice. Stir it.
Close the lid and cook the mass for 5 minutes over the medium heat.
Then add shredded Cheddar cheese and heavy cream.
Mix up well and stir it until cheese is melted.
Close the lid and simmer mash for 5 minutes more over the low heat.
Switch off the heat and close the lid.
Let the lemon onion mash chill for 10 minutes.
Nutrition: calories 179, fat 13.3, fiber 2.1, carbs 7.6, protein 8.5

262) **Keto Chopped Ragu**

PREPARATION TIME: 10 minutes
COOKING TIME: 25 minutes
SERVINGS: 5
INGREDIENTS:
1 bell pepper, chopped
2 oz green beans, chopped
1 oz bok choy, chopped
2 oz collard greens, chopped
½ white onion, chopped
3 oz kale, chopped
2 oz jicama, chopped
3 oz asparagus
½ cup of coconut milk
1/3 cup water
1 teaspoon salt
½ teaspoon ground black pepper
½ teaspoon cayenne pepper
1 teaspoon marinara sauce
DIRECTIONS:
Take the big pan and add water inside.
Bring water to boil and add chopped bell pepper, green beans, bok choy, collard greens, onion, kale, jicama, and asparagus.
Then add salt, ground black pepper, cayenne pepper, and marinara sauce.
Add coconut milk and carefully stir the vegetable ragu.
Preheat the oven to 365F.
Close the lid of the pan.
Transfer the pan in the preheated oven and bake ragu for 25 minutes.
When the ragu is cooked, remove it from the oven and remove the lid.
Don't stir ragu anymore!
If ragu will chill for 10-15 minutes, you will get the most delicious taste of ragu.
Nutrition: calories 93, fat 6, fiber 3.2, carbs 9.5, protein 2.5

263) **Easy Cauliflower Fritters**

PREPARATION TIME: 15 minutes
SERVINGS: 5
Nutrition: 173 Calories; 10.7g Fat; 6.9g Carbs; 10.8g Protein; 2.9g Fiber
Ingredients
1 cup parmesan cheese, shredded
1 egg, beaten
1/2 cup almond meal
1 ½ pounds cauliflower florets
1 celery stalk, chopped
Directions
Process the cauliflower florets and celery in your food processor until they have broken down into rice-sized pieces.
Add in parmesan, egg, and almond meal. Mix until everything is well combined. Season with the salt and black pepper to taste.
Form the mixture into 5 equal patties.
In a nonstick skillet, heat 2 tablespoons of sesame oil. Once hot, fry the patties for 3 to 4 minutes per side. Serve warm and enjoy!

264) **Avocado and Cucumber Salad**

PREPARATION TIME: 5 minutes
SERVINGS: 4
Nutrition: 149 Calories; 14.3g Fat; 5.8g Carbs; 1.4g Protein; 3.6g Fiber
Ingredients
1 Lebanese cucumber, sliced
3 teaspoons fresh lemon juice
2 tablespoons extra-virgin olive oil
1 avocado, peeled, pitted and sliced
1/2 white onion, chopped
Directions
Combine avocado, onion, and cucumber in a salad bowl.
Drizzle lemon juice and extra-virgin olive oil over everything.
Taste, adjust seasonings, and serve well chilled. Bon appétit!

265) **Greek Autumn Casserole**

PREPARATION TIME: 1 hour 25 minutes
SERVINGS: 5
Nutrition: 226 Calories; 14.1g Fat; 6.8g Carbs; 16.3g Protein; 2.8g Fiber
Ingredients
1 cup Greek-style yogurt
5 eggs, beaten
1 ½ cups feta cheese, grated

1 pound aubergine cut into rounds
2 vine-ripe tomatoes, sliced
Directions
Toss the aubergine with 1 teaspoon of sea salt; let it sit for 25 minutes. Discard excess water and pat your aubergine dry with kitchen towel.

Now, place aubergine rounds in a lightly greased baking pan. Brush them with a non-stick oil and roast them at 380 degrees F for about 35 to 40 minutes or until tender.

Lay the roasted aubergine rounds on the bottom of a lightly greased casserole dish. Top with sliced tomatoes.

Then, whisk Greek yogurt with eggs. Pour the mixture over the roasted aubergine rounds. Top with feta cheese and continue to bake in the preheated oven at 365 degrees F for about 15 minutes. Enjoy!

266) Creamy Swiss Chard with Cheese

PREPARATION TIME: 15 minutes
SERVINGS: 6
Nutrition: 149 Calories; 11.1g Fat; 6.6g Carbs; 5.4g Protein; 2.2g Fiber
Ingredients
1 ½ pounds Swiss chard
1/2 cup vegetable broth
1 cup sour cream
1 yellow onion, chopped
2 garlic cloves, minced
Directions
Melt 2 tablespoons of butter in a sauté pan over medium-high heat. Sauté the onion for 3 to 4 minutes until tender and translucent.

Stir in the garlic and continue to cook until aromatic or about 30 seconds. Season with the salt and black pepper.

Stir in the Swiss chard and broth; continue to cook, partially covered, for 5 to 6 minutes over medium-low heat. Fold in the sour cream.

Ladle into individual bowls and serve warm.

267) Chanterelle Omelet with Peppers

PREPARATION TIME: 20 minutes
SERVINGS: 4
Nutrition: 239 Calories; 17.5g Fat; 6.1g Carbs; 12.3g Protein; 1.8g Fiber
Ingredients
6 eggs
1 cup Chanterelle mushrooms, chopped
1 white onion, chopped
2 bell peppers, chopped
2 tablespoons olive oil
Directions
In a frying pan, heat olive oil over moderate flame. Now, cook the mushrooms, onion, and peppers for 3 to 4 minutes until they are tender and fragrant.

Whisk the eggs until pale and frothy. Pour the eggs into the skillet and turn the heat to medium-low.

Let it cook for 4 to 5 minutes until the eggs are done and center of the omelet starts to look dry.

Serve warm and enjoy!

268) Japanese-Style Shirataki Noodle Ramen

PREPARATION TIME: 20 minutes
SERVINGS: 4
Nutrition: 76 Calories; 5g Fat; 5.3g Carbs; 3.8g Protein; 0.9g Fiber
Ingredients
1 ½ tablespoons ghee, melted
1 pound brown mushrooms, chopped
2 tablespoons green onions, chopped
4 cups roasted vegetable broth
8 ounces shirataki noodles
Directions
In a heavy-bottomed pot, melt the ghee over medium-high heat. Sauté the mushrooms for about 3 minutes or until they release liquid.

Add in green onions and continue sautéing an additional 2 minutes. Season with black pepper and salt to taste.

Add in the vegetable broth and bring to a boil. Turn the heat to simmer.

Continue to cook for about 10 minutes. Fold in the shirataki noodles and cook according to package directions. Bon appétit!

269) Vegetables in Creamy Sauce

PREPARATION TIME: 15 minutes
SERVINGS: 3
Nutrition: 256 Calories; 24g Fat; 6.5g Carbs; 3g Protein; 2.9g Fiber
Ingredients
1 white onion, chopped
1 bell pepper
1/2 pound cauliflower florets
1/2 pound savoy cabbage, shredded
1 cup double cream
Directions
Heat 2 tablespoons of olive oil in a saucepan over medium-high heat. Cook the onion until tender and fragrant about 4 minutes.

Stir in the bell pepper, cauliflower, and savoy cabbage; pour in 1 cup of water or mushroom soup.

Turn the heat to medium-low and let it cook for about 10 minutes until everything is heated through.

Fold in the double cream and let it simmer, partially covered, for about 3 minutes. Taste, adjust seasonings and serve warm.

270) Asparagus Frittata with Halloumi Cheese

PREPARATION TIME: 25 minutes
SERVINGS: 4
Nutrition: 376 Calories; 29.1g Fat; 4g Carbs; 24.5g Protein; 1g Fiber
Ingredients
5 whole eggs, beaten
10 ounces Halloumi cheese, crumbled
1/2 red onion, sliced
1 tomato, chopped
4 ounces asparagus, cut into small chunks
Directions

Heat 1 tablespoon of oil in a frying pan over medium-high heat; then, sauté the onion and asparagus for 3 to 4 minutes, stirring periodically to ensure even cooking.

Stir in tomato and cook for 2 to 3 minutes more. Place the sautéed vegetables in a lightly greased casserole dish.

Combine the eggs with cheese and pour the mixture over the vegetables. Bake in the preheated oven at 360 degrees F for 13 to 15 minutes.

Garnish with 2 tablespoons of Greek olives if desired. Enjoy!

271) Cheese and Kale Casserole

PREPARATION TIME: 35 minutes
SERVINGS: 4
Nutrition: 384 Calories; 29.1g Fat; 5.9g Carbs; 25.1g Protein; 1.5g Fiber
Ingredients
1 cup Cheddar cheese, grated
1 cup Romano cheese
4 eggs, whisked
2 tablespoons sour cream
6 ounces kale, torn into pieces
Directions
Begin by preheating your oven to 360 degrees F. Brush the sides and bottom of a casserole dish with a nonstick cooking spray.

Thoroughly combine the ingredients and pour the mixture into the casserole dish.

Bake in the preheated oven for about 35 minutes or until the top is golden brown. Salt to taste. Bon appétit!

272) Spicy Peppery Eggs

PREPARATION TIME: 15 minutes
SERVINGS: 2
Nutrition: 439 Calories; 36.7g Fat; 3.8g Carbs; 22.9g Protein; 0.1g Fiber
Ingredients
4 eggs, whisked
4 tablespoons full-fat yogurt
2 bell peppers, chopped
1 onion, sliced

3 ounces cheddar cheese, shredded
Directions
In a frying pan, heat 2 tablespoons of olive oil over medium-high heat. Sauté the peppers and onion for about 3 minutes until they have softened.

Whisk the eggs with yogurt. Pour the egg mixture into the frying pan. Season with pepper and salt to taste.

Cook the eggs for 5 to 6 minutes until they are set. Top with cheddar cheese and serve warm.

273) Old-Fashioned Green Chowder

PREPARATION TIME: 25 minutes
SERVINGS: 4
Nutrition: 85 Calories; 5.9g Fat; 3.8g Carbs; 3.7g Protein; 1.3g Fiber
Ingredients
1/2 cup scallions, chopped
2 zucchinis, sliced
1 celery stalk, chopped
4 ounces baby spinach
1 egg, beaten
Directions
In a heavy-bottomed pot, heat 1 tablespoon of oil over medium-high flame. Now, cook the scallions for about 3 minutes until tender and aromatic.

Add in 4 cups of water, zucchini, and celery; add in 1 tablespoons of vegetable bouillon powder, if desired.

Let it cook, partially covered, for about 15 minutes. Fold in spinach and continue to cook for 5 to 6 minutes more.

Afterwards, add in the egg and stir to combine well. Serve immediately, drizzled with melted butter, if desired.

274) Tofu Salad with Peppers

PREPARATION TIME: 15 minutes
SERVINGS: 4
Nutrition: 155 Calories; 11.4g Fat; 6.4g Carbs; 8.6g Protein; 1.1g Fiber
Ingredients

1 (14-ounce tofu block, pressed and cubed
2 tablespoons fresh lemon juice
2 tablespoons extra-virgin olive oil
4 bell peppers, deveined and halved
2 scallions, chopped
Directions
Brush a frying pan with cooking spray. Cook the tofu cubes for about 3 minutes over medium-high heat; reserve.

Then, cook the peppers for 4 to 5 minutes, stirring periodically to ensure even cooking. Toss the scallions and peppers with lemon juice and and olive oil. Top your salad with tofu cubes and enjoy!

275) Cheese and Zucchini Bake

PREPARATION TIME: 50 minutes
SERVINGS: 5
Nutrition: 371 Calories; 32g Fat; 5.2g Carbs; 15.7g Protein; 0.3g Fiber
Ingredients
2 zucchini, sliced
1/2 medium-sized leek, sliced
10 large eggs
3 tablespoons yogurt
2 cups Swiss cheese, shredded
Directions
Preheat your oven to 350 degrees F. Brush an oven-proof skillet with a nonstick cooking spray.

Place 1/2 of the zucchini in the skillet; place the leek slices on zucchini layer. Season with salt, and black pepper to your liking.

Add the remaining zucchini and leek.

Whisk the eggs and yogurt until well combined and frothy. Add the egg mixture and top with cheese.

Bake in the preheated oven for 35 to 40 minutes, until the top is hot and bubbly. Enjoy!

276) Dad's Keto Crêpes

PREPARATION TIME: 50 minutes
SERVINGS: 5

Nutrition: 248 Calories; 21.7g Fat; 5.7g Carbs; 9.1g Protein; 0.6g Fiber
Ingredients
2 tablespoons coconut oil
2 tablespoons toasted coconut
3 tablespoons peanut butter
4 eggs, well whisked
4 ounces cream cheese
Directions
In a mixing bowl, whisk the eggs and cream cheese until well combined.
Melt coconut oil in a frying pan over medium-high flame.
Cook each crêpe for 3 to 4 minutes per side. Serve with peanut butter and toasted coconut. Bon appétit!

277) Graded Broccoli and Cheese Bake

PREPARATION TIME: 35 minutes
SERVINGS: 6
Nutrition: 241 Calories; 16.3g Fat; 5.5g Carbs; 16.4g Protein; 1.5g Fiber
Ingredients
3/4 pounds broccoli florets
6 eggs
6 ounces sour cream
1 cup vegetable broth
6 ounces Swiss cheese, shredded
Directions
Parboil broccoli in a pot of lightly-salted water for 2 to 3 minutes.
Brush the sides and bottom of a casserole dish with nonstick cooking spray. In a mixing bowl, combine the eggs, sour cream, and broth.
Place the broccoli florets on the bottom of the casserole dish. Pour the egg mixture over the broccoli. Top with Swiss cheese.
Bake in the preheated oven at 370 degrees for about 25 minutes. Bon appétit!

278) Authentic Zuppa alla Marinara with Broccoli

PREPARATION TIME: 30 minutes
SERVINGS: 3
Nutrition: 130 Calories; 9.4g Fat; 8.8g Carbs; 2.9g Protein; 2.2g Fiber
Ingredients
1 cup spinach leaves, torn into pieces
1 cup marinara sauce
4 ounces broccoli
2 tablespoons sesame oil
1 small-sized onion, chopped
Directions
Chopp the broccoli into small grain sized pieces; reserve.
Heat sesame oil in a frying pan over a moderate heat. Sauté the onion until tender and aromatic.
Stir in broccoli and cook for 2 to 3 minutes more. Add in marinara sauce along with 3 cups of water or vegetable broth. Season with Italian spice mix, if desired.
Bring to a boil; turn the heat to medium-low and continue to simmer for 20 to 25 minutes.
Fold in spinach leaves, cover, and let it sit in the residual heat for 10 minutes. Bon appétit!

279) Mexican Stuffed Peppers

PREPARATION TIME: 45 minutes
SERVINGS: 3
Nutrition: 194 Calories; 13.9g Fat; 3.5g Carbs; 13.3g Protein; 0.7g Fiber
Ingredients
1 ripe tomato, pureed
1 cup Mexican cheese blend
1 garlic clove, minced
3 bell peppers, halved, seeds removed
3 eggs, whisked
Directions
Preheat your oven to 380 degrees F. Brush the bottom and sides of a baking dish with a nonstick cooking spray.

Then, combine the eggs, cheese, and garlic; add in chili powder, if desired. Stuff the peppers and place them in the baking pan.

Pour the tomato puree into the baking dish. Bake, covered, for 35 to 40 minutes, until everything is thoroughly cooked. Bon appétit!

280) Pan-Fried Tofu with Vegetables

PREPARATION TIME: 15 minutes
SERVINGS: 2
Nutrition: 217 Calories; 17g Fat; 7.5g Carbs; 11.5g Protein; 4.5g Fiber
Ingredients
6 ounces firm tofu, pressed and cubed
1/2 avocado, pitted, peeled and sliced
2 cups enoki mushrooms
1 red bell pepper, sliced
4 tablespoons scallions, chopped
Directions
In a frying pan, heat 1 teaspoon of the olive oil over a moderate heat. Once hot, fry the tofu cubes for 3 to 4 minutes, stirring periodically; reserve.

In the same frying pan, heat the remaining teaspoon of olive oil. Now, sauté the scallions, peppers, and mushrooms for about 3 minutes or until they have softened.

Sprinkle the sautéed vegetables with salt and black pepper. Top with the reserved tofu. Garnish with avocado and serve.

281) Baked Avocado Egg Cups

PREPARATION TIME: 20 minutes
SERVINGS: 4
Nutrition: 300 Calories; 24.6g Fat; 5.4g Carbs; 14.9g Protein; 4.6g Fiber
Ingredients
1 cup Asiago cheese, grated
1/2 teaspoon dried rosemary
1 tablespoon fresh chives, chopped
2 avocados, pitted and halved
4 eggs
Directions

Start by preheating your oven to 410 degrees F.

Crack an egg into each avocado half. Season with salt and black pepper to taste.

Top with cheese and rosemary.

Bake in the preheated oven for 15 to 17 minutes. Garnish with fresh chives and enjoy!

282) Breakfast Keto Veggies

PREPARATION TIME: 25 minutes
SERVINGS: 4
Nutrition: 172 Calories; 11.1g Fat; 8g Carbs; 8.2g Protein; 2.8g Fiber
Ingredients
4 eggs
1 cup green cabbage, shredded
2 cups broccoli florets
1 shallot, sliced
2 bell peppers, deseeded and sliced
Directions
In a large skillet, heat 2 tablespoons of olive oil over medium-high heat. Cook the shallots and peppers until they've softened.

Fold in the cabbage and broccoli; pour in 1/2 cup of onion soup (preferably homemade. Turn the temperature to medium-low.

Continue to simmer for 10 to 13 minutes or until cooked through. Create four indentations in the vegetable mixture. Crack an egg into each indentation.

Cook for 8 to 11 minutes more until the eggs are cooked to desired doneness. Enjoy!

283) Green Cabbage with Tofu

PREPARATION TIME: 20 minutes
SERVINGS: 3
Nutrition: 167 Calories; 11.8g Fat; 5.1g Carbs; 10.6g Protein; 2.4g Fiber
Ingredients
1 (1.5-pounds head green cabbage, cut into strips
1/2 cup vegetable broth
6 ounces tofu, diced
1/2 shallot, chopped

2 garlic cloves, finely chopped
Directions
Spritz a saucepan with a nonstick cooking oil. Fry the tofu in the preheated saucepan for about 5 minutes until crisp; reserve, keeping it warm.
Then, cook the shallot and garlic for 3 minutes longer until tender and aromatic. Stir in cabbage and beef bone broth.
Turn the temperature to simmer and let it cook, partially covered, for 10 to 12 minutes. Season with salt and pepper to taste.
Serve with reserved fried tofu and enjoy!

284) Roasted Asparagus Salad

PREPARATION TIME: 25 minutes
SERVINGS: 3
Nutrition: 159 Calories; 12.3g Fat; 6.1g Carbs; 5.8g Protein; 3.9g Fiber
Ingredients
3 tablespoons extra-virgin olive oil
1 cup cherry tomatoes, sliced
1 tablespoon Dijon mustard
1/2 lime, freshly squeezed
1 pound asparagus, trimmed
Directions
Place the asparagus spears on a lightly greased baking sheet and roast them at 390 degrees F for about 15 minutes.
In a small mixing dish, whisk the mustard, lime juice, and olive oil; add in minced garlic, if desired.
Cut the asparagus spears into small chunks and toss them with the prepared dressing. Top with cherry tomatoes and serve well-chilled.

285) Traditional Indian Saar

PREPARATION TIME: 30 minutes
SERVINGS: 4
Nutrition: 113 Calories; 5.5g Fat; 9.3g Carbs; 5.4g Protein; 2.5g Fiber
Ingredients
2 cups Indian masala sauce
1 cup full-fat yogurt

1 ½ tablespoons ghee
1 medium-sized leek, sliced
1 bell pepper, roughly chopped
Directions
Melt the ghee in a soup pot over a moderate heat. Now, cook the leek and peppers until they've softened.
Stir in Indian masala sauce and water, bringing to a boil; reduce the heat to medium-low. Let it simmer, covered, for 20 to 23 minutes.
Puree your soup in a blender and serve warm with yogurt on the side. Enjoy!

286) Roasted Cauliflower with Feta Cheese

PREPARATION TIME: 45 minutes
SERVINGS: 4
Nutrition: 194 Calories; 15g Fat; 5.7g Carbs; 7.4g Protein; 2.5g Fiber
Ingredients
1 pound cauliflower, halved
1 tablespoon Greek seasoning blend
1 cup feta cheese, crumbled
1 medium-sized leek, cut into 2-inch pieces
2 tablespoons olive oil
Directions
Pat cauliflower dry with paper towels.
Brush cauliflower and leeks with olive oil; sprinkle your veggies with Greek seasoning blend.
Place the cauliflower and leeks on a foil-lined baking sheet.
Roast in the predated oven at 380 degrees F for about 40 minutes, turning them over halfway through cooking. Serve with feta cheese and enjoy!

287) Broccoli Salad with Horseradish Mayo

PREPARATION TIME: 30 minutes
SERVINGS: 6
Nutrition: 170 Calories; 14.1g Fat; 7g Carbs; 3.1g Protein; 2.8g Fiber
Ingredients
1 tablespoon prepared horseradish
1 shallot, sliced

1/2 cup mayonnaise
6 cups broccoli florets
2 tablespoons balsamic vinegar
Directions
Roast the broccoli florets in the preheated oven at 420 degrees F for about 20 minutes until little charred.

Toss the roasted broccoli florets with the remaining ingredients; toss to combine well.

Serve at room temperature or well-chilled. Bon appétit!

288) Vegetable Noodles with Avocado Sauce

PREPARATION TIME: 10 minutes
SERVINGS: 3
Nutrition: 181 Calories; 16.2g Fat; 6.9g Carbs; 2.1g Protein; 4.1g Fiber
Ingredients
1 avocado, peeled and pitted
1/2 lemon, juiced and zested
1 zucchini
1 cucumber
2 garlic cloves, peeled
Directions
Spiralize the zucchini and cucumber.

In a frying pan, heat 2 tablespoons of olive oil over medium-high heat. Once hot, cook vegetable noodles for 5 to 6 minutes.

Meanwhile, puree the remaining ingredients until creamy and smooth. Pour the sauce over vegetable noodles and serve immediately.

289) Cream of Cauliflower and Ginger Soup

PREPARATION TIME: 20 minutes
SERVINGS: 4
Nutrition: 69 Calories; 1.5g Fat; 7g Carbs; 6.2g Protein; 3g Fiber
Ingredients
1 pound cauliflower florets
1/2 teaspoon ginger-garlic paste
3 cups vegetable broth
2 green onions, chopped
1 celery stalk, chopped

Directions
Preheat a heavy-bottomed pot over a medium-high heat. Sauté green onions until they are just tender and aromatic.

Stir in the celery, ginger-garlic paste, cauliflower, and vegetable broth, bringing to a boil. Immediately reduce heat to simmer.

Let it simmer for 15 to 16 minutes more or until everything is thoroughly cooked; remove from heat.

Puree the soup in your food processor and serve warm!

290) Cheesy Broccoli Casserole

PREPARATION TIME: 30 minutes
SERVINGS: 5
Nutrition: 194 Calories; 14.2g Fat; 7.2g Carbs; 9.3g Protein; 2.7g Fiber
Ingredients
1/2 cup heavy cream
1 pound broccoli florets
1 cup yellow onion, sliced
1 cup Colby cheese, shredded
2 cloves garlic, smashed
Directions
Start by preheating your oven to 380 degrees F. Brush the sides and bottom of a casserole dish with a nonstick cooking oil.

Parboil broccoli florets for about 3 minutes until just tender. Place the broccoli in the prepared casserole dish.

Stir in yellow onion and garlic. Now, whisk the heavy cream with the 1 cup of vegetable broth. Season with salt and black pepper to taste.

Pour the cream/broth mixture over the vegetables and bake at 390 degrees F for about 20 minutes.

Top with Colby cheese and continue to bake for 5 to 6 minutes more or until the top is hot and bubbly. Bon appétit!

291) **Peppery Red Cabbage Soup**

PREPARATION TIME: 30 minutes
SERVINGS: 6
Nutrition: 82 Calories; 4.1g Fat; 6g Carbs; 2.1g Protein; 2.6g Fiber
Ingredients
1 cup broccoli florets
1 pound red cabbage, shredded
1 cup tomato puree
2 tablespoons canola oil
2 bell peppers, chopped
Directions
Ina stockpot, heat the canola oil over medium-high heat. Sauté the bell peppers and broccoli for 4 to 5 minutes or until they are just tender and fragrant.
Stir in red cabbage and tomato puree along with 5 cups of water (or vegetable broth. Reduce heat to simmer.
Partially cover and let it simmer for 25 to 30 minutes. Enjoy!

292) **Mediterranean-Style Zucchini Salad**

PREPARATION TIME: 15 minutes
SERVINGS: 5
Nutrition: 186 Calories; 13.5g Fat; 6.6g Carbs; 11.2g Protein; 2.2g Fiber
Ingredients
1 ½ pounds zucchini, sliced
2 tomatoes, sliced
4 ounces goat cheese, crumbled
4 tablespoons extra-virgin olive oil, divided
1 red onion, sliced
Directions
Begin by preheating your oven to 420 degrees F.
Toss zucchini slices with 2 tablespoons of olive oil; season with Mediterranean spice mix. Place them on a baking sheet.
Roast in the preheated for about 11 minutes.
Gently stir roasted zucchini with red onion and tomatoes.

Drizzle remaining 2 tablespoons of olive oil along with 2 tablespoons of vinegar. Top with goat cheese and serve immediately!

293) **Mediterranean-Style Cauliflower Au Gratin**

PREPARATION TIME: 1 hour
Servings 2
Nutrition: 342 Calories; 23.3g Fat; 8g Carbs; 21.3g Protein; 2.7g Fiber
Ingredients
5 ounces sour cream
2 eggs, whisked
3 ounces Provolone cheese, freshly grated
1/2 pound small cauliflower florets
2 scallions, chopped
Directions
Start by prehating your oven to 365 degrees F.
In a saucepan, barboil the cauliflower florets over medium-low heat until just tender. Place the cauliflower florets in a lightly oiled baking dish.
Thoroughly combine the scallions, eggs, sour cream, salt, and black pepper. Pour the cream/egg mixture over the cauliflower florets.
Top with grated Provolone cheese and cover with a piece of foil.
Bake for 40 to 45 minutes or until everything is thoroughly cooked. Bon appétit!

294) **Cauliflower Tabbouleh Salad**

PREPARATION TIME: 15 minutes
SERVINGS: 2
Nutrition: 180 Calories; 16.1g Fat; 7g Carbs; 2.7g Protein; 2.7g Fiber
Ingredients
1/2 cup cherry tomatoes, halved
1 Lebanese cucumber, diced
2 tablespoons extra-virgin olive oil
1 cup cauliflower florets
1/2 white onion, thinly sliced
Directions

Process the cauliflower in your food processor until it has broken into rice-sized chunks. Cook cauli rice in a lightly-oiled frying pan over a moderate flame for about 9 minutes. Toss cauliflower rice with onion, tomatoes, cucumber, and olive oil. Enjoy!

295) Classic Mushroom Stew

PREPARATION TIME: 20 minutes
SERVINGS: 4
Nutrition: 108 Calories; 7.5g Fat; 7g Carbs; 3.14g Protein; 2.5g Fiber
Ingredients
1 pound brown mushrooms, chopped
1/2 cup leeks, chopped
2 ripe tomatoes, pureed
1 teaspoon garlic, minced
1 medium-sized zucchini, diced
Directions
Heat a lightly-oiled soup pot over medium-high heat. Sauté the leeks and mushrooms until they are softened and mushrooms release liquid.
Now, stir in the garlic and zucchini, and continue to sauté for 2 to 3 minutes more or until they've softened.
Add in tomatoes along with 2 cups of water. Season with Sazón spice, if desired.
Cover part-way and continue to simmer for about 10 minutes. Enjoy!

296) Mediterranean Cauliflower Chowder

PREPARATION TIME: 30 minutes
SERVINGS: 4
Nutrition: 172 Calories; 14.7g Fat; 7g Carbs; 3.1g Protein; 2.9g Fiber
Ingredients
1 pound cauliflower florets
1 white onion, chopped
1 cup half and half
1 tablespoon butter, softened at room temperature
1/2 stalk celery, chopped
Directions

In a heavy-bottomed pot, melt the butter over medium-high flame. Sauté the celery and onion until they've softened.
Stir in the cauliflower; season with sea salt, black pepper, and Mediterranean spice mix, if desired; continue to sauté for a further 2 minutes.
Pour in 4 cups of water (or vegetable broth, bringing to a boil. Turn the heat to medium-low and continue to simmer for 20 to 25 minutes
Puree the chowder in your food processor and stir in the half and half. Continue to cook for 5 minutes more or until your chowder is thoroughly cooked. Enjoy!

297) Neufchatel Cheese Balls with Nuts

PREPARATION TIME: 10 minutes
SERVINGS: 6
Nutrition: 183 Calories; 15.9g Fat; 2.9g Carbs; 8.4g Protein; 0.9g Fiber
Ingredients
4 ounces Neufchatel cheese
4 ounces blue cheese
2 tablespoons fresh parsley, chopped
2 tablespoons fresh cilantro, chopped
8 tablespoons walnuts, finely chopped
Directions
In a mixing bowl, combine the cheese, parsley, and cilantro; season with the salt and black pepper to your liking.
Shape the mixture into 8 balls; roll them over the chopped walnuts until well coated. Serve well-chilled.

298) Mushroom Stroganoff with Sour Cream

PREPARATION TIME: 25 minutes
SERVINGS: 5
Nutrition: 166 Calories; 13g Fat; 7g Carbs; 6g Protein; 1.6g Fiber
Ingredients
2 tablespoons olive oil
1/2 cup onion, minced
1 ½ pounds button mushrooms, sliced

2 tablespoons marinara sauce
1 cup sour cream
Directions
Heat the olive oil in a large stockpot over the highest setting. Then, sauté the onion for 3 to 4 minutes until just tender and translucent.

Now, melt 1 tablespoon of butter in the same pot and cook the mushrooms for about 4 minutes until they release liquid. Add in marinara sauce and 4 cups of water (or vegetable stock.

Reduce the heat to simmer; cover part-way and continue to cook for a further 15 to 20 minutes.

Serve with sour cream and enjoy!

299) **Keto Seed and Nut Granola**

PREPARATION TIME: 30 minutes
SERVINGS: 10
Nutrition: 162 Calories; 15.5g Fat; 4.6g Carbs; 3.2g Protein; 2.9g Fiber
Ingredients
1/3 cup sunflower seeds
1/3 cup flaxseed meal
1 cup coconut, shredded, unsweetened
1 cup pecans, chopped
1/2 stick butter
Directions
Start by preheating your oven to 300 degrees F.

In a mixing bowl, combine all ingredients until everything is well incorporated. Pour in 1/4 cup water and stir again. Add in vanilla and cinnamon, if desired.

Spread the mixture in a thin layer on a parchment-lined cookie sheet. Bake in the preheated oven for 25 to 28 minutes.

Transfer to wire racks to cool completely. Devour!

300) **Chinese Stir-Fry**

PREPARATION TIME: 15 minutes
SERVINGS: 5
Nutrition: 108 Calories; 8.5g Fat; 7.5g Carbs; 2.2g Protein; 2.3g Fiber
Ingredients
1 ½ pounds Chinese cabbage, shredded
2 garlic cloves, minced
1 tablespoon Shaoxing wine
3 tablespoons sesame oil
1 shallot, sliced
Directions
In a wok, warm the sesame oil until sizzling. Once hot, cook the shallot and garlic for 2 to 3 minutes until they've softened. Add in Shaoxing wine to deglaze the pan.

Stir in Chinese cabbage and stir-fry for 5 to 6 minutes more. Season with salt and Sichuan peppercorns, if desired.

Serve in individual bowls and enjoy!

301) **Breakfast Green Salad with Eggs**

PREPARATION TIME: 15 minutes
SERVINGS: 3
Nutrition: 156 Calories; 10g Fat; 7g Carbs; 10.4g Protein; 2.6g Fiber
Ingredients
1 roasted pepper in oil, drained and chopped
1 tomato, diced
2 tablespoons extra-virgin olive oil
4 eggs
1/2 pound spinach
Directions
Place eggs in a saucepan and cover them with water by 1 inch. Let it boil for about 7 minutes over medium-high heat.

Toss the spinach, red pepper, tomato, and olive oil in a salad bowl. Drizzle 2 tablespoons of vinegar and olive oil over your vegetables.

Garnish with sliced eggs and enjoy!

302) Italian Insalata Caprese

PREPARATION TIME: 10 minutes
SERVINGS: 4
Nutrition: 245 Calories; 22.7g Fat; 3.9g Carbs; 6.3g Protein; 1.7g Fiber
Ingredients
1/2 cup mayonnaise
1/2 cup mozzarella cheese
8 ounces arugula
1 tomato, sliced
1/2 cup olives, pitted and halved
Directions
Toss the arugula, tomato, and olives in a salad bowl. Add in mayonnaise and toss again to combine well.
Top with mozzarella. Taste and adjust seasonings.
Serve garnished with fresh basil and enjoy!

303) Vegetable Stir Fry with Cheese

PREPARATION TIME: 20 minutes
SERVINGS: 3
Nutrition: 338 Calories; 28.4g Fat; 9.2g Carbs; 13g Protein; 2.2g Fiber
Ingredients
3 eggs
3 ounces Asiago cheese, shredded
2 cups white mushrooms, sliced
1 cup cauliflower rice
2 tomatoes, pureed
Directions
In a wok, heat 1 tablespoon of the sesame oil over medium-high flame. Sauté the mushrooms for 3 to 4 minutes until they release liquid; reserve.
Heat another 2 tablespoons of sesame oil. Now, cook the cauliflower rice for about 4 minutes or until tender. Return the reserved mushrooms to the wok.
Add in tomatoes and continue to cook for 2 to 3 minutes longer; season with Five-spice powder, if desired.
Heat 1 tablespoon of sesame oil; now, cook the eggs over a moderate flame for 4 to 5 minutes to desired doneness.

Top the vegetables with the fried eggs, garnish with cheese, and serve warm. Enjoy!

304) Greek-Style Zucchini Lasagna

PREPARATION TIME: 1 hour 20 minutes
SERVINGS: 2
Nutrition: 338 Calories; 23.3g Fat; 7.9g Carbs; 17.7g Protein; 3g Fiber
Ingredients
1/2 pound chestnut mushrooms, chopped
1/2 cup Greek-style yogurt
1/2 cup Provolone cheese, grated
1 large-sized zucchini, sliced lengthwise
1 cup tomato sauce with onion and garlic, no sugar added
Directions
Place the zucchini slices and 1 teaspoon of salt in a bowl with a colander; let it sit for 15 minutes and gently squeeze to discard the excess water.
Grill your zucchini for about 5 minutes and reserve.
Heat 1 tablespoon of olive oil in a frying pan over medium-high flame. Sauté the mushrooms until they are tender and fragrant. Add in the Greek spice mix if desired.
Stir in tomato sauce and continue to cook for 5 to 6 minutes longer.
Spread the mushroom sauce on the bottom of a lightly oiled casserole dish. Place the zucchini slices on top.
Mix Greek yogurt and Provolone cheese. Top your casserole with the cheese mixture.
Bake in the preheated oven at 380 degrees F for 42 to 45 minutes until the edges are hot and bubbly.

305) Braised Cabbage with Brown Mushrooms

PREPARATION TIME: 15 minutes
SERVINGS: 3
Nutrition: 133 Calories; 9.4g Fat; 7.5g Carbs; 3.9g Protein; 4.3g Fiber
Ingredients

2 tablespoons canola oil
2 cups brown mushrooms, sliced
3/4 pound green cabbage, shredded
1/2 cup cream of mushroom soup
1/2 cup onion, chopped
Directions
In a soup pot, heat canola oil over a moderate heat. Sauté the onion for about 4 minutes until translucent.

Fold in the mushrooms and continue sautéing for 3 to 4 minutes, stirring continuously to ensure even cooking.

Add in the cabbage and soup. Continue to simmer for about 9 minutes until cooked through. Bon appétit!

306) <u>**Festive Keto Coleslaw**</u>

PREPARATION TIME: 15 minutes
SERVINGS: 5
Nutrition: 121 Calories; 8.5g Fat; 6.8g Carbs; 3.3g Protein; 2.3g Fiber
Ingredients
4 tablespoons shallots, chopped
1 teaspoon garlic, minced
1 cup fresh cauliflower, chopped
1 cup green cabbage, shredded
1/3 cup mayonnaise
Directions
Place the shallots, garlic, cauliflower, and cabbage in a salad bowl.

Toss the vegetables with mayonnaise; you can add salt, pepper, and fresh lemon juice to taste.

Serve well chilled and enjoy!

307) <u>**Easy Family Ratatouille**</u>

PREPARATION TIME: 1 hour 10 minutes
SERVINGS: 6
Nutrition: 104 Calories; 7.2g Fat; 6.7g Carbs; 1.6g Protein; 2.7g Fiber
Ingredients
2 yellow onions, sliced
1 cup tomato sauce with onion and garlic, no sugar added
3 bell peppers, sliced

1 medium-sized Japanese eggplant, cut into rounds
2 medium-sized zucchinis, cut into rounds
Directions
Preheat your oven to 380 degrees F. Toss the vegetables with 3 tablespoons of extra-virgin olive oil.

Arrange the vegetables in the casserole dish. Add in tomato sauce along with Herbes de Provence, if used.

Cover with foil and bake for 30 to 35 minutes. Remove the foil and continue to bake an additional 25 minutes or until heated through.

Allow Ratatouille to rest for a couple of minutes before serving. Enjoy!

308) <u>**Middle Eastern Eggplant with Tahini**</u>

PREPARATION TIME: 30 minutes
SERVINGS: 7
Nutrition: 94 Calories; 6g Fat; 6.7g Carbs; 2.5g Protein; 4.1g Fiber
Ingredients
1 avocado, pitted, peeled and mashed
2 tablespoons tahini
1 teaspoon garlic paste
2 pounds eggplant, sliced
3 teaspoons avocado oil
Directions
Start by preheating your oven to 410 degrees F.

Brush the bottom of a baking sheet pan with nonstick cooking oil. Place the eggplant slices on the prepared pan; drizzle 2 teaspoons of avocado oil over eggplant slices.

Roast in the preheated oven approximately 20 minutes.

In the meantime, mix tahini with garlic paste; add in brown mustard, if desired.

Divide the tahini mixture between the eggplant slices and place under the preheated broiler for 4 to 5 minutes. Top with the mashed avocado and enjoy!

309) Skinny Avocado Smoothie Bowl

PREPARATION TIME: 5 minutes
SERVINGS: 2
Nutrition: 286 Calories; 28g Fat; 7.4g Carbs; 4.7g Protein; 2.4g Fiber
Ingredients
1/2 ripe avocado, peeled and pitted
2 teaspoons sunflower seeds
2 tablespoons sesame seeds
1 teaspoon ground cinnamon
1/2 cup canned coconut milk
Directions
Place all ingredients in a bowl of your food processor; add in 1/2 cup of water and process until creamy and smooth.
Divide your smoothie between two serving bowls and enjoy!

310) Swiss Cauliflower and Cheese Dip

PREPARATION TIME: 10 minutes
SERVINGS: 8
Nutrition: 129 Calories; 10.4g Fat; 3.4g Carbs; 5.7g Protein; 0.7g Fiber
Ingredients
5 ounces Swiss cheese, grated
1/2 teaspoon dried oregano
1/2 teaspoon dried basil
1 cup double cream
1/2 pound cauliflower
Directions
Parboil the cauliflower until crisp-tender; mash with a potato masher and season with the salt and black pepper to your liking.
Add in oregano and basil and stir to combine.
In a sauté pan, melt the cream and cheese over low heat. Stir in the mashed cauliflower and let it simmer for 5 minutes or until everything is heated through.
Bon appétit!

311) Classic Vegetable Chowder

PREPARATION TIME: 40 minutes
SERVINGS: 5
Nutrition: 131 Calories; 12.8g Fat; 2.5g Carbs; 2.2g Protein; 0.6g Fiber
Ingredients
1/4 cup dry white wine
1 cup heavy cream
1 cup celery, chopped
5 cups vegetable broth
1/2 cup shallots, chopped
Directions
Warm 1 tablespoon of olive oil in a soup pot until sizzling. Cook the shallots and celery until they've softened.
Stir in vegetable broth and wine and bring to a rolling boil. Turn the heat to simmer and continue to cook, partially covered, for 25 to 30 minutes.
Fold in the cream and continue to simmer for about 7 minutes. Enjoy!

312) Zucchini Noodles with Cheese (Zoodles

PREPARATION TIME: 20 minutes
SERVINGS: 3
Nutrition: 241 Calories; 17.4g Fat; 6.2g Carbs; 13g Protein; 2.6g Fiber
Ingredients
2 green onions, chopped
2 vine-ripe tomatoes, pureed
3/4 pound zucchini, spiralized
1 cup Asiago cheese, shredded
2 green garlic stalks, chopped
Directions
Melt 1 tablespoon of butter in a saucepan over medium-high flame. Sauté green onions and garlic until they've softened.
Stir in pureed tomatoes, bringing the sauce to just below boiling point. Season with the salt and black pepper to your taste.
Continue to cook over low heat for about 15 minutes. Afterwards, fold in zucchini noodles and continue to cook for 3 to 4 minutes longer.

Garnish with Asiago cheese and serve warm.

313) Cream of Green Vegetable Soup

PREPARATION TIME: 25 minutes
SERVINGS: 4
Nutrition: 111 Calories; 10.4g Fat; 4.4g Carbs; 1.9g Protein; 1.5g Fiber
Ingredients
1 green bell pepper, chopped
1 medium zucchini, cut into chunks
4 cups vegetable broth
3 tablespoons olive oil
2 cups broccoli florets
Directions
Warm the olive oil in a stockpot over a moderate heat. Sauté the broccoli, pepper, and zucchini until tender and aromatic.
Pour in vegetable broth and cook until it comes to a boil. Turn the heat to medium-low.
Continue to simmer, partially covered, for 20 to 23 minutes. Puree your soup with an immersion blender and serve in individual bowls.

314) One-Skillet Keto Vegetables

PREPARATION TIME: 15 minutes
SERVINGS: 3
Nutrition: 118 Calories; 9.5g Fat; 6.1g Carbs; 1.9g Protein; 1.4g Fiber
Ingredients
2 bell pepper, deseeded and sliced
1 cup tomato sauce with herb and garlic, no sugar added
2 tablespoons sesame oil
1 yellow onion, sliced
1/2 cup cream of mushroom soup
Directions
Heat the sesame oil in a nonstick skillet over medium-high flame. Sweat yellow onion and peppers for about 4 minutes or until they are just tender.

Stir in tomato sauce and mushrooms soup; continue to simmer, partially covered, for 7 to 8 minutes.
Salt to taste and serve. Bon appétit!

315) Creamed Tahini and Broccoli Soup

PREPARATION TIME: 15 minutes
SERVINGS: 2
Nutrition: 220 Calories; 19g Fat; 8.4g Carbs; 4.4g Protein; 2.7g Fiber
Ingredients
2 tablespoons tahini butter
1/2 small-sized leek, chopped
1 cup spinach leaves
1/3 cup yogurt
1 2/3 cups broccoli florets
Directions
Melt 1 tablespoon of butter in a soup pot over a moderate heat. Sauté the leeks until tender and aromatic or about 4 minutes.
Add in the broccoli along with 2 cups of vegetable broth. When your mixture reaches boiling, reduce the temperature to a simmer. Continue to cook, covered, for about 7 minutes.
Fold in the spinach; season with the salt and black pepper to taste; let it simmer for 2 to 3 minutes or until spinach leaves have wilted completely.
Puree your soup along with tahini butter. Serve with yogurt and enjoy!

316) Cheese Stuffed Peppers

PREPARATION TIME: 35 minutes
SERVINGS: 2
Nutrition: 387 Calories; 30.3g Fat; 5.3g Carbs; 22.7g Protein; 0.9g Fiber
Ingredients
3 bell peppers, deseeded and sliced in half
3 eggs
2 scallions, chopped
6 ounces cream cheese
4 Kalamata olives, pitted and sliced
Directions

Begin by preheating your oven to 380 degrees F. Brush a baking pan with a nonstick cooking oil.

Thoroughly combine the, scallions, cream cheese, and eggs; season with Greek spice mix, if desired.

Stuff the peppers with the cheese filling.

Bake in the preheated oven for 27 to 30 minutes until cooked through. Garnish with olives and serve warm.

317) <u>Summer Vegetable Stew</u>

PREPARATION TIME: 30 minutes
SERVINGS: 4
Nutrition: 67 Calories; 3.8g Fat; 6g Carbs; 2.1g Protein; 1.7g Fiber
Ingredients
4 tablespoons sour cream, well-chilled
1 summer zucchini, chopped
2 vine-ripe tomatoes
2 bell peppers, deseeded and chopped
1 small-sized shallot, chopped
Directions
Heat 2 teaspoons of sesame oil in a heavy-bottomed pot over medium-high flame. Sauté the bell peppers and shallot until they are just starting to lightly brown.

Stir in the zucchini, broth, tomatoes, and stir to combine. Bring to a rolling boil. Immediately reduce the heat to medium-low and let it simmer for 25 minutes until everything is thoroughly cooked.

Ladle into individual bowls and garnish with sour cream and fresh chives. Enjoy!

318) <u>Cremini Mushroom Medley</u>

PREPARATION TIME: 25 minutes
SERVINGS: 5
Nutrition: 156 Calories; 11.9g Fat; 6.2g Carbs; 4.9g Protein; 2g Fiber
Ingredients
1 pound cremini mushrooms, sliced
2 garlic cloves
2 cup tomato sauce with herbs, no sugar added

1 red onion, chopped
2 sweet Italian peppers, chopped
Directions
Heat 2 tablespoons of canola oil in a large stockpot over a moderate flame. Once hot, cook the onion and peppers until fragrant.

Add in the mushrooms and garlic and continue to sauté for 2 to 3 minutes or until just tender and fragrant.

Add in tomato sauce long with 2 cups of water (or cream of mushroom soup; reduce heat to medium-low and partially cover.

Continue to cook for 20 to 22 minutes or until thoroughly warmed. Ladle into soup bowls and serve. Bon appétit!

319) <u>Italian Zoodles with Parmesan Cheese</u>

PREPARATION TIME: 10 minutes
SERVINGS: 2
Nutrition: 164 Calories; 13.3g Fat; 8.7g Carbs; 5.5g Protein; 4.9g Fiber
Ingredients
1 medium-sized zucchini, sliced
1 ripe tomato, quartered
1/2 avocado, pitted and peeled
2 tablespoons sunflower seeds, hulled
2 tablespoons parmesan cheese, preferably freshly grated
Directions
Puree the avocado, sunflower seeds, and tomato until well combined. Add in 2 tablespoons of water if needed.

Season with salt and black pepper to taste. You can add Italian slice mix, if desired.

Spiralize your zucchini and divide zucchini noodles (zoodles among two serving plates. Top your zoodles with avocado sauce.

Garnish with parmesan cheese and serve right away!

320) <u>Creamed Broccoli Slaw</u>

PREPARATION TIME: 10 minutes
SERVINGS: 2
Nutrition: 323 Calories; 25.3g Fat; 6.8g Carbs; 15.7g Protein; 3.4g Fiber

Ingredients
2 ounces mozzarella cheese
1/4 cup tahini dressing
1 cup broccoli florets
1 bell pepper, seeded and sliced
1 shallot, thinly sliced
Directions
Toss all ingredients, except for mozzarella cheese, in a salad bowl.
Top with the mozzarella cheese and serve well chilled. Enjoy!

321) Tom Kha Kai

PREPARATION TIME: 20 minutes
SERVINGS: 2
Nutrition: 273 Calories; 27.3g Fat; 5.7g Carbs; 5.2g Protein; 0.5g Fiber
Ingredients
1 cup vegetable broth
1 shallot, chopped
1/2 celery stalk, chopped
1/2 bell pepper, chopped
1 cup coconut milk, full-fat
Directions
Heat 1 teaspoon of coconut oil in a small pot; now, sauté the shallot, celery, and pepper until they've softened.
Pour in a splash of broth to scrape up the browned bits that stick to the bottom of the pot.
Pour in the remaining broth along with salt and pepper to taste and bring to a boil.
Turn the heat to simmer; continue to cook for 15 to 17 minutes or until thoroughly cooked. Pour in the coconut milk and stir for 2 minutes.
Garnish with fresh Thai basil, if desired. Enjoy!

322) Asparagus with Tangy Mayo Sauce

PREPARATION TIME: 15 minutes
SERVINGS: 5
Nutrition: 296 Calories; 28.4g Fat; 7g Carbs; 3.9g Protein; 3.3g Fiber
Ingredients
4 tablespoons sour cream
4 tablespoons shallots, minced
1/2 cup mayonnaise
1 ½ pounds asparagus, trimmed
4 tablespoons olive oil
Directions
Preheat your oven to 385 degrees F.
Drizzle the asparagus spears with olive oil. Season with sea salt and black pepper to taste. Roast in the preheated oven for about 10 minutes.
Whisk the shallots, mayonnaise, and sour cream until well combined. Serve the asparagus with the mayo sauce.

323) Cocoa Smoothie with Mint

PREPARATION TIME: 5 minutes
SERVINGS: 2
Nutrition: 140 Calories; 9g Fat; 6.6g Carbs; 3.7g Protein; 2.8g Fiber
Ingredients
1/4 teaspoon grated nutmeg
2 teaspoons granulated erythritol
1 cup milk
1/3 ripe avocado, peeled and pitted
3 teaspoons cacao powder, unsweetened
Directions
Place all ingredients in a bowl of your food processor; pour in 1/2 cup of water.
Blend until creamy and smooth.
Spoon into chilled glasses and serve right away!

Soups and stews

324) Carrot Soup

SERVINGS: 8
PREPARATION TIME: 15 minutes
COOKING TIME: 1 hour 40 minutes
INGREDIENTS:
2-pounds carrots, peeled and cut into slices
7 tablespoons extra-virgin essential olive oil, divided
2 large fennel bulbs, sliced
Salt, to taste
¼ cup pumpkin seeds
1 medium yellow onion, chopped
6 garlic cloves, minced
1 tablespoon fresh ginger, grated
1 tablespoon ground turmeric
½ teaspoon red pepper cayenne
2 tablespoons fresh lime juice
1½ cups coconut milk
4-6 cups water
¼ cup scallion (green part, minced
DIRECTIONS:
Preheat the oven to 375 degrees F.
In a baking sheet, place the carrot and drizzle with 2 tablespoons of oil.
Roast approximately one hour.
Remove the carrots from oven and make aside.
Now, raise the temperature of oven to 400 degrees F.
In a skillet, heat 3 tablespoons of oil on medium heat.
Add fennel bulbs and pinch of salt and sauté for about 4-5 minutes.
Transfer the fennel bulb onto a baking sheet and roast approximately 20-a half-hour.
Meanwhile, heat a nonstick skillet on medium heat. Keep aside.
Add pumpkin seeds and stir fry for around 3-4 minutes or till toasted. Keep aside.
Meanwhile in a very soup pan, heat remaining oil on medium heat.
Add onion and sauté for around 12 minutes.
Add garlic and sauté for approximately 1 minute.

In a blender, add onion mixture, carrots, ginger, spices, lime juice and coconut milk and pulse till well combined.
Add required amount of water and pulse till smooth.
Return the soup in the pan on medium heat.
Bring to some boil and cook approximately 3-5 minutes.
Serve hot with all the topping of fennel and pumpkin seeds.
Nutrition:
Calories: 230, Fat: 16g, Carbohydrates: 20g, Fiber: 6g, Protein: 5g

325) Carrot & Ginger Soup

SERVINGS: 4
PREPARATION TIME: 15 minutes
COOKING TIME: 30 minutes
INGREDIENTS:
1 tablespoon coconut oil
1 medium brown onion chopped
2 minced garlic cloves
1 long red chili, chopped
1 (1/3-inch fresh turmeric piece, peeled and sliced
1 (¾-inch fresh galangal piece, peeled and sliced
1 (¾-inch fresh ginger piece, peeled and sliced
4 cups carrots, peeled and chopped
2 lemongrass stalks
2 cups water
2 cups vegetable broth
Coconut cream, as required
DIRECTIONS:
In a substantial soup pan, heat oil on medium heat.
Add onion and sauté for about 5 minutes.
Add garlic, red chili, turmeric and sauté for approximately 5 minutes.
Add carrots, lemongrass stalks, water and broth and produce to some boil.
Reduce the warmth to low and simmer for about 15-20 minutes.
Remove from heat and aside to chill slightly.
Discard the lemongrass stalks.
In a blender, add soup in batches and pulse till smooth.

Serve immediately with the topping of coconut cream.
Nutrition:
Calories: 299, Fat: 7g, Carbohydrates: 25g, Fiber: 12g, Protein: 18g

326) **Curried Carrot & Sweet Potato Soup**

SERVINGS: 5
PREPARATION TIME: 15 minutes
COOKING TIME: 37 minutes
INGREDIENTS:
2 teaspoons olive oil
½ cup shallots, chopped
1½ cups carrots, peeled and sliced into ¼-inch size
3 cups sweet potato, peeled and cubed into ½-inch size
1 tablespoon fresh ginger, grated
2 teaspoons curry powder
3 cups Fat-free chicken broth
Salt, to taste
DIRECTIONS:
In a sizable soup pan, heat oil on medium heat.
Add shallots and sauté for approximately 3 minutes.
Add carrot, sweet potato, ginger and curry powder and sauté for around 3-4 minutes.
Add broth and bring to a boil.
Reduce heat to low.
Cover and simmer approximately 25-thirty minutes.
Stir in salt and black pepper and remove from heat.
Keep aside to cool down the slightly.
In a blender, add soup in batches and pulse till smooth.
Serve immediately.
Nutrition:
Calories: 131, Fat: 2.1g, Carbohydrates: 23.1g, Fiber: 3.9g, Protein: 5.7g

327) **Creamy Broccoli Soup**

SERVINGS: 3-4
PREPARATION TIME: 15 minutes

COOKING TIME: 35 minutes
INGREDIENTS:
1 tablespoon virgin coconut oil
1 celery stalk, chopped
½ cup white onion, chopped
Salt, to taste
1 teaspoon ground turmeric
2 minced garlic cloves
1 large head broccoli, cut into florets
¼ teaspoon fresh ginger, grated
1 bay leaf
1/8 teaspoon cayenne pepper
Freshly ground black pepper, to taste
5 cups vegetable broth
1 small avocado, peeled, pitted and chopped
1 tablespoon fresh lemon juice
DIRECTIONS:
In a substantial soup pan, heat oil on medium heat.
Add celery, onion and several salt and sauté for around 3-4 minutes.
Add turmeric and garlic and sauté for approximately 1 minute.
Add desired mount of salt and remaining ingredients except avocado and lemon juice and provide with a boil
Reduce heat to medium-low.
Cover and simmer for about 25-thirty minutes.
Remove from heat and keep aside to cool down the slightly.
In a blender, add soup and avocado in batches and pulse till smooth.
Serve immediately with the drizzling of freshly squeezed lemon juice.
Nutrition:
Calories: 275, Fat: 3g, Carbohydrates: 20g, Fiber: 13g, Protein: 28g

328) **Pumpkin Soup**

SERVINGS: 2
PREPARATION TIME: 15 minutes
COOKING TIME: 18 minutes
INGREDIENTS:
2 teaspoons coconut oil
1 brown onion, chopped
1 (¾-inch fresh turmeric piece
1 (¾-inch fresh galangal piece

1 long red chili, seeded and chopped
2 tablespoons fresh cilantro, chopped
4 kefir lime leaves
3 cups pumpkin, peeled and cubed
1 teaspoon fresh lime peel piece
1 large garlic oil, chopped
4 cups vegetable broth
2 tablespoons fish sauce
½ cup coconut cream
2 tablespoons fresh lime juice

DIRECTIONS:
In a substantial soup pan, heat oil on medium heat.
Add onion, turmeric, galangal, red chili, cilantro and lime leaves and sauté for approximately 2-3 minutes.
Add pumpkin, lime peel, garlic, broth and fish sauce and convey to your boil
Reduce the heat to low.
Cover and simmer approximately 15 minutes.
Remove from heat whilst aside to chill slightly.
Discard the turmeric, galangal and lemon peel.
In a blender, add soup mixture with coconut cream and lemon juice in batches and pulse till smooth.

Nutrition:
Calories: 322, Fat: 3g, Carbohydrates: 28g, Fiber: 14g, Protein: 15g

329) **Butternut Squash Soup**

SERVINGS: 6
PREPARATION TIME: 15 minutes
COOKING TIME: 33 minutes a few seconds
INGREDIENTS:
3 tablespoons extra virgin olive oil
1 large onion, chopped finely
1 cup raw cashews
1 garlic herb, minced
2 tablespoons fresh ginger, minced
1 (2-pound butternut squash, peeled and cubed into ½-inch size
2 teaspoons ground coriander
2 tsps. ground cumin
1 teaspoon ground turmeric

1 teaspoon curry powder
Freshly ground black pepper and salt, to taste
5 cups vegetable broth
1 cup coconut milk

DIRECTIONS:
In a large soup pan, heat oil on medium heat.
Add onion and sauté for approximately 5 minutes.
Add cashews and sauté for around 3 minutes.
Add garlic and ginger and sauté approximately 30 seconds.
Add remaining ingredients except coconut milk and bring to some boil
Reduce the temperature to low.
Cover and simmer for around 20-25 minutes.
Remove from heat and make aside to cool down the slightly.
In a blender, add soup mixture with coconut milk in batches and pulse till smooth.
Serve immediately.

Nutrition:
Calories: 323, Fat: 18g, Carbohydrates: 39g, Fiber: 6g, Protein: 7g

330) **Butternut Squash Soup**

SERVINGS: 4
PREPARATION TIME: 15 minutes
COOKING TIME: 20 minutes
INGREDIENTS:
1 small butternut squash, peeled, seeded and cubed
2 tablespoons coconut oil, melted
Salt, to taste
4 cups reduced-sodium vegetable broth, divided
14-ounces coconut milk
1 small shallot, sliced thinly
2 lemongrass stalks, cut into 6-inch pieces
3 tablespoons fresh ginger, grated
½ of Serrano pepper, chopped
1 cup fresh mushrooms, sliced
Freshly ground black pepper, to taste
2 tablespoons fresh lime juice
Chopped fresh cilantro, for garnishing
DIRECTIONS:

Preheat the oven to 400 degrees F.

Place the butternut squash in a baking sheet.

Drizzle with oil and sprinkle with salt and roast approximately 12-15 minutes.

Remove from oven whilst aside to chill completely.

In a big soup pan, add 3 cups from the broth, coconut milk, shallot, lemongrass, ginger and Serrano pepper and bring to a boil.

Reduce the warmth to simmer.

In a blender, add roasted butternut squash and remaining broth and pulse till smooth.

Add squash puree and mushrooms in simmering broth and stir to combine.

Simmer for about 5 minutes.

Stir in salt, black pepper and lime juice and take away from heat.

Serve hot with all the garnishing of cilantro.

Nutrition:

Calories: 165, Fat: 7.5g, Carbohydrates: 19g, Fiber: 2.5g, Protein: 4.3g

331) Cauliflower Soup

SERVINGS: 2
PREPARATION TIME: 15 minutes
COOKING TIME: 46 minutes
INGREDIENTS:
2 teaspoons essential olive oil
½ cup onion, chopped
1 large head cauliflower, cut into small florets
1 (1-inch piece fresh ginger, chopped
Salt and freshly ground black pepper, to taste
3 cups chicken broth
DIRECTIONS:
In a big soup pan, heat oil on medium heat.

Add onion and sauté for approximately 1 minute.

Add cauliflower and cook, covered approximately 10 min, stirring occasionally.

Add remaining ingredients and provide with a boil

Reduce the warmth to low.

Cover and simmer for approximately 30 minutes.

Remove from heat and make aside for cooling slightly.

In a blender, add soup mixture in batches and pulse till smooth.

Return the soup inside the pan on low heat.

Simmer for approximately 4-5 minutes or till heated completely.

Serve immediately.

Nutrition:

Calories: 183, Fat: 6.2g, Carbohydrates: 28.4g, Fiber: 11.5g, Protein: 9.8g

332) Cauliflower & Zucchini Soup

SERVINGS: 4-6
PREPARATION TIME: 15 minutes
COOKING TIME: 45 minutes
INGREDIENTS:
2-3 cups cauliflower, chopped into large pieces
2 tablespoons coconut oil, divided
1 medium yellow onion, chopped
1 tablespoon garlic, minced
1 teaspoon fresh ginger, minced
1 teaspoon dried ginger
1½ teaspoons ground coriander
Salt and freshly ground black pepper, to taste
1½ pound zucchini, peeled and chopped
4 cups chicken broth
½ cup coconut milk
Chopped chives, for garnishing
DIRECTIONS:
Preheat the oven to 375 degrees F.

Place the cauliflower in a baking sheet and drizzle with 1 tablespoon of oil

Roast approximately half an hour, stirring once in the middle way.

Meanwhile in a large soup pan, heat remaining oil on medium heat.

Add onion and sauté approximately 5 minutes.

Add garlic, ginger, coriander, salt and black pepper and sauté for around 1 minute.

Add zucchini and cook for around 1 minute.

Add broth and produce to your boil.

Reduce the temperature to simmer.

Add the cauliflower and stir to combine.

Simmer approximately 15 minutes.

Remove in the heat and stir in coconut milk. With an immersion blender, puree the soup completely.

Serve hot with the topping of chives.

Nutrition:

Calories: 305, Fat: 3g, Carbohydrates: 15g, Fiber: 10g, Protein: 26g

333) <u>Cauliflower & Apple Soup</u>

SERVINGS: 5
PREPARATION TIME: 15 minutes
COOKING TIME: 42 minutes
INGREDIENTS:
½ cup pistachios
2 tablespoons extra-virgin olive oil
2 cups carrots, peeled and sliced
1 large onion, chopped
1 teaspoon fresh ginger, minced
1 tablespoon garlic, minced
3 cups cauliflower, cut into small florets
3 cups apples, cored and chopped roughly
1 teaspoon ground cumin
1 tablespoon ground cinnamon
¼ teaspoon paprika
1/8 teaspoon allspice
Salt and freshly ground black pepper, to taste
2 cups low-sodium vegetable broth
7 tablespoons water
Chopped fresh cilantro, for garnishing
DIRECTIONS:
Preheat the oven to 400 degrees F.
Place the pistachios in to a baking sheet and bake for about 5-7 minutes or till toasted.
Transfer the pistachios in a very pan of water on medium heat.
Bring to some gentle boil and simmer for about 35 minutes.
Meanwhile in a substantial soup pan, heat oil on medium heat.
Add carrot, onion, ginger and garlic and sauté for around 2 minutes.
Add cauliflower, apples and spices and cook, stirring occasionally for around 5 minutes.
Add broth and produce to your boil, then simmer, covered for about 20 minutes.

Remove from heat and keep aside for cooling slightly.

Drain the pistachios and transfer into a higher speed blender, then pulse till creamy and smooth.

Add the soup mixture in batches and pulse till smooth.

Serve immediately while using garnishing of cilantro.

Nutrition:

Calories: 272, Fat: 15g, Carbohydrates: 33.7g, Fiber: 8.4g, Protein: 6g

334) <u>Kabocha Squash Soup</u>

SERVINGS: 8
PREPARATION TIME: 15 minutes
COOKING TIME: 65 minutes
INGREDIENTS:
1 (4-5-pound kabocha squash, stemmed, peeled, seeded and chopped
Coconut oil, as required
1 large sweet onion, chopped
6-10 garlic cloves, chopped
6 cups chicken broth
1 (14-ounce can coconut milk
¼ teaspoon ground cumin
¼ teaspoon ground ginger
¼ teaspoon ground turmeric
Pinch of freshly ground white pepper
Salt and freshly ground black pepper, to taste
Pumpkin seeds, for garnishing
DIRECTIONS:
Preheat the oven to 350 degrees F.
Place the squash into a baking sheet and drizzle with a few melted oil
Roast for around 30-45 minutes or till tender.
Remove from oven and make aside.
In a substantial soup pan, heat some oil on medium heat.
Add onion and garlic and sauté for around 4-5 minutes.
Add squash and remaining ingredients and simmer approximately 10-15 minutes.
Remove from heat and by having an immersion blender, puree the soup completely.

Serve hot using the topping of pumpkin seeds.
Nutrition:
Calories: 337, Fat: 4g, Carbohydrates: 20g, Fiber: 6g, Protein: 19g

335) **Collard Greens Soup**

SERVINGS: 6
PREPARATION TIME: 15 minutes
COOKING TIME: 50 minutes
INGREDIENTS:
2 tablespoons olive oil
1 large onion, chopped
Salt, to taste
2 large leeks, sliced
2 tablespoons fresh ginger, minced
1 bunch collard greens, chopped
8 cups chicken broth
1 tablespoon fresh lemon juice
DIRECTIONS:
In a substantial soup pan, heat oil on low heat.
Add onion and salt and cook for approximately twenty minutes.
Stir in leeks and cook approximately 10 minutes.
Stir in ginger and greens and cook for approximately 5 minutes.
Add broth and provide to a boil on medium heat.
Cook approximately 10 min.
Remove from heat and make aside to chill slightly.
In a blender, add the soup mixture and pulse till smooth.
Return the soup in pan on medium heat.
Cook approximately 5 minutes.
Stir in freshly squeezed lemon juice and serve hot.
Nutrition:
Calories: 316, Fat: 2g, Carbohydrates: 16g, Fiber: 11g, Protein: 21g

336) **Mixed Veggie Soup**

SERVINGS: 4
PREPARATION TIME: 20 minutes
COOKING TIME: 31 minutes
INGREDIENTS:
1 tbsp extra virgin olive oil
½ of small onion, chopped
1 tablespoon fresh ginger herb, chopped finely
2-3 garlic cloves, minced
¼ teaspoon ground turmeric
2 celery stalks, chopped
½ head of cauliflower, chopped
2 small potatoes, peeled and chopped
2 large carrots, peeled and chopped
1 medium zucchini, chopped
Salt and freshly ground black pepper, to taste
2 tablespoons fresh lemon juice
¼-½ teaspoon cayenne
4 cups vegetable broth
DIRECTIONS:
In a substantial soup pan, heat oil on medium heat.
Add onion, ginger, garlic and turmeric and sauté for approximately 4-5 minutes.
Add vegetables, salt and black pepper and cook, stirring occasionally approximately 5-7 minutes.
Stir in fresh lemon juice.
Add red pepper cayenne and broth and produce to a boil.
Simmer, covered for about 10-15 minutes.
Remove from heat and with an immersion blender, puree the soup completely.
Return the soup in pan on medium-low heat and simmer for around 3-4 minutes or till heated completely.
Serve immediately.
Nutrition:
Calories: 274, Fat: 1g, Carbohydrates: 17g, Fiber: 13g, Protein: 19g

337) Citrus Acorn Squash Soup

SERVINGS: 3-4
PREPARATION TIME: 10 minutes
COOKING TIME: 1 hour 5 minutes
INGREDIENTS:
1 large acorn squash, halved and seeded
½ teaspoon essential olive oil
Salt and freshly ground black pepper, to taste
1 teaspoon fresh orange zest, grated finely
¾ teaspoon ground ginger
2 pinches of cayenne pepper
2 cups vegetable broth
¼ cup fresh orange juice
¼ cup coconut milk
1 tablespoon coconut aminos
Fresh pomegranate seeds, for garnishing
DIRECTIONS:
Preheat the oven to 400 degrees F. Line a baking sheet with foil paper.
Coat the squash halves with oil evenly and sprinkle with salt and black pepper.
Arrange the squash halves, cut side up within the prepared baking sheet.
Roast approximately one hour.
Remove from oven and allow it to go cool slightly.
Scoop the flesh from roasted squash and transfer right into a blender.
Add remaining all ingredients except pomegranate seeds and pulse till smooth.
Transfer the soup in a very pan on medium heat.
Cook approximately 3-5 minutes or till heated completely.
Serve hot while using garnishing of pomegranate seeds.
Nutrition:
Calories: 300, Fat: 0g, Carbohydrates: 21g, Fiber: 11g, Protein: 22g

338) Tangy Mushroom Soup

SERVINGS: 3-4
PREPARATION TIME: 15 minutes
COOKING TIME: 15-20 minutes

INGREDIENTS:
For Soup:
4 cups low-sodium vegetable broth
1 cup button mushrooms, sliced
1 cup cherry tomatoes, chopped
½ of white onion, sliced
3 slices lemongrass
3 fresh ginger pieces
5 fresh kaffir lime leaves
5 Thai chile peppers, seeded and mashed
¼ cup fresh lime juice
2 tablespoons tamari
For Garnishing:
1 cu bean sprouts
¼ cup scallion, chopped
½ cup fresh cilantro, chopped
DIRECTIONS:
In a sizable pan, add broth on medium-high heat.
Bring with a boil reducing the temperature to medium.
Add remaining soup ingredients and again bring to some gentle simmer.
Simmer approximately 15-20 min.
Remove from heat and discard lemongrass, ginger and lime leaves.
Serve hot while using ingredients of garnishing.
Nutrition:
Calories: 295, Fat: 4g, Carbohydrates: 21g, Fiber: 8g, Protein: 23g

339) Butternut Squash & Lentil Soup

SERVINGS: 6-8
PREPARATION TIME: 15 minutes
Cooking Time 1 hour 40 minutes
INGREDIENTS:
1 medium butternut squash, halved and seeded
2/3 cup celery, divided
¼ cup onion, chopped and divided
3 teaspoons garlic, minced and divided
2 teaspoons dried parsley, crushed and divided
2 teaspoons dried basil, crushed and divided
2 fresh thyme pieces, divided

Salt, to taste
2 tablespoons extra-virgin essential olive oil
½ cup carrot, peeled and chopped
1 medium tomato, chopped
1 teaspoon ground turmeric
1 bay leaf
1 teaspoon freshly squeezed lemon juice
1 vegetable bouillon cube
6 cups water, divided
½ cup split red lentil, soaked and drained
Freshly ground black pepper, to taste

DIRECTIONS:

Preheat the oven to 375 degrees F. Line a baking sheet with foil paper.

Arrange the squash halves within the prepared baking sheet, cut side up.

Place about ¼ cup from the celery, 2 tablespoons of onion, 1 teaspoon garlic, 1 teaspoon of every dried herbs, 1 thyme piece and salt.

Roast for around 50-60 minutes or till squash becomes tender.

Remove from heat whilst aside to cool completely.

Chop the three cups of flesh and aside.

Meanwhile in a soup pan, heat oil on medium-low heat.

Add carrot, remaining celery, onion and garlic and sauté for approximately 5-7 minutes.

Add tomato, turmeric, bay leaf, fresh lemon juice, bouillon cube, remaining herbs and 1 cup of water and simmer, covered for around 15 minutes.

In the center way, add 1 cup of more water.

Stir in lentils, squash and remaining water and provide to some boil.

Reduce heat to low.

Cover partially and simmer approximately 30-40 minutes.

Remove through the heat and by having an immersion blender, puree the soup completely.

Serve hot together with your desired topping.

Nutrition:

Calories: 317, Fat: 3g, Carbohydrates: 17g, Fiber: 9g, Protein: 22g

340) <u>**Tomatoes & Quinoa Soup**</u>

SERVINGS: 4
PREPARATION TIME: 15 minutes
COOKING TIME: 22 minutes
INGREDIENTS:

5 tablespoons extra-virgin coconut oil
1 brown onion, chopped
1 (3-inch piece fresh ginger, chopped
4 garlic cloves, chopped
2 teaspoons ground cumin
1 teaspoon ground turmeric
1 teaspoon dried sage
1 teaspoon dried thyme
1/8 teaspoon red pepper cayenne
Salt and freshly ground black pepper, to taste
1½ cups quinoa
4 tomatoes, chopped
1 red bell pepper, seeded and chopped
3 celery stalks, chopped
¾ cup fresh cilantro, chopped and divided
6 cups water
2 tablespoons fresh lemon juice
2 tablespoons extra-virgin extra virgin olive oil
1 avocado, peeled, pitted and sliced
1 lemon, cut into 4 wedges

DIRECTIONS:

In a big soup pan, heat coconut oil on medium heat.

Add onion, ginger and garlic and sauté for around 4 minutes.

Add cumin, turmeric, sage and thyme and sauté for about 1 minute.

Add cayenne pepper, salt and black pepper and sauté approximately 2 minutes.

Add quinoa, tomatoes, bell pepper, celery, ¼ cup of cilantro, and water and produce with a boil on high heat.

Reduce the warmth to medium-low

Simmer, covered for around 15 minutes.

Stir in remaining cilantro and lemon juice and remove from heat.

Transfer the soup into serving bowls and drizzle with organic olive oil.

Serve hot using the garnishing of avocado lemon wedges.
Nutrition:
Calories: 437, Fat: 10g, Carbohydrates: 79g, Fiber: 5g, Protein: 8g

341) **Tomato & Lentil Soup**

SERVINGS: 4
PREPARATION TIME: 15 minutes
COOKING TIME: 33 minutes
INGREDIENTS:
2 garlic cloves, peeled
2 tablespoons extra-virgin extra virgin olive oil
1 large yellow onion, sliced
1 cup red lentils
2 carrots, peeled and chopped
1 (28-ounce can tomatoes
2 teaspoons ground coriander
2 teaspoons ground cumin
1 teaspoon ground ginger
Salt and freshly ground black pepper, to taste
6 cups vegetable broth
DIRECTIONS:
Crush the garlic cloves whilst in a very bowl for about 5-10 min.
In a large soup pan, heat oil on medium heat.
Add onion and sauté for approximately 3 minutes.
Add lentils, carrots, tomatoes, spices and broth and bring to some boil.
Simmer, covered for around 25 minutes.
Stir in garlic and simmer approximately 5 minutes more.
Remove from heat and having an immersion blender, puree the soup completely.
Serve immediately.
Nutrition:
Calories: 343, Fat: 2g, Carbohydrates: 26g, Fiber: 10g, Protein: 28g

342) **Sweet Potato, Spinach & Lentil Soup**

SERVINGS: 4
PREPARATION TIME: 15 minutes

COOKING TIME: 31 minutes
INGREDIENTS:
1 tbsp extra virgin olive oil
1 large onion, minced
6 garlic cloves, minced
1½ teaspoons garam masala
½ teaspoon ground turmeric
2 pinches red pepper flakes, crushed
4 cups vegetable broth
1 cup lentil
2 sweet potatoes, peeled and cubed into ½-inch size
4 cups fresh spinach, chopped
DIRECTIONS:
In a substantial soup pan, heat oil on medium heat.
Add onion and garlic and sauté for approximately 2-4 minutes.
Stir in garam masala, turmeric and red pepper flakes and sauté approximately 2 minutes.
Add broth and lentil and provide with a boil.
Reduce heat to low and simmer, covered approximately fifteen minutes.
Stir in sweet potatoes and simmer approximately 10 min.
Stir in spinach and simmer for approximately 3-5 minutes.
Stir in salt and serve hot.
Nutrition:
Calories: 361, Fat: 4.9g, Carbohydrates: 23.7g, Fiber: 20.9g, Protein: 16.9g

343) **Carrot & Lentil Soup**

SERVINGS: 2
PREPARATION TIME: 15 minutes
COOKING TIME: 30 minutes
INGREDIENTS:
For Soup:
6 carrots, peeled and sliced
3 tablespoons olive oil, divided
1 tablespoon herbs de Provence
Salt and freshly ground black pepper, to taste
¼ cup split red lentils
1 teaspoon mustard seeds
1 teaspoon ground cumin
1 teaspoon ground turmeric

3 garlic cloves, chopped
1/3 cup coconut milk
1½ cups water
For Topping:
1 tbsp organic olive oil
12 chestnut mushrooms, sliced thinly
1 (14-ounce can cannellini beans, drained
2 minced garlic cloves
1 tablespoon mixed dried herbs

DIRECTIONS:

Preheat the oven to 355 degrees F.

Arrange the carrot slices inside a baking dish in the single layer.

Drizzle with 1 tablespoon of oil and sprinkle with herbs de Provence, salt and black pepper.

Roast for around 25 minutes.

Meanwhile in a very pan of boiling water, add lentils and cook for approximately 10 min.

Drain well.

In a sizable frying pan, heat remaining oil on medium heat.

Add mustard seeds, cumin and turmeric and sauté for approximately 30 seconds.

In a blender, add carrots, lentils, mustard seeds mixture, coconut milk and water and pulse till smooth.

Transfer the soup mixture inside a pan on medium heat and cook approximately 4-5 minutes or till heated completely.

For mushroom mixture inside same frying pan, of spices, heat oil on medium heat.

Add mushrooms, beans, garlic and herbs and sauté for about 3-4 minutes.

Transfer soup in serving bowls and top with mushroom mixture and serve.

Nutrition:

Calories: 354, Fat: 3.4g, Carbohydrates: 25.2g, Fiber: 5.3g, Protein: 32g

344) **Barley, Beans & Veggie Soup**

SERVINGS: 6
PREPARATION TIME: 20 minutes
COOKING TIME: 48 minutes
INGREDIENTS:

3 tablespoons extra virgin olive oil
¼ cup pearl barley
1 onion, chopped
2 celery stalks, chopped
2 carrots, peeled and chopped
1 garlic clove, minced
½ teaspoon ground turmeric
½ teaspoon curry powder
Salt and freshly ground black pepper, to taste
6 cups chicken broth
1 small sweet potato, peeled and chopped
1 (14-ounce can diced tomatoes, drained
1 (19-ounce can mixed beans, rinsed and drained

DIRECTIONS:

In a substantial soup pan, heat oil on medium heat.

Add barley, onion, celery, carrots, garlic, turmeric and curry powder and sauté for around 6-8 minutes.

Add salt, black pepper and broth and bring to a boil.

Reduce the heat and simmer, covered for approximately 30 minutes.

Stir in the remaining ingredients and again bring to some boil.

Simmer, covered for around 10 minutes.

Serve hot.

Nutrition:

Calories: 337, Fat: 2.6g, Carbohydrates: 29g, Fiber: 9g, Protein: 32g

345) **Carrot Soup with Chickpeas**

SERVINGS: 4
PREPARATION TIME: 15 minutes
COOKING TIME: 30 minutes
INGREDIENTS:

1 (15-ounce can chickpeas, drained
½ teaspoon ground allspice
½ teaspoon ground cinnamon
1 teaspoon extra virgin olive oil
2 tablespoons coconut oil
2-3 teaspoons fresh ginger, chopped finely
2 garlic cloves, chopped finely
1 teaspoon ground turmeric

5 cups carrots, peeled and chopped
1½ cups vegetable broth
Freshly ground black pepper and salt, to taste
½ cup coconut milk
DIRECTIONS:
Preheat the oven to 375 degrees F.
In a bowl, add chickpeas, allspice, cinnamon and olive oil and toss to coat well.
Transfer a combination in to a baking dish and bake approximately 30 minutes.
In a substantial soup pan, melt coconut oil on medium heat.
Add ginger, garlic and turmeric and sauté for approximately 5 minutes.
Add remaining ingredients except coconut milk and produce with a boil.
Reduce the temperature and simmer approximately 20-25 minutes.
Stir in coconut milk and take off from heat.
With an immersion blender, puree the soup completely.
Serve immediately with all the topping of chickpeas.
Nutrition:
Calories: 301, Fat: 4.7g, Carbohydrates: 25g, Fiber: 7g, Protein: 27g

346) <u>Black Beans Soup</u>

SERVINGS: 4
PREPARATION TIME: 15 minutes
COOKING TIME: 30-45 minutes
INGREDIENTS:
2 (15-ounce cans black beans, rinsed and drained
1 (14½-ounce can diced tomatoes
1 cup vegetable broth
1 (14-ounce can coconut milk
2 scallions, chopped
2 minced garlic cloves
1 tablespoon ground cumin
1 tablespoon ground ginger
1 tablespoon ground turmeric
Salt, to taste
DIRECTIONS:
In a large soup pan, mix together all ingredients except salt on medium-high heat.
Bring to your boil and reduce the heat.

Simmer for approximately 30-45 minutes.
Stir in salt and serve hot.
Nutrition:
Calories: 436, Fat: 22.2g, Carbohydrates: 46.3g, Fiber: 17.8g, Protein: 16.6g

347) <u>Veggies & Quinoa Soup</u>

SERVINGS: 4-6
PREPARATION TIME: 15 minutes
COOKING TIME: 43 minutes
INGREDIENTS:
2 tablespoons extra-virgin essential olive oil
1 medium shallot, chopped
1 medium onion, chopped
2 medium turnips, peeled and chopped
5 large carrots, peeled and chopped
2 teaspoons fresh ginger, minced
½ cup uncooked quinoa
3 cups water
3 cups vegetable broth
½ teaspoon ground turmeric
¼ tsp cayenne
Salt and freshly ground black pepper, to taste
DIRECTIONS:
In a large soup pan, heat oil on medium-high heat.
Add shallot, onion, turnips and carrots and sauté for about 5-7 minutes.
Stir in ginger and sauté for approximately 1 minute.
Stir in remaining ingredients and bring to some boil.
Reduce the heat to low and simmer, covered for around 20-a half-hour.
Remove from heat and make aside to chill slightly.
In an increased speed blender, add soup mixture in batches and pulse till smooth.
Return the soup in pan on medium heat.
Simmer approximately 4-5 minutes or till heated completely.
Nutrition:
Calories: 376, Fat: 5.3g, Carbohydrates: 25g, Fiber: 6g, Protein: 30g

348) Chicken & Veggies Soup

SERVINGS: 10-12
PREPARATION TIME: 15 minutes
COOKING TIME: 33 minutes
INGREDIENTS:
1½ tablespoons extra virgin olive oil
1 large onion, chopped
2 large potatoes, peeled and chopped
4 parsnips, peeled and chopped
1-2 zucchinis, chopped
1 cup fresh peas, shelled
2 large raw chicken breasts
2 teaspoons ground cumin
1 tablespoon ground turmeric
4 cups chicken broth
6 cups water
Chopped fresh cilantro, for garnishing
DIRECTIONS:
In a large soup pan, heat oil on medium heat. Add onion and sauté approximately 3 minutes.
Stir in vegetables and cook for around 5 minutes.
Stir in remaining ingredients and produce with a boil.
Reduce the heat to medium-low.
Simmer for around 10-fifteen minutes
Remove the chicken breasts from soup with forks, shred them
Return the shredded chicken into soup and simmer for approximately 10 min.
Serve hot while using garnishing of cilantro.
Nutrition:
Calories: 359, Fat: 3.2g, Carbohydrates: 25g, Fiber: 9.1g, Protein: 32.4g

349) Halibut, Quinoa & Veggies Soup

SERVINGS: 8-10
PREPARATION TIME: 15 minutes
COOKING TIME: 1 hour 10 minutes
INGREDIENTS:
2 cups onions, chopped
1 cup celeriac root, chopped
2 garlic cloves, chopped
2 tablespoons fresh ginger herb, chopped finely
1 cup shiitake mushrooms, sliced
1 cup quinoa
8 cups vegetable broth
14-ounces halibut fillets
6 cups fresh baby spinach
1cup fresh cilantro, chopped
1 cup coconut milk
Salt, to taste
2 scallions, chopped
DIRECTIONS:
In a sizable soup pan, onions, celeriac root, garlic, ginger root, mushrooms, quinoa and broth and provide to your boil.
Reduce heat to low and simmer, covered approximately 45 minutes.
Arrange the halibut fillets over soup mixture.
Simmer, covered for around 15 minutes.
Stir in remaining ingredients except scallions and simmer for around 5 minutes.
Serve hot using the garnishing of scallions.
Nutrition:
Calories: 300, Fat: 3g, Carbohydrates: 27g, Fiber: 11g, Protein: 30g

350) Beef, Mushroom & Broccoli Soup

SERVINGS: 8
PREPARATION TIME: 15 minutes
COOKING TIME: 13 minutes
INGREDIENTS:
8 cups beef broth
2-3 cups broccoli, chopped
8-ounces mushrooms, sliced
1 bunch scallion, chopped (reserve dark green part for garnishing
1 (1-inch piece fresh ginger, minced
5 garlic cloves, minced
1-pound cooked beef, sliced thinly
½ teaspoon red pepper flakes, crushed
3 tablespoons coconut aminos
1 lemon, sliced
DIRECTIONS:
In a soup pan, add broth and provide to a boil.

Add broccoli and cook for approximately 2 minutes.

Stir in mushroom, scallions, ginger and garlic and simmer for around 7-8 minutes.

Stir in beef, red pepper flakes and coconut aminos minimizing heat to low.

Simmer approximately 2-3 minutes.

Serve hot while using garnishing of reserved green part of scallion and lemon slices.

Nutrition:

Calories: 374, Fat: 7.4g, Carbohydrates: 29g, Fiber: 10.2g, Protein: 30.6g

351) **Butternut Squash & Chickpeas Stew**

SERVINGS: 6
PREPARATION TIME: 15 minutes
COOKING TIME: 36 minutes
INGREDIENTS:

1 tbsp olive oil

1 medium sweet onion, chopped

1½ teaspoons fresh ginger, grated

2 minced garlic cloves

½ tablespoon coconut sugar

¼ teaspoon ground cumin

¾ teaspoon ground cinnamon

1-2 teaspoons red chili flakes, crushed

3½ cups butternut squash, peeled and chopped

Salt and freshly ground black pepper, to taste

1½ cups water, divided

Salt and freshly ground black pepper, to taste

¼ cup creamy natural almond butter

1½ cups cooked chickpeas

3 cups fresh kale, trimmed and chopped

½ cup raw almonds, chopped

DIRECTIONS:

In a big soup pan, heat oil on medium heat.

Add onion and cook, covered for about 5 minutes, stirring occasionally.

Stir in ginger, garlic, coconut sugar and spices and sauté approximately 1 minute.

Add squash and stir to mix well.

Add 1¼ glasses of water, salt and black pepper and bring with a boil.

Reduce heat to low.

In a bowl, mix together remaining water and peanut butter.

Add peanut butter mixture in pan and stir to mix.

Simmer, covered for approximately twenty minutes.

Stir in chickpeas, kale and almonds and simmer for around 10 min more.

Nutrition:

Calories: 393, Fat: 10.4g, Carbohydrates: 23g, Fiber: 8.3g, Protein: 27g

352) **Mixed Veggies Stew**

SERVINGS: 4
PREPARATION TIME: 15 minutes
COOKING TIME: 21 minutes
INGREDIENTS:

2 tablespoons coconut oil

1 large onion, chopped

1 teaspoon ground turmeric

1 teaspoon ground cumin

Salt and freshly ground black pepper, to taste

1-2 cups water, divided

1 cup cabbage, shredded

1 bunch broccoli, chopped

2 large carrots, peeled and sliced

2 teaspoons fresh ginger, grated

DIRECTIONS:

In a large soup pan, melt coconut oil on medium heat.

Add onion and sauté approximately 5 minutes.

Stir in spices and sauté for about 1 minute.

Add 1 cup of water and convey to some boil.

Simmer approximately 10 min.

Add vegetables and enough water that covers the 50 % of vegetables mixture.

Simmer, covered for about 10-fifteen minutes, stirring occasionally.

Serve hot.

Nutrition:

Calories: 274, Fat: 3.2g, Carbohydrates: 23g, Fiber: 14.1g, Protein: 22g

353) Root Veggies Stew

SERVINGS: 6-8
PREPARATION TIME: 15 minutes
COOKING TIME: 33 minutes
INGREDIENTS:
2 tablespoons coconut oil
1 large sweet onion, chopped
1 medium parsnips, peeled and chopped
3 tablespoons tomato paste
2 large garlic cloves, minced
½ teaspoon ground cinnamon
½ teaspoon ground ginger
1 teaspoon ground cumin
¼ tsp red pepper cayenne
Salt, to taste
2 medium carrots, peeled and chopped
2 medium purple potatoes, peeled and chopped
2 medium sweet potatoes, peeled and chopped
4 cups vegetable broth
2 tablespoons freshly squeezed lemon juice
2 cups fresh kale, kale, trimmed and chopped
¼ cup fresh cilantro leaves, chopped
Slivered almonds, for garnishing
DIRECTIONS:
In a sizable soup pan, melt coconut oil on medium-high heat.
Add onion and sauté for approximately 5 minutes.
Add parsnip and sauté for approximately 3 minutes.
Stir in tomato paste, garlic and spices and sauté approximately 2 minutes.
Add carrots, potatoes and sweet potatoes and stir to mix well.
Add broth and produce with a boil and reduce the temperature to medium-low.
Simmer for about twenty or so minutes.
Stir in freshly squeezed lemon juice and kale and simmer approximately 2-3 minutes.
Serve using the garnishing of cilantro and almonds.
Nutrition:
Calories: 366, Fat: 2g, Carbohydrates: 21g, Fiber: 7.5g, Protein: 20g

354) Chicken & Tomato Stew

SERVINGS: 6-8
PREPARATION TIME: 15 minutes
COOKING TIME: 31 minutes
INGREDIENTS:
2 tablespoons olive oil
1 onion, chopped
½ tablespoon fresh ginger, grated finely
1 tablespoon fresh garlic, minced
1 teaspoon ground turmeric
1 teaspoon ground cumin
1 teaspoon ground coriander
1 teaspoon paprika
1 teaspoon red pepper cayenne
6 skinless, boneless chicken thighs, trimmed and cut into 1-inch pieces
3 Roma tomatoes, chopped
1 (14-ounce coconut milk
Salt and freshly ground black pepper, to taste
1/3 cup fresh cilantro, chopped
DIRECTIONS:
In a substantial pan, heat oil on medium heat.
Add onion and sauté for around 8-10 minutes.
Add ginger, garlic and spices and sauté for approximately 1 minute.
Add chicken and cook for around 4-5 minutes.
Add tomatoes, coconut milk, salt and black pepper and brig to gentle simmer.
Reduce the heat to low and simmer, covered for around 10-15 minutes or till desired doneness.
Stir in cilantro and take away from heat.
Nutrition:
Calories: 347, Fat: 3.7g, Carbohydrates: 23.3g, Fiber: 7.7g, Protein: 20g

355) Chicken, Chickpeas & Olives Stew

SERVINGS: 10-12
PREPARATION TIME: 15 minutes
COOKING TIME: 1 hour 9 minutes
INGREDIENTS:

6-pound skinless, boneless grass-fed chicken thighs, trimmed
Salt and freshly ground black pepper, to taste
¼ cup extra-virgin essential olive oil
3 large yellow onions, sliced thinly
8 garlic cloves, crushed
3 small red chiles, stemmed
2 fresh bay leaves
1 tablespoon ground turmeric
2 teaspoon ground coriander
2 teaspoons ground cumin
2 (3-inch cinnamon sticks
4 teaspoons fresh lemon zest, grated finely
½ cup fresh lemon juice, divided
4 cups low-sodium chicken broth
2 cups small green olives, pitted
2 cups canned chickpeas, rinsed and drained
3 tablespoons fresh cilantro, chopped
DIRECTIONS:
Sprinkle the chicken thighs with salt and black pepper evenly.
In a sizable pan, heat oil on medium-high heat.
Add the chicken thighs in 4 batches and cook for around 3 minutes from each party.
Transfer the chicken into a bowl and make aside.
Reduce the warmth to medium and sauté the onion for about 5-6 minutes.
Add garlic, red chiles, bay leaves and spices and sauté for about 1 minute.
Add lemon zest, 1/3 cup with the lemon juice and broth and produce to your boil.
Reduce the warmth to medium-low and simmer, covered approximately a half-hour.
Stir inside the cooked chicken, olives and chickpeas and boost the heat to medium-high.
Cook, stirring occasionally for about 6-8 minutes.
Stir in remaining fresh lemon juice, salt and black pepper and remove from heat.
Serve hot while using garnishing of cilantro.
Nutrition:
Calories: 490, Fat: 25g, Carbohydrates: 18g, Fiber: 4g, Protein: 48g

356) **Beef & Squash Stew**

SERVINGS: 4-6
PREPARATION TIME: 15 minutes
COOKING TIME: 1 hour 17 minutes
INGREDIENTS:
1½ tablespoons coconut oil, divided
2-3-pound stew meat, trimmed and cubed into 1½-inch size
1 onion, chopped
1 (2-inch piece fresh ginger, minced
5 garlic cloves, minced
2 cups bone broth
1 butternut squash, peeled and cubed
¼ teaspoon ground cinnamon
2 pears, cored and chopped
1 cup fresh mushrooms, sliced
1 tablespoon fresh thyme, chopped
DIRECTIONS:
In a big heavy bottomed pan, heat 1 tablespoon of oil on medium-high heat
Add beef and sear for around 8-10 minutes or till browned completely.
With a slotted spoon, transfer the beef in to a bowl.
Now, decrease the heat to medium.
Add onion and sauté for approximately 5 minutes.
Add ginger and garlic and sauté for about 2 minutes.
Add cooked beef and broth and provide with a boil.
Reduce the warmth to low and simmer, covered approximately 15 minutes.
Stir in squash, cinnamon and salt and simmer, covered for around fifteen minutes.
Stir in pears and simmer, covered for approximately half an hour.
Meanwhile in the small skillet, heat the remainder oil on high heat.
Add mushrooms and cook for approximately 5 minutes or till browned.
Serve the stew with the topping f mushrooms and thyme.
Nutrition:
Calories: 298, Fat: 6.66g, Carbohydrates: 27g, Fiber: 3.4g, Protein: 31g

357) **Baked Lamb Stew**

SERVINGS: 4
PREPARATION TIME: 15 minutes
COOKING TIME: 1 hour 10 minutes
INGREDIENTS:
For Lamb Marinade:
3 large garlic cloves, minced
1 tablespoon fresh ginger, minced
1 lemongrass stalk, minced
2 tablespoons coconut aminos
2 tablespoons tapioca starch
Salt and freshly ground black pepper, to taste
2-3-pound boneless lamb shoulder, trimmed and cubed into 2-inch pieces
For Stew:
2 tablespoons coconut oil
4 shallots, minced
2 Thai chilies, minced
2 tablespoons tomato paste
4 large tomatoes, chopped
4 carrots, peeled and chopped
1 butternut squash, peeled and cubed
2-star anise
1 cinnamon stick
1 teaspoon Chinese 5-spice powder
2½ cups hot beef broth
DIRECTIONS:
For lamb marinade in a substantial glass bowl, add all ingredients and mix well.
Cover and refrigerate to marinate for around 2-8 hours.
Preheat the oven to 325 degrees F.
In an oven proof casserole dish, heat oil on medium-high heat.
Add lamb and cook for around 4-5 minutes. Reduce heat to medium.
Add shallots and chilies and cook for around 2-3 minutes.
Stir in tomato paste and tomatoes and cook approximately 1-2 minutes.
Add remaining ingredients and stir to combine well.
Cover the casserole dish and immediately, transfer into oven.
Bake for approximately one hour or till desired doneness.

Nutrition:
Calories: 291, Fat: 5.6g, Carbohydrates: 23g, Fiber: 5.3g, Protein: 26g

358) **Haddock & Potato Stew**

SERVINGS: 4
PREPARATION TIME: 15 minutes
COOKING TIME: 13 minutes
INGREDIENTS:
2 large Yukon Gold potatoes, sliced into ¼-inch size
1 tbsp. olive oil
1 (2-inch piece fresh ginger, chopped finely
1 (16-ounce can whole tomatoes, crushed
½ cup water
1 cup clam juice
¼ teaspoon red pepper flakes, crushed
Salt, to taste
1½ pound boneless haddock, cut into 2inch pieces
2 tablespoons fresh parsley, chopped
Direction:
Arrange a steamer basket in a big pan of water and produce to your boil.
Place the potatoes in steamer basket and cook, covered approximately 8 minutes.
Meanwhile in the pan, heat oil on medium heat.
Add ginger and sauté for about 1 minute.
Add tomatoes and cook, stirring continuously approximately 2 minutes.
Add water, clam juice, red pepper flakes and produce to a boil.
Simmer for around 5 minutes, stirring occasionally.
Gently, stir in haddock pieces and simmer, covered for about 5 minutes or till desired doneness.
In serving bowls, divide potatoes and top with haddock mixture.
Garnish with parsley and serve.
Nutrition:
Calories: 421, Fat: 3g, Carbohydrates: 14g, Fiber: 9g, Protein: 24g

359) Adzuki Beans & Carrot Stew

SERVINGS: 4
PREPARATION TIME: 15 minutes
COOKING TIME: 1 hour 18 minutes
INGREDIENTS:
2 tablespoons extra virgin olive oil
1 large yellow onion, chopped
5 (½-inch fresh ginger slices
Salt, to taste
3 cups water
1 cup dried adzuki beans, soaked for overnight, rinsed and drained
4 large carrots, peeled and sliced into ¾-inch pieces
2 tablespoons brown rice vinegar
3 tablespoons tamari
½ cup fresh parsley, minced
DIRECTIONS:
In a sizable pan, heat oil on medium heat.
Add onion, ginger and salt and sauté for around 2-3 minutes.
Add water and beans and convey to a boil.
Reduce heat to low and simmer, covered for around 45 minutes.
Arrange carrot slices over beans and simmer, covered for around 20-thirty minutes.
Stir in vinegar and tamari and remove from heat.
Discard the ginger slices before serving.
Serve hot with garnishing of parsley.
Nutrition:
Calories: 309 Fat: 3g, Carbohydrates: 22g, Fiber: 7g, Protein: 27g

360) Black-Eyed Beans Stew

SERVINGS: 4-5
PREPARATION TIME: 15 minutes
COOKING TIME: 2 hours 20 minutes
INGREDIENTS:
2 cups dried black eyed beans, soaked for overnight, rinsed and drained
2 medium onions, chopped and divided
1 (4-inch piece fresh ginger chopped
4 garlic cloves, chopped
¼ cup essential olive oil

2 scotch bonnet peppers
2 (14-ounce cans plum tomatoes
½-¾ cup water
1 vegetable bouillon cube
Salt, to taste
DIRECTIONS:
In a big pan of boiling water, add beans and cook, covered approximately 60-90 minutes or till bens become soft.
In a blender, add 1 onion, ginger and garlic and pulse till a puree form.
In a big pan, heat oil on medium heat.
Add onion and sauté for around 2-5 minutes.
Stir in 5 tablespoons of onion puree and cook for approximately 5 minutes.
Meanwhile in blender, add bonnet peppers and tomatoes and pulse till smooth.
Add tomato mixture and stir to blend.
Reduce the warmth to low and simmer, covered for about 30 minutes, stirring occasionally.
Stir in beans, cube and salt and simmer for approximately 10 minutes.
Nutrition:
Calories: 300, Fat: 4g, Carbohydrates: 15g, Fiber: 14g, Protein: 26g

361) Creamy Chickpeas Stew

SERVINGS: 4-6
PREPARATION TIME: 15 minutes
COOKING TIME: 56 minutes
INGREDIENTS:
¼ cup coconut oil
1 medium yellow onion, chopped
2 teaspoons fresh ginger, chopped finely
2 minced garlic cloves
1 teaspoon ground cumin
1 teaspoon ground coriander
¾ teaspoon ground turmeric
¼ teaspoon yellow mustard seeds
¼ tsp cayenne
1 (19-ounce can chickpeas, rinsed and drained
2 large sweet potatoes, peeled and cubed into 1-inch size
1-pound fresh kale, trimmed and chopped
5 cups vegetable broth
Salt, to taste

1 cup coconut milk
¼ cup red bell pepper, seeded and julienned
2 tablespoons fresh cilantro, chopped
DIRECTIONS:
In a substantial pan, heat oil on medium heat.

Add onion and sauté for around 3 minutes.

Add ginger and garlic and sauté for about 2 minutes.

Add spices and sauté for around 1 minute.

Add chickpeas, sweet potato, kale and broth and bring with a boil on medium-high heat.

Reduce the temperature to medium-low and simmer, covered for about 35 minutes.

Stir in coconut milk and simmer for about fifteen minutes or till desired thickness of stew.

Serve hot with garnishing of bell pepper and cilantro.

Nutrition:

Calories: 323, Fat: 3g, Carbohydrates: 15g, Fiber: 9g, Protein: 25g

Snacks

362) Turmeric Bars

PREPARATION TIME: 2 hours and 5 minutes
COOKING TIME: 10 minutes
SERVINGS: 6
INGREDIENTS:
1 cup shredded coconut
10 dates, pitted
1 tablespoon coconut oil
1 teaspoon cinnamon
1 ¼ cup coconut butter
1 ½ teaspoon turmeric powder
2 teaspoons honey
1/8 teaspoon black pepper
DIRECTIONS:
Prepare a baking pan and line with parchment paper.
Place the coconut and dates in a food processor and pulse until well-combined. Add in the coconut oil and cinnamon.
Press the dough at the bottom of the pan and allow to set in the fridge for 2 hours.
Make the filling by melting the coconut butter in a double boiler. Stir in turmeric powder and honey.
Pour in the mixture into the pan with the crust.
Allow to set in the fridge for at least 2 hours.
Nutrition:
Calories 410, Total Fat 41g, Saturated Fat 6g, Total Carbs 13g, Net Carbs11 g, Protein 1g, Sugar: 11g, Fiber: 2g, Sodium: 208mg, Potassium 347mg

363) Anti-Inflammatory Turmeric Gummies

PREPARATION TIME: 4 hours
COOKING TIME: 10 minutes
SERVINGS: 6
INGREDIENTS:
1 teaspoon ground turmeric
6 tablespoons maple syrup
8 tablespoons unflavored gelatin powder
3 ½ cups water
DIRECTIONS:
In a pot, combine the water, turmeric, and maple syrup.
Bring to a boil for 5 minutes.
Remove from the heat and sprinkle with gelatin powder. Mix to hydrate the gelatin.
Turn on the heat and bring to a boil until the gelatin is completely dissolved.
Pour the mixture in a dish and chill the mixture in the fridge for at least 4 hours.
Once set, slice into small squares.
Nutrition:
Calories 68, Total Fat 0.03g, Saturated Fat 0g, Total Carbs 17g, Net Carbs 16.9g, Protein 0.2g, Sugar: 15g, Fiber: 0.1g, Sodium: 19mg, Potassium 53mg

364) Ginger Spiced Mixed Nuts

PREPARATION TIME: 5 minutes
COOKING TIME: 40 minutes
SERVINGS: 4
INGREDIENTS:
2 large egg whites, pasture-raised
2 cups mixed nuts (raw almond, pumpkin seeds, cashew, etc.
1 teaspoon grated ginger
½ teaspoon salt
DIRECTIONS:
Preheat the oven to 2500F.
Whip the egg whites until frothy. Add in ginger and salt.
Add in the mixed nuts into the egg mixture. Stir to coat everything.
Place parchment paper in a baking tray and spread the nuts evenly on to the sheet.
Bake for 40 minutes.
Allow the mixture to cool and harden.
Break into pieces and store in the fridge until ready to consume
Nutrition:
Calories 423, Total Fat 36g, Saturated Fat 3g, Total Carbs 16g, Net Carbs 7g, Protein 17g, Sugar: 3g, Fiber: 9g, Sodium: 28mg, Potassium 553mg

365) **Spicy Tuna Rolls**

PREPARATION TIME: 10 minutes
COOKING TIME: 0 minutes
SERVINGS: 6
INGREDIENTS:
1 medium cucumber
1 can yellowfin tuna, wild-caught
2 slices avocado, diced
1/8 teaspoon salt
1/8 teaspoon pepper
DIRECTIONS:
Use a mandolin to thinly slice the cucumber lengthwise.
In a mixing bowl, combine the tuna and avocado. Season with salt and pepper to taste.
Spoon the tuna and avocado mixture and spread evenly on cucumber slices.
Roll the cucumber slices and secure the ends with toothpicks.
Allow to chill in the fridge before serving.
Nutrition:
Calories 135, Total Fat 10g, Saturated Fat 1g, Total Carbs 6g, Net Carbs 1g, Protein 7g, Sugar:0.9 g, Fiber: 5g, Sodium: 73mg, Potassium 420mg

366) **Veggie Burrito**

PREPARATION TIME: 10 minutes
COOKING TIME: 5 minutes
SERVINGS: 2
INGREDIENTS:
4 medium collard greens, stalks trimmed
1 teaspoon avocado oil
1/3 cup bell pepper, julienned
1/3 cup chopped tomatoes
1/3 cup red onions, sliced thinly
¼ cup avocado meat
1 cup cooked quinoa
¼ cup cilantro leaves, chopped
¼ teaspoon salt
DIRECTIONS:
Bring water to a boil and blanch the collard greens. Set aside.
In a skillet, heat the avocado oil over medium flame and sauté the bell pepper for 1 minute. Set aside.

Assemble the burrito by placing the blanched collard greens on a flat surface.
Place the bell pepper, tomatoes, onions, avocado meat, and quinoa in the center. Add in the cilantro leaves.
Roll the collard greens to create a burrito.
Nutrition:
Calories 175, Total Fat 7g, Saturated Fat 0.8g, Total Carbs 25g, Net Carbs 20g, Protein 5g, Sugar: 3g, Fiber: 5g, Sodium:11 mg, Potassium 372mg

367) **Spicy Kale Chips**

PREPARATION TIME: 10 minutes
COOKING TIME: 20 minutes
SERVINGS: 4
INGREDIENTS:
1 bunch curly kale, rinsed
¼ teaspoon ground cayenne pepper
1/8 teaspoon garlic powder
spray oil for greasing
¼ teaspoon salt
1/8 teaspoon black pepper
DIRECTIONS:
Preheat the oven to 3000F.
Pat dry the kale to remove water.
Tear the kale leaves into bite-sized pieces and place on a baking sheet lined with foil.
Spray with cooking oil and season with garlic powder, season, and black pepper.
Bake in the oven for 20 minutes or until crunchy.
Nutrition:
Calories 5, Total Fat 0.08g, Saturated Fat 0g, Total Carbs 1g, Net Carbs 0.7g, Protein 0.4g, Sugar: 0.3g, Fiber: 0.3g, Sodium: 3mg, Potassium 50mg

368) **Ginger Date Bars**

PREPARATION TIME: 10 minutes
COOKING TIME: 20 minutes
SERVINGS: 8
INGREDIENTS:
1 ½ cups almond, soaked in water overnight then drained
¾ cup dates, pitted

¼ cup almond milk
1 teaspoon ground ginger
DIRECTIONS:
Preheat the oven to 3500F.
Place the almond in a food processor. Pulse a thick dough is formed.
Press the dough in a baking dish lined with parchment paper. Set aside.
Make the date mix by combining the rest of the ingredients in a food processor. Pulse until smooth.
Pour the date mixture on to the almond crust.
Bake for 20 minutes.
Allow to cool before slicing.
Nutrition:
Calories 45, Total Fat 0.3g, Saturated Fat 0.01g, Total Carbs 11g, Net Carbs 10 g, Protein 0.5g, Sugar: 9g, Fiber: 1g, Sodium: 6mg, Potassium 101mg

369) **Vanilla Turmeric Orange Juice**

PREPARATION TIME: 2 hours
COOKING TIME: 0 minutes
SERVINGS: 2
INGREDIENTS:
3 oranges, peeled and quartered
1 cup almond milk, unsweetened
1 teaspoon vanilla extract
½ teaspoon cinnamon
¼ teaspoon turmeric
a pinch of pepper
DIRECTIONS:
Place all ingredients in a blender.
Pulse until smooth.
Pour into glasses and allow to chill in the fridge before serving.
Nutrition:
Calories 188, Total Fat 5g, Saturated Fat 2g, Total Carbs 33g, Net Carbs 27g, Protein 5g, Sugar: 27g, Fiber: 6g, Sodium: 53mg, Potassium 558mg

370) **Hibiscus Ginger Gelatin**

PREPARATION TIME: 2 hours

COOKING TIME: 20 minutes
SERVINGS: 5
INGREDIENTS:
3 tablespoons dried hibiscus flower
1 ½ tablespoons honey
1 teaspoon ginger juice
2 tablespoons gelatin powder
1 cup water
DIRECTIONS:
Bring water to a boil.
Once the water boils, remove from the heat and add the hibiscus flowers.
Allow to infuse for 5 minutes.
Remove the flowers and discard.
Heat the liquid and add the honey, ginger, and gelatin.
Allow the gelatin to dissolve.
Pour the mixture into a baking sheet.
Place in the fridge and allow to set.
Slice the gelatin once it hardens.
Nutrition:
Calories 27, Total Fat 0.06g, Saturated Fat 0.03g, Total Carbs 7g, Net Carbs 7g, Protein 0.2g, Sugar: 7g, Fiber: 0g, Sodium: 6mg, Potassium 6mg

371) **Turmeric Nuggets**

PREPARATION TIME: 15 minutes
COOKING TIME: 25;4
INGREDIENTS:
2 cups cauliflower florets
2 cups broccoli florets
1 cup carrots, chopped
1 teaspoon garlic, minced
½ teaspoon ground turmeric
½ cup almond meal
2 egg, pasture-raised
¼ teaspoon salt
¼ teaspoon black pepper
DIRECTIONS:
Preheat the oven to 4000F and line a baking sheet with parchment paper.
In a food processor, combine all ingredients and pulse until smooth.
Scoop a tablespoon of mixture and place on the baking sheet.
Bake for 25 minutes.
Nutrition:

Calories 97, Total Fat 5g, Saturated Fat 1g, Total Carbs 7g, Net Carbs 4g, Protein 7g, Sugar: 3g, Fiber: 3g, Sodium: 93mg, Potassium 377mg

372) **Coconut Flour Muffins**

PREPARATION TIME: 10 minutes
COOKING TIME: 25 minutes
SERVINGS: 6
INGREDIENTS:
6 large eggs, pasture raised
½ cup unsweetened coconut milk
1/3 cup maple syrup
1 teaspoon vanilla extract
¾ cup + 2 tablespoons coconut flour
½ teaspoon baking soda
2 teaspoon turmeric powder
½ teaspoon ginger powder
salt and pepper to taste
DIRECTIONS:
Preheat the oven to 3500F.
Prepare a muffin tin and line with muffin liners.
In a mixing bowl, combine the eggs, milk, maple syrup, and vanilla.
In another bowl, sift the coconut flour, baking soda, turmeric, and ginger powder. Season with salt and pepper to taste.
Gradually pour the wet ingredients into the dry ingredients until well-combined.
Pour into the prepared muffin tins.
Bake for 25 minutes or until a toothpick inserted in the middle comes out clean.
Nutrition:
Calories 157, Total Fat 9g, Saturated Fat 2g, Total Carbs 15g, Net Carbs 14g, Protein 3g, Sugar: 12g, Fiber: 1g, Sodium: 150mg, Potassium 205mg

373) **No Bake Golden Energy Bites**

PREPARATION TIME: 60 minutes
COOKING TIME: 0 minutes
SERVINGS: 6
INGREDIENTS:
1 cup almond butter

¾ cup coconut flakes, unsweetened
6 tablespoons protein powder
1 teaspoon coconut oil
½ teaspoon maple syrup
2 teaspoons turmeric
DIRECTIONS:
In a bowl, combine all ingredients until a thick dough is formed.
Place dough in a pan lined with parchment paper and spread evenly.
Place in the refrigerator for at least an hour to set.
Remove the bars from the pan and slice to 16 pieces.
Nutrition:
Calories 376, Total Fat 36g, Saturated Fat 5g, Total Carbs 9g, Net Carbs 7g, Protein 6g, Sugar: 5g, Fiber: 2g, Sodium: 194mg, Potassium 310mg

374) **Banana Ginger Bars**

PREPARATION TIME: 10 minutes
COOKING TIME: 40 minutes
SERVINGS: 5
INGREDIENTS:
2 large ripe bananas, peeled and mashed
1 cup coconut flour
1/3 cup coconut oil
1/3 cup raw honey
6 eggs, pasture-raised
1 tablespoon grated fresh ginger
2 teaspoons cinnamon powder
1 teaspoon ground cardamom powder
1 teaspoon baking soda
2 teaspoons apples cider vinegar
DIRECTIONS:
Preheat the oven to 3500F.
Grease a baking dish or line with parchment paper.
In a food processor, combine the bananas, coconut flour, coconut oil, honey, eggs, ginger, cinnamon, and cardamom. Pulse until smooth.
Add the baking soda and apple cider vinegar last and quickly blend.
Pour into the prepared pan.

Bake in the oven for 40 minutes or until a toothpick inserted in the middle comes out clean.

Allow to cool before slicing.

Nutrition:

Calories 364, Total Fat 26g, Saturated Fat 3g, Total Carbs 23g, Net Carbs 22g, Protein 12g, Sugar: 20g, Fiber: 1g, Sodium: 187mg, Potassium 334mg

375) **Kombucha Gummies**

PREPARATION TIME: 3 hours
COOKING TIME: 10 minutes
SERVINGS: 5
INGREDIENTS:
1 teaspoon grated ginger
1 ½ cups plain kombucha
½ cup grapefruit juice
1 tablespoon grapefruit zest
6 tablespoons honey
1/3 cup gelatin powder
DIRECTIONS:
Line the bottom of a glass pan with plastic wrap. Set aside.

In a pot, add the ginger and a cup of water. Bring to a boil for 5 minutes. Drain and save the grated ginger.

In another saucepan, combine the kombucha, grapefruit juice, zest, and honey. Sprinkle with the gelatin powder and allow to hydrate for 5 minutes.

Turn on the heat and bring to a boil until the gelatin dissolves. Add in the grated ginger.

Pour into the mixture the prepared glass and chill for 3 hours until the gelatin has set.

Slice into small squares.

Nutrition:

Calories 99, Total Fat 0.03g, Saturated Fat 0g, Total Carbs 26g, Net Carbs 25.9g, Protein 0.4g, Sugar: 26g, Fiber: 0.1g, Sodium: 15mg, Potassium 57mg

376) **Cacao Coffee Protein Bars**

PREPARATION TIME: 10 minutes
COOKING TIME: 0 minutes
SERVINGS: 6
INGREDIENTS:
2 cups mixed nuts (almond, pecans, cashew and walnuts
1 cup egg white protein powder
¼ cup cacao powder
3 tablespoons powdered coffee
18 large medjool dates, pitted
¼ cup raw cacao nibs
5 tablespoons water
DIRECTIONS:
Line a baking pan with parchment paper. Set aside

In a food processor, pulse the nuts, protein powder, cacao powder, and powdered coffee. Add in the pitted dates and process until fine crumbs form. If dry, add a tablespoon of water until a sticky dough is formed.

Place in a bowl and stir in the cacao nibs.

Transfer the mixture into the pan and spread evenly.

Place inside the fridge and allow to set for 30 minutes before slicing.

Nutrition:

Calories 493, Total Fat 25g, Saturated Fat 3g, Total Carbs 67g, Net Carbs 55g, Protein 12g, Sugar: 50g, Fiber: 12g, Sodium: 2mg, Potassium 956mg

377) **Spicy Taro Crunch**

PREPARATION TIME: 10 minutes
COOKING TIME: 20 minutes
SERVINGS: 2
INGREDIENTS:
2 cups taro, sliced thinly
1 teaspoon cayenne pepper powder
1 tablespoon olive oil
a pinch of salt
DIRECTIONS:
Preheat the oven to 3500F.

In a bowl, combine all ingredients. Toss to coat the taro with the spices and seasoning.

Place the taro slices on a baking rack.

Bake for 20 minutes or until the taro becomes crispy.

Nutrition:

Calories 179, Total Fat 7g, Saturated Fat 1g, Total Carbs 28g, Net Carbs 23g, Protein 2g,

Sugar: 0.5g, Fiber: 5g, Sodium: 12mg, Potassium 633mg

378) **White Beans Hummus**

PREPARATION TIME: 10 minutes
COOKING TIME: 5 minutes
SERVINGS: 7
INGREDIENTS:
¼ cup olive oil
1 teaspoon fresh rosemary, chopped
2 cups cooked white beans
¼ cup pure almond butter, unsweetened
1 clove garlic, minced
1 tablespoon lemon juice
¼ cup hot water
¼ teaspoon salt
DIRECTIONS:
Heat oil in a skillet over medium heat and fry the rosemary for a few minutes. Remove from heat and allow to cool before removing the rosemary leaves. Set aside.
In a food processor, combine the white beans, almond butter, garlic, and lemon juice. Season with salt to taste.
Pulse until smooth. Gradually drizzle with oil and water to adjust the consistency. Save a quarter of the oil.
Place in a bowl and drizzle the remaining olive oil on top.
Serve with vegetable sticks.
Nutrition:
Calories 195, Total Fat 13g, Saturated Fat 2g, Total Carbs 15g, Net Carbs 11g, Protein 7g, Sugar: 0.8g, Fiber: 4g, Sodium: 28mg, Potassium 358mg

379) **Mushroom Pizza**

Prep time:10 minutes
Cooking time:15 minutes
SERVINGS: 4
INGREDIENTS:
2 tablespoons olive oil
¾ pound portobello mushrooms, stems removed
½ cup tomato puree
2 cloves of garlic, minced

½ cup mozzarella cheese, shredded
Salt and pepper to taste
DIRECTIONS:
Preheat the oven to 3500F.
Brush oil on the inverted side of the mushrooms.
Brush with tomato puree and sprinkle with garlic and mozzarella cheese on top.
Place on a baking pan and bake for 15 minutes.
Nutrition:
Calories 112, Total Fat 7g, Saturated Fat 0.9g, Total Carbs 7g, Net Carbs 5g, Protein 7g, Sugar: 4g, Fiber: 2g, Sodium: 122mg, Potassium 468mg

380) **Quinoa and Beet Kale Dolmades**

PREPARATION TIME: 20 minutes
COOKING TIME: 50 minutes
SERVINGS: 1
INGREDIENTS:
¼ cup uncooked quinoa
4 leaves dinosaur kale
½ cup beets, grated
1 tablespoons lemon juice
1 teaspoon balsamic vinegar
½ teaspoon orange zest
1 tablespoons olive oil
½ cup water
Instructions
Bring water to a boil over medium flame and cook the quinoa according to package instruction. Drain and allow to cool. Save the warm water.
Place the kale leaves in warm water and blanch for 10 minutes. Set aside and allow water to drain.
In a bowl, combine the quinoa, beets, lemon juice, balsamic vinegar and orange zest.
Place the kale leaves stem side up and add 2 tablespoons of the quinoa mixture. Fold the edges as you would a burrito or spring roll.
Place them in a pan with olive oil and pour ½ cup water.
Cover and bring to a gentle boil over medium low heat. Cook for 45 minutes.

Once the leaves have darkened, remove from the pan and transfer to a plate.
Serve with hummus.
Nutrition:
Calories 490, Total Fat 19g, Saturated Fat 2g, Total Carbs 71g, Net Carbs 55g, Protein 18g, Sugar: 23g, Fiber: 16g, Sodium: 406mg, Potassium 1750mg

381) Salted Raw Caramel Dip

PREPARATION TIME: minutes
COOKING TIME: minutes
SERVINGS: 2
INGREDIENTS:
1 cup soft medjool dates, pitted
1 teaspoon fresh lemon juice
¼ cup almond milk
1 teaspoon vanilla extract
1 tablespoon coconut oil
¼ teaspoon salt
DIRECTIONS:
Combine all ingredients in a blender or food processor.
Pulse until smooth.
Place in a container and allow to chill before serving.
Nutrition:
Calories 113, Total Fat 7.2g, Saturated Fat 0.01g, Total Carbs 12g, Net Carbs 11.1g, Protein 0.4g, Sugar: 11g, Fiber: 0.9g, Sodium:22 mg, Potassium 112mg

382) Roasted Red Pepper Hummus with Garlic

PREPARATION TIME: 5 minutes
Cooking time:0 minutes
SERVINGS: 4
INGREDIENTS:
1 cup chickpea, cooked
2 whole roasted red pepper, seeded and peeled
2 teaspoons minced garlic
4 tablespoons lemon juice
3 tablespoons olive oil
1 teaspoon salt
1 teaspoon black pepper

DIRECTIONS:
Place all ingredients in a food processor and pulse until smooth.
Place in a bowl and serve with grain-free chips or vegetable chips.
Nutrition:
Calories 293, Total Fat 12g, Saturated Fat 2g, Total Carbs 35g, Net Carbs 28g, Protein 11g, Sugar: 7g, Fiber: 7g, Sodium: 91mg, Potassium 441mg

383) Zucchini and Black Beans Enchiladas

PREPARATION TIME: 10 minutes
COOKING TIME: 20 minutes
SERVINGS: 6
INGREDIENTS:
3 large zucchini, diced
3 teaspoons extra virgin olive oil
1 ¼ teaspoon garlic salt
½ small red onion, chopped
1 cup black beans, cooked
¼ cup goat cheese, diced
1 cup tomatoes, diced
A handful of coriander, chopped
salt and pepper to taste
DIRECTIONS:
Preheat the oven to 3750F.
Place zucchini in a baking tray and drizzle with olive oil. Season with garlic salt.
Bake for 20 minutes or until the edges have browned.
Allow to cool.
Mix all ingredients in a bowl and toss to coat everything.
Serve with vegetable chips.
Nutrition:
Calories 225, Total Fat 9g, Saturated Fat 2g, Total Carbs 22g, Net Carbs 17g, Protein 14g, Sugar: 2g, Fiber: 5g, Sodium: 121mg, Potassium 601mg

384) Greek Yogurt with Fresh Toppings

PREPARATION TIME: 5 minutes
COOKING TIME: 0 minutes

SERVINGS: 1
INGREDIENTS:
1 cup plain Greek yogurt
¼ cup fresh strawberries
1teaspoon organic raw hone
¼ teaspoon cinnamon
DIRECTIONS:
Combine all ingredients in a bowl.
Chill in the fridge before serving.
Nutrition:
Calories 164, Total Fat 8g, Saturated Fat 1g, Total Carbs 15g, Net Carbs 14g, Protein 9g, Sugar: 14g, Fiber: 1g, Sodium: 150mg, Potassium 348mg

385) <u>Simple Guacamole</u>

PREPARATION TIME: 5 minutes
COOKING TIME: 0 minutes
SERVINGS: 2
INGREDIENTS:
2 tablespoons chopped onion
2 tablespoons chopped cilantro
1 medium chopped avocado
1/8 teaspoon salt
Instructions
Place all ingredients in a food processor.
Pulse until smooth.
Nutrition:
Calories 165, Total Fat 15g, Saturated Fat 2g, Total Carbs 10g, Net Carbs 3g, Protein 2g, Sugar: 1g, Fiber: 7g, Sodium: 8mg, Potassium 507mg

386) <u>Pumpkin Spiced Apple Chips</u>

PREPARATION TIME: 10 minutes
COOKING TIME: 1 hour and 30 minutes
SERVINGS: 3
INGREDIENTS:
2 tablespoons ground cinnamon
1 tablespoons ground ginger
1 ½ teaspoon ground nutmeg
1 ½ teaspoon ground cloves
3 apples, cored and sliced thinly
DIRECTIONS:
Preheat the oven to 2000F.

Line a baking sheet with parchment paper.
In a bowl, toss all ingredients together to coat the apples.
Arrange the seasoned apple slices on the baking sheet.
Place in the oven and bake for 1 ½ hours until the apples are crispy.
Nutrition:
Calories 119, Total Fat 0.9g, Saturated Fat 0.4g, Total Carbs 31g, Net Carbs 23g, Protein 0.9g, Sugar: 19g, Fiber: 8g, Sodium: 3mg, Potassium 244mg

387) <u>Cranberry Pistachio Energy Bars</u>

PREPARATION TIME: 10 minutes
COOKING TIME: 20 minutes
SERVINGS: 5
INGREDIENTS:
1 cup uncooked rolled oat
¾ cup cooked quinoa
¾ cup dried cranberries, chopped
½ cup dry roasted pistachios
1/3 cup unsweetened coconut flakes
2 tablespoons flaxseed meal
1-ounce bittersweet chocolate, chopped
½ cup creamy almond butter
6 tablespoons honey
1 tablespoon olive oil
¼ teaspoon salt
DIRECTIONS:
Preheat the oven to 3500F.
Spread the oats and quinoa on a baking sheet and bake for 8 minutes until lightly browned.
Place the mixture in a bowl and add in the cranberries, pistachios, coconut flakes, flaxseed, and chocolate.
In a saucepan, combine the almond butter, honey, and olive oil. Mix over low heat for one minute.
Pour the butter mixture into the dry ingredients. Toss to coat.
Press the mixture into a baking dish.
Place the oven and bake for 15 minutes until lightly browned.
Nutrition:

Calories 487, Total Fat 27g, Saturated Fat 4g, Total Carbs 60g, Net Carbs 51g, Protein 13g, Sugar: 33g, Fiber: 9g, Sodium: 135mg, Potassium 550 mg

388) Orange Mango Gritty with Turmeric and Walnuts

PREPARATION TIME: 5 minutes
COOKING TIME: 0 minutes
SERVINGS: 2
INGREDIENTS:
¾ cup plain Greek yogurt
1 cup ice cubes
¾ cup chopped peeled ripe mango
½ cup fresh orange slices
¼ cup chopped toasted walnuts
¼ cup fresh orange juice
1 tablespoon ground flaxseed
2 teaspoons grated fresh turmeric
A dash of grated nutmeg
DIRECTIONS:
Place all ingredients in a blender and pulse until smooth.
Pour in glasses and serve chilled.
Nutrition:
Calories 245, Total Fat 13g, Saturated Fat 2.3g, Total Carbs 25g, Net Carbs 21g, Protein 11g, Sugar: 19g, Fiber: 4g, Sodium: 91mg, Potassium 731mg

389) Thai Sesame Edamame

PREPARATION TIME: 10 minutes
Cooking time:1 hour and 10 minutes
SERVINGS: 6
INGREDIENTS:
4 cups edamame pods
1 tablespoon dark sesame oil
1 tablespoon rice vinegar
1 teaspoon toasted sesame seeds
3 tablespoons water
½ teaspoon salt
½ teaspoon ground black pepper
DIRECTIONS:
Preheat the oven to 300ºF.

Line a baking sheet with aluminum foil. Set aside.
Place all ingredients in a bowl and toss to coat the edamame pods with the seasoning.
Arrange the seasoned edamame pods in the baking sheet.
Bake for 1 hour and 10 minutes until the pods are crispy.
Nutrition:
Calories 149, Total Fat 8g, Saturated Fat 0.9g, Total Carbs 10g, Net Carbs 5g, Protein 11g, Sugar: 2g, Fiber: 5g, Sodium:9 mg, Potassium 454mg

390) Sweet Potato Anti-Inflammatory Muffins

PREPARATION TIME: 15 minutes
COOKING TIME: 35 minutes
SERVINGS: 6
INGREDIENTS:
1 small sweet potato, cooked
1 egg, pasture-raised
¾ cup coconut milk
2 tablespoons olive oil
½ cup pure maple syrup
1 cup brown rice flour
¼ cup coconut flour
1 tablespoon baking powder
1 tablespoon ground cinnamon
1 teaspoon ground ginger
1 teaspoon ground turmeric
1/8 teaspoon ground cloves
1/8 teaspoon ground nutmeg
½ teaspoon salt
DIRECTIONS:
Preheat the oven to 400ºF.
Peel the cooked potato and place in a bowl. Mash gently with fork or masher.
Add in the eggs, coconut milk, olive oil, and maple syrup. Mix until well combined.
In a separate bowl, mix the rice flour, coconut flour, baking powder, cinnamon, ginger, turmeric, cloves, and nutmeg.
Gradually add the milk mixture into the flour mixture. Fold until well-combined.
Grease muffin cups then pour batter into the pan until ¾ full.

Bake in the oven for 35 minutes.
Nutrition:
Calories 311, Total Fat 14g, Saturated Fat 2g, Total Carbs 43g, Net Carbs 40g, Protein 5g, Sugar: 18g, Fiber: 3g, Sodium: 41mg, Potassium 329mg

391) **Beet Chips**

PREPARATION TIME: 10 minutes
COOKING TIME: 1 hour and 30 minutes
SERVINGS: 2
INGREDIENTS:
3 medium beets, peeled and sliced thinly
1 tablespoon olive oil
Salt to taste
DIRECTIONS:
Preheat the oven to 3500F.
Place all ingredients in a bowl and toss to coat.
Arrange the seasoned beet slices on a baking tray lined with aluminum foil.
Bake in the oven for 1 hour and 30 minutes.
Make sure to flip the beets halfway through the cooking time.
Nutrition:
Calories 120, Total Fat 7g, Saturated Fat 1g, Total Carbs 12g, Net Carbs 9g, Protein 2g, Sugar: 8g, Fiber: 3g, Sodium: 210mg, Potassium 921mg

Desserts

392) Dark Chocolate Almond Butter Crunch Balls

PREPARATION TIME: 15 minutes
COOKING TIME: 10 minutes
SERVINGS: 20
INGREDIENTS:
1 cup almond butter, organic and unsweetened
4 tablespoons raw honey
3 tablespoons coconut flour
6 tablespoons rolled oats
½ tablespoon coconut oil
¾ cup dark chocolate chips
DIRECTIONS:
In a bowl, mix the almond butter and honey until well combined.
Stir in the coconut flour and add oats. Season with salt to taste.
Shape into small balls and place in the fridge to allow to set.
Meanwhile, place the coconut oil in a double boiler and allow to melt. Add in the chocolate chips.
Once melted, dip the balls into the melted chocolate.
Place on a parchment lined tray and allow to set in the fridge for 20 minutes.
Nutrition:
Calories 141, Total Fat 9g, Saturated Fat 3g, Total Carbs 11g, Net Carbs 9g, Protein 4g, Sugar: 7g, Fiber: 2g, Sodium: 27mg, Potassium 321mg

393) Easy Peach Cobbler

PREPARATION TIME: 15 minutes
Cooking time:20 minutes
SERVINGS: 6
INGREDIENTS:
5 organic peaches, pitted and chopped
¼ cup coconut palm sugar, divided
½ teaspoon cinnamon
¾ cup chopped pecans
½ cup gluten-free oats
¼ cup ground flaxseeds
¼ brown rice flour
¼ cup extra virgin olive oil
DIRECTIONS:
Preheat the oven to 3500F.
Grease the bottom of 6 ramekins.
In a bowl, mix the peaches, ½ of the coconut sugar, cinnamon and pecans.
Distribute the peach mixture into the ramekins.
In the same bowl, mix the oats, flaxseed, rice flour, and oil. Add in the remaining coconut sugar. Mix until a crumbly texture is formed.
Top the mixture over the peaches.
Place for 20 minutes.
Nutrition:
Calories 266, Total Fat 11g, Saturated Fat 2g, Total Carbs 28g, Net Carbs 22 g, Protein 10g, Sugar: 12g, Fiber: 6g, Sodium: 127mg, Potassium 440mg

394) Avocado Chocolate Mousse

PREPARATION TIME: 10 minutes
COOKING TIME: 0 minutes
SERVINGS: 9
INGREDIENTS:
3 ripe avocado, pitted and flesh scooped out
6 ounces plain Greek yogurt
1 bar dark chocolate
1/8 cup unsweetened almond milk
¼ cup ground espresso beans
2 tablespoons raw honey
1 teaspoon vanilla extract
¼ cup cocoa powder
½ teaspoon salt
DIRECTIONS:
Place all ingredients in a food processor.
Pulse until smooth.
Chill in the fridge before serving.
Nutrition:
Calories 208, Total Fat 15g, Saturated Fat 4g, Total Carbs 17g, Net Carbs 11g, Protein 5g, Sugar: 8g, Fiber: 6g, Sodium: 16mg, Potassium 500mg

395) Anti-Inflammatory Easy Brownies

PREPARATION TIME: 15 minutes
COOKING TIME: 35 minutes
SERVINGS: 12
INGREDIENTS:
¼ cup ground flaxseed meal
½ cup almond butter
1 ½ cups raw honey
1 teaspoon vanilla extract
¾ cup cocoa powder
1 cup almond flour
1 teaspoon baking powder
¾ cup water
½ teaspoon salt
DIRECTIONS:
Preheat the oven to 3500F.
In a bowl, mix the flaxseed meal and water. Set aside for 5 minutes.
In a bigger bowl, combine the almond butter, honey, and vanilla extract. Stir to combine.
In another bowl, combine the cocoa powder, almond flour, baking powder, and salt.
Gradually add the wet ingredients to the dry ingredients. Fold until well combined.
Transfer the batter into greased baking pan and spread evenly.
Bake for 35 minutes or until the sides are coming away from the pan.
Allow to cool before slicing.
Nutrition:
Calories 225, Total Fat 8g, Saturated Fat 1g, Total Carbs 41g, Net Carbs 37g, Protein 4g, Sugar: 36g, Fiber: 4g, Sodium: 27mg, Potassium 265mg

396) Banana Coconut Foster

PREPARATION TIME: 5 minutes
COOKING TIME: 1 hour and 30 minutes
SERVINGS: 6
INGREDIENTS:
10 small cooking bananas, peeled and sliced into quarters
½ cup chopped walnuts
1 cup coconut flakes
1 teaspoon cinnamon
¼ cup honey
½ cup coconut oil, melted
2 teaspoons lemon zest
¼ cup lemon juice
1 teaspoon vanilla extract
Coconut cream for serving
DIRECTIONS:
Place the bananas in a slow cooker and top with walnuts and coconuts.
In a bowl, combine the cinnamon, honey, coconut oil, lemon zest, lemon juice, and vanilla extract.
Pour the wet mixture over the bananas.
Cook for 1 ½ hour in the slow cooker until the bananas are tender.
Serve with coconut cream on top.
Nutrition:
Calories 463, Total Fat 27g, Saturated Fat 5g, Total Carbs 60g, Net Carbs 53g, Protein 3g, Sugar: 38g, Fiber:7 g, Sodium:43 mg, Potassium 706mg

397) Antioxidant Chocolate Bites

PREPARATION TIME: 40 minutes
COOKING TIME: 0 minutes
SERVINGS: 6
INGREDIENTS:
½ cup organic unrefined coconut oil
½ cup organic and unsweetened cocoa powder
½ cup organic maple syrup
1 teaspoon vanilla
¼ cup crushed macadamia nuts
¼ cup shredded coconut flakes
¼ cup goji berries
DIRECTIONS:
In a stove, melt the coconut oil. Set aside.
Put the cocoa powder, maple syrup, vanilla, and melted coconut. Blend well.
Pour into a bowl. Add in the rest of the ingredients.
Mix to combine and form small balls using your hands.
Allow to chill before serving.
Nutrition:

149

Calories 303, Total Fat 24g, Saturated Fat 5g, Total Carbs 24g, Net Carbs 21g, Protein 2g, Sugar: 18g, Fiber: 3g, Sodium: 15mg, Potassium 270mg

398) Anti-Inflammatory Apricot Squares

PREPARATION TIME: 60 minutes
COOKING TIME: 0 minutes
SERVINGS: 8
INGREDIENTS:
1 cup dried shredded coconut
1 cup dried apricot, chopped
1 cup raw macadamia nuts, chopped
1 tablespoons coconut oil, melted
1/3 cup turmeric powder
1 teaspoon vanilla extract
DIRECTIONS:
Combine all ingredients in a food processor until slightly smooth.
Pour mixture into a square pan and press evenly.
Refrigerate for an hour before cutting into squares.
Nutrition:
Calories 201, Total Fat 15g, Saturated Fat 4g, Total Carbs 18g, Net Carbs 14g, Protein 3g, Sugar: 11g, Fiber: 4g, Sodium: 36mg, Potassium 455mg

399) Anti-Inflammatory Lemon Pudding

PREPARATION TIME: 60 minutes
COOKING TIME: 5minutes
SERVINGS: 6
INGREDIENTS:
2 tablespoons agar flakes
1 cup organic yogurt
½ cup flax oil
¾ cup softened coconut butter
Zest from 3 lemons
1 tablespoon vanilla extract
2 tablespoons coconut oil, melted
½ teaspoon ground cardamom
½ cup raw honey
¼ cup water

1/8 teaspoon salt
DIRECTIONS:
Heat water in a saucepan until it boils. Remove from the heat and add the agar flakes. Turn on the heat and boil until agar dissolves. Set aside.
In a small bowl, mix everything until well combined.
Pour into glasses.
Place in the fridge to set before serving.
Nutrition:
Calories 521, Total Fat 47g, Saturated Fat 5g, Total Carbs 26g, Net Carbs 25.9g, Protein 2g, Sugar: 25g, Fiber: 0.1g, Sodium: 94mg, Potassium 203mg

400) Rustic Flourless Strawberry and Chocolate Cake

PREPARATION TIME: 10 minutes
COOKING TIME: 40 minutes
SERVINGS: 1
INGREDIENTS:
1 egg, pasture raised
2 teaspoons cocoa unsweetened
¼ cup coconut sugar
1 ½ tablespoons pecans, ground
1ounce bittersweet chocolate, melted
1 cup strawberries, hulled
1 tablespoon water
DIRECTIONS:
Preheat the oven to 3500F.
Line a baking pan with parchment paper.
Combine all ingredients in a food processor and pulse until smooth.
Place in a small baking dish and tap the bottom to release air.
Bake in the oven for 30 to 40 minutes or until a toothpick inserted in the middle comes out clean.
Nutrition:
Calories 434, Total Fat 19g, Saturated Fat 4g, Total Carbs 59g, Net Carbs 53g, Protein 12g, Sugar: 47g, Fiber: 6g, Sodium:166 mg, Potassium 571mg

401) Raw Black Forest Brownies

PREPARATION TIME: 2 hours and 10 minutes
COOKING TIME: 0 minutes
SERVINGS: 6
INGREDIENTS:
1 ½ cups dried cherries, pitted and chopped
2 cups walnuts, copped
1 cup raw cacao powder
½ cup dates, pitted
½ cup almonds, chopped
¼ teaspoon salt
DIRECTIONS:
Put all ingredients in a food processor.
Pulse until small crumbs are formed.
Press the brownie batter in a pan and freeze for two hours.
Slice before serving.
Nutrition:
Calories 294, Total Fat 18g, Saturated Fat 2g, Total Carbs 33g, Net Carbs 26g, Protein 7g, Sugar: 14g, Fiber: 6g, Sodium: 18mg, Potassium 440mg

402) Anti-Inflammatory Spice Cookies

PREPARATION TIME: 15 minutes
Cooking time:15 to 20 minutes

SERVINGS: 18
INGREDIENTS:
8 tablespoons coconut butter
3 eggs, pasture raised
2/3 cup coconut sugar
1 tablespoon blackstrap molasses
1 tablespoon ground turmeric
1 tablespoon ground ginger
2 teaspoons ground cinnamon
5 drops orange essential oil or ½ teaspoon orange extract
½ teaspoon baking soda
1 ½ cups cassava flour
1 tablespoon black pepper
½ teaspoon salt
DIRECTIONS:
Preheat the oven to 3500F.
Line a baking sheet with parchment paper.
In a mixing bowl, combine the coconut butter, eggs, coconut sugar, and molasses. Stir until well-combined.
Stir in the rest of the ingredients. Mix until well-combined.
Pour into the prepared baking sheet.
Use a spoon to scoop a tablespoon of the batter and place on the baking sheet.
Bake for 15 to 20 minutes until golden brown.
Nutrition:
Calories 115, Total Fat 7g, Saturated Fat 4g, Total Carbs 12g, Net Carbs 11.5g, Protein 2g, Sugar: 5g, Fiber: 0.5g, Sodium: 96mg, Potassium 108mg

4-Week Meal Plan

DAY	BREAKFAST	MAIN	DESSERT
1.	Rhubarb Vanilla Muffins	Poached Cod	Dark Chocolate Almond Butter Crunch Balls
2.	Winter Fruit Salad	Beans and Cauliflower Stew	Easy Peach Cobbler
3.	Cocoa Buckwheat Granola	Squash and Chickpea Stew	Avocado Chocolate Mousse
4.	Mushroom Frittata	Chicken Salad	Anti-Inflammatory Easy Brownies
5.	Almond Breakfast Crepes	Zucchini Mix	Banana Coconut Foster
6.	Millet Muffins	Spicy Cauliflower Stew	Antioxidant Chocolate Bites
7.	Kale and Pears Smoothie	Green Bean Mix	Anti-Inflammatory Apricot Squares
8.	Apple Muesli	Chickpea Stew	Spiced Apples and Raisins
9.	Veggie Mix	Spicy Eggplant Stew	Mango Turmeric Chia Pudding
10.	Sweet Potato Cakes	Turkey Burgers	Date Brownies
11.	Green Salad with Pine Nuts	Veggie and Egg Burrito Bowls	Mixed Berry Crumb Cake
12.	Bean Sprout Breakfast Salad	Lemony Lentil Soup	Healthy Chocolate Bread
13.	Breakfast Beef Casserole	Chard Soup	Anti-Inflammatory Lemon Pudding
14.	Seafood Omelette	Black Rice with Hemp Seeds Mix	Rustic Flourless Strawberry and Chocolate Cake
15.	Nutritious Avocado Smoothie	Shrimp Stir-Fry	Raw Black Forest Brownies
16.	Coconut Porridge	Veggie Tangine	Raw Carrot Cake
17.	Brussel Sprout Eggs	Mushroom and Tomato Cream	Sweet Potato Brownie
18.	Morning Fritters	Tomato Cream with Celery	Anti-Inflammatory Spice Cookies
19.	Egg Muffins	Grape Gazpacho	Tropical Fruit Parfaits
20.	Avocado Eggs in Bacon	Garlic Mushroom Cream	Dark Chocolate Almond Butter Crunch Balls
21.	Kale Egg Ramekins	Creamy Asparagus Soup	Easy Peach Cobbler

22.	Broccoli Muffins	Greek Sea Bass Mix	Avocado Chocolate Mousse
23.	Breakfast Chai Latte	Black Beans Chili	Anti-Inflammatory Easy Brownies
24.	Cauliflower-Meat Skillet	Black Bean and Corn Soup	Banana Coconut Foster
25.	Croque Madame	Barley Soup with Mushrooms	Antioxidant Chocolate Bites
26.	Stuffed Avocado	Spicy Sweet Potato Soup	Anti-Inflammatory Apricot Squares
27.	Fruit and Veggie Mix	Beet and Carrot Soup	Spiced Apples and Raisins
28.	Rosemary Oats	Turkey Soup	Mango Turmeric Chia Pudding
29.	Garlic Swiss Chard Bowls	Spicy Chicken and Zucchini Meatballs	Date Brownies
30.	Breakfast Pizza	Crispy Cod	Mixed Berry Crumb Cake

Conclusion

Thank you for making it to the end of Anti-Inflammatory Diet. Let's hope it was informative and able to provide you with all of the tools you need to achieve your goals whatever it is that they may be. This book provided a lot of information about a nutritious diet that will provide many health benefits and may even save someone's life. It is up to you if you would like to follow it in order to live a healthier lifestyle to prevent chronic illnesses and have a better quality of life.

Quality of life is what we are promoting the most with the anti-inflammatory diet. The next step is to start using the information presented in this book and begin incorporating it into your everyday life. We spoke extensively in this eBook about the inflammatory disease and how to prevent or resolve it with a proper diet.

The anti-inflammatory diet will provide you with nutritious and delicious meals. Include it in your own meal prep and create a daily, weekly, or monthly meal schedule so you can stay ahead of the game. Avoiding serious health consequences is an important part of living a long and productive life. A proper diet is instrumental in creating that life for all of us. We know that we were oftentimes blunt when going over information in this book. But we want to make sure people understand the risks of inflammatory disease and the importance of an anti-inflammatory diet.

If you write it down, you are more likely to do it. You are more likely to do something if you get some type of enjoyment out of it. Enjoy it then. Try the recipes in this book, get creative with your own recipes, do even more research, and just have fun eating great food. It may seem like a chore at first. Change is never easy, but oftentimes, it is for the better, especially with matters regarding our health. Chronic inflammatory disease is no laughing matter. It is a disease that causes much suffering and can lead to many health problems down the line. Avoid these at all costs by sticking to an anti-inflammatory diet. The benefits will be tremendous.

Lightning Source UK Ltd.
Milton Keynes UK
UKHW030803100521
383461UK00013B/867

9 781802 671131

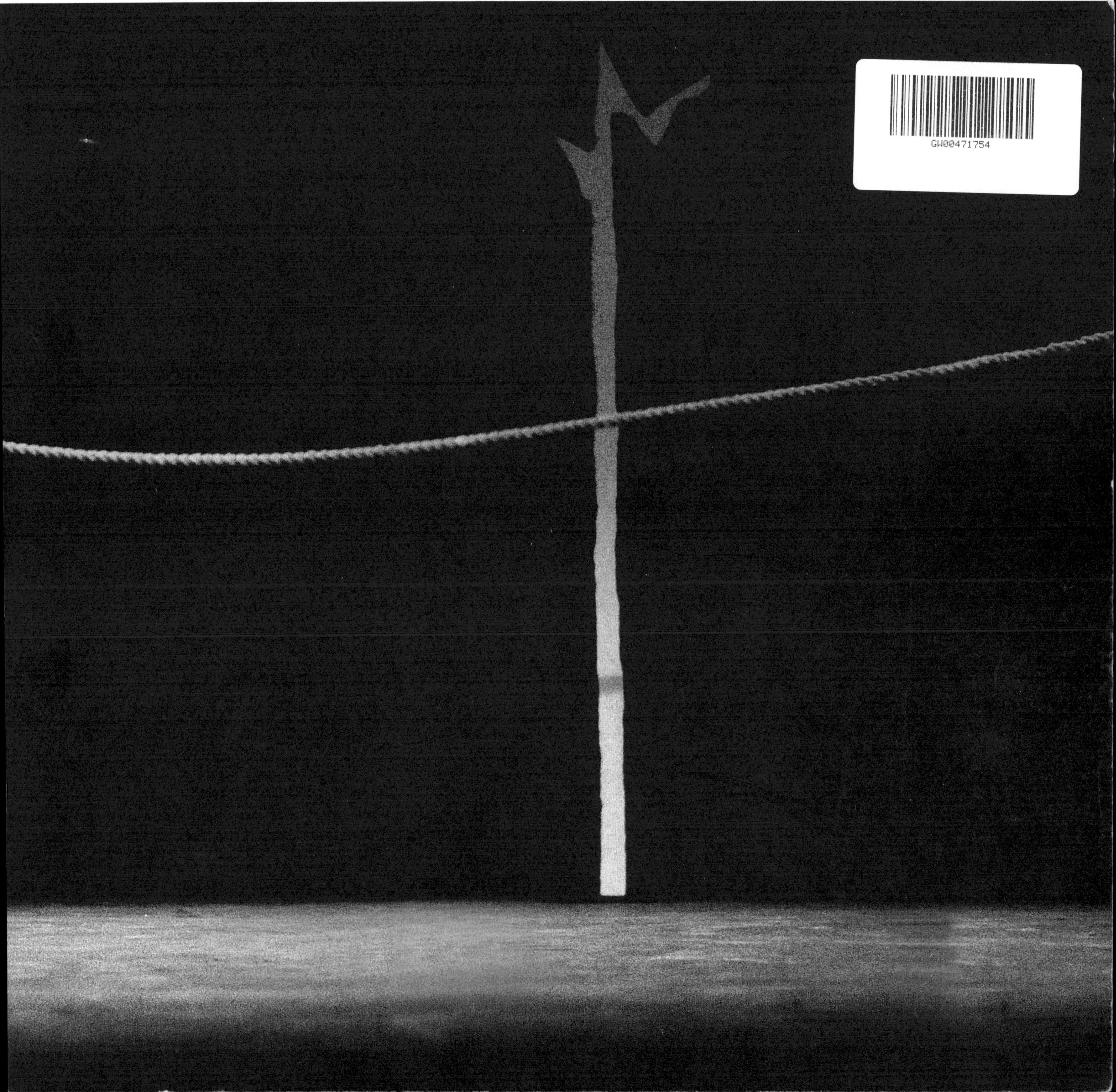

Tom Lawlor At the Gate

Tom Lawlor at the Gate

First published in 1997 by Design Inc, Killegar House, Carrigallen, Co Leitrim

By kind permission of the Gate Theatre

Photographs © Tom Lawlor 1985-1997

Editorial advisor: Marie Rooney

Design: Tony Fahy

Printed in Ireland by Inkspot

Reproduction by: Irish Platemaking Services

ISBN 0 9531452 0 4

Design Inc would like to thank the Leitrim County Enterprise Board and John Kilbracken for their support

www.designinc.ie

Opposite: **Olwen Fouéré** as **Salomé** in *Salomé* by **Oscar Wilde**
Endpapers: **Stephen Brennan** as **Lucky** and **Alan Stanford** as **Pozzo** in *Waiting for Godot* by **Samuel Beckett**

tom Lawlor
at the gate

COMMEMORATING
TOM LAWLOR'S PHOTOGRAPHS AT
THE GATE THEATRE, DUBLIN, IRELAND

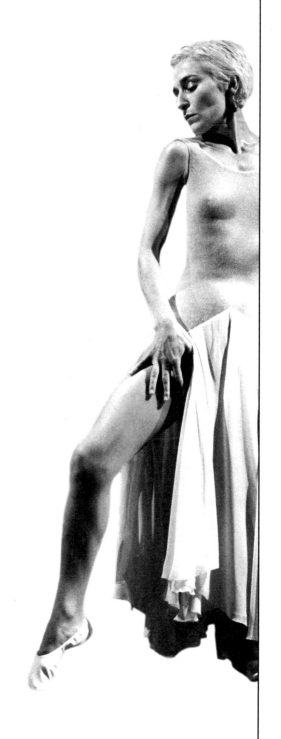

PUBLISHED BY DESIGN INC

For Fran, Jenny and Deirdre

For detailed captions to all the photographs, see end of book, pages 135-139

foreword

michael colgan DIRECTOR, GATE THEATRE

Good theatre comes from creating moments, and good photography from capturing them.

These photographs were taken at the Gate over the twelve years since 1985 and I was privileged, simply by being there a lot, to witness many special moments. But theatre is ephemeral, and even now some are only half-remembered, and some may be forgotten. Still, there are few that will never go away and thankfully, because of Tom Lawlor and this collection, we now have a record that can never be lost.

It is a record that presents striking images with technical brilliance and all of us—actors, directors, designers—are happy in the knowledge that there will always remain this lasting evidence of the work we did.

I am grateful to Marie Rooney for her inspiration and persuasion in getting Tom into our theatre, and I will always be grateful to him, not only for his art, but for the sensitivity with which he creates it.

The Gate Theatre is proud to be associated with this collection of Tom Lawlor's remarkable work.

introduction

Joe Dowling ARTISTIC DIRECTOR, THE GUTHRIE THEATRE, MINNEAPOLIS, USA

If, as some cultures suggest, the camera steals the soul of those it photographs, it also has the power to illuminate its deeper recesses and explore emotional responses in a more immediate way than any other form of communication. A great photographer not only captures a particular moment forever but also helps us witness the human spirit in all its forms. While words can reflect a more complex and layered human response, a good photograph cuts to the emotional quick and reveals lasting truths in moments of joy or sorrow. We use photographs to evoke memories of people long gone and places well forgotten. They can also startle us with the frozen image of ourselves looking like other people! The yellowing album in the attic, with portraits of fashions that now make us laugh or cringe, forces us to accept the unrelenting march of time more completely than any mirror.

A posed photograph from a distant time tells only part of the story. The formal wedding picture, a reminder of a special day, often looks stilted and unnatural because the focus of our attention is the camera. We strain to make this a significant moment in our lives and memory. It is no coincidence that the best photos are taken when the subject is unaware of the camera and when the focus is on something other than being recorded for posterity.

This is specially true of the theatre photograph. When theatre photos are set up in a formal way, with actors conscious of performing for the camera, they look mummified and the production seems utterly devoid of vitality and personality. The very act of photographing a scene from a play can kill it and reduce the immediacy of the experience unless the actors perform unaware of the clicking camera. The art of theatrical photography is a special skill, The great theatre photographers always shoot during a dress rehearsal or performance. In this way, the action of the scene is preserved and, often, great photos are produced.

Directors and actors greatly appreciate the skill of the photographer who, against the very nature of theatre itself, can preserve the essence of our work for future generations. Theatre is a wholly ephemeral art. That is its attraction. Unless you are actually in the room sharing in the event, you can never know the power of the moment or the electricity of the atmosphere. Filming the event can create a false sense of the power of the moment because acting for film is so different from acting on the stage. A dramatic photograph is often the most important record of a special theatrical moment. It can be cherished both by those who created the magic and by those who witnessed it.

To capture that split second when theatrical alchemy happens requires a particular skill and a real sensitivity to the human beings onstage. Tom Lawlor is a leader in the field. He possesses both the talent and the humanity that are hallmarks of a great photographer. His Gate Theatre pictures will have a resonance for many beyond the pages of this book. They serve as memories, as reminders of achievements, a record of triumphs and disappointments. Above all, they celebrate the diversity and quality of the Gate Theatre under Michael Colgan's inspired leadership.

Tom Lawlor brings to his theatrical work the same focus and concentration that he brought to his award-winning journalistic career. When following a story for a newspaper, the photographer has to be a master of timing, Blink and the moment will be lost. The same focus is required during a dress rehearsal. An actor moves in a particular way and makes a gesture that holds for only a second. A good photographer knows instinctively when to move in and capture the gesture or reaction. Often during a Gate dress rehearsal, I have watched Tom move around the theatre with stealth and purpose, as a predator sizes up his prey. He follows the scene with acute interest and concentration and, seizing his moment with the accuracy of a master hunter, he captures the perfect image, which, for all time, reflects the actors' spontaneous creativity.

One of the qualities that make Tom a great theatre photographer is his sense of humour. As a production nears its public unveiling, actors and directors sink into wells of insecurity. The final dress rehearsal is a particularly tense time. One of my favourite sounds is that of Tom Lawlor's infectious laugh rising up from the darkness as he clicks away happily. Before critics or word-of-mouth, his approval is needed. Tom Lawlor is a true artist whose contribution to the theatre in Ireland will be a lasting one. This collection, which so magnificently records and immortalizes great actors and performances, is a treasured testimonial to a remarkable time in the history of the Gate Theatre and to the continuing vitality of our art form.

Johnny Murphy as **Estragon** in *Waiting for Godot* by **Samuel Beckett**

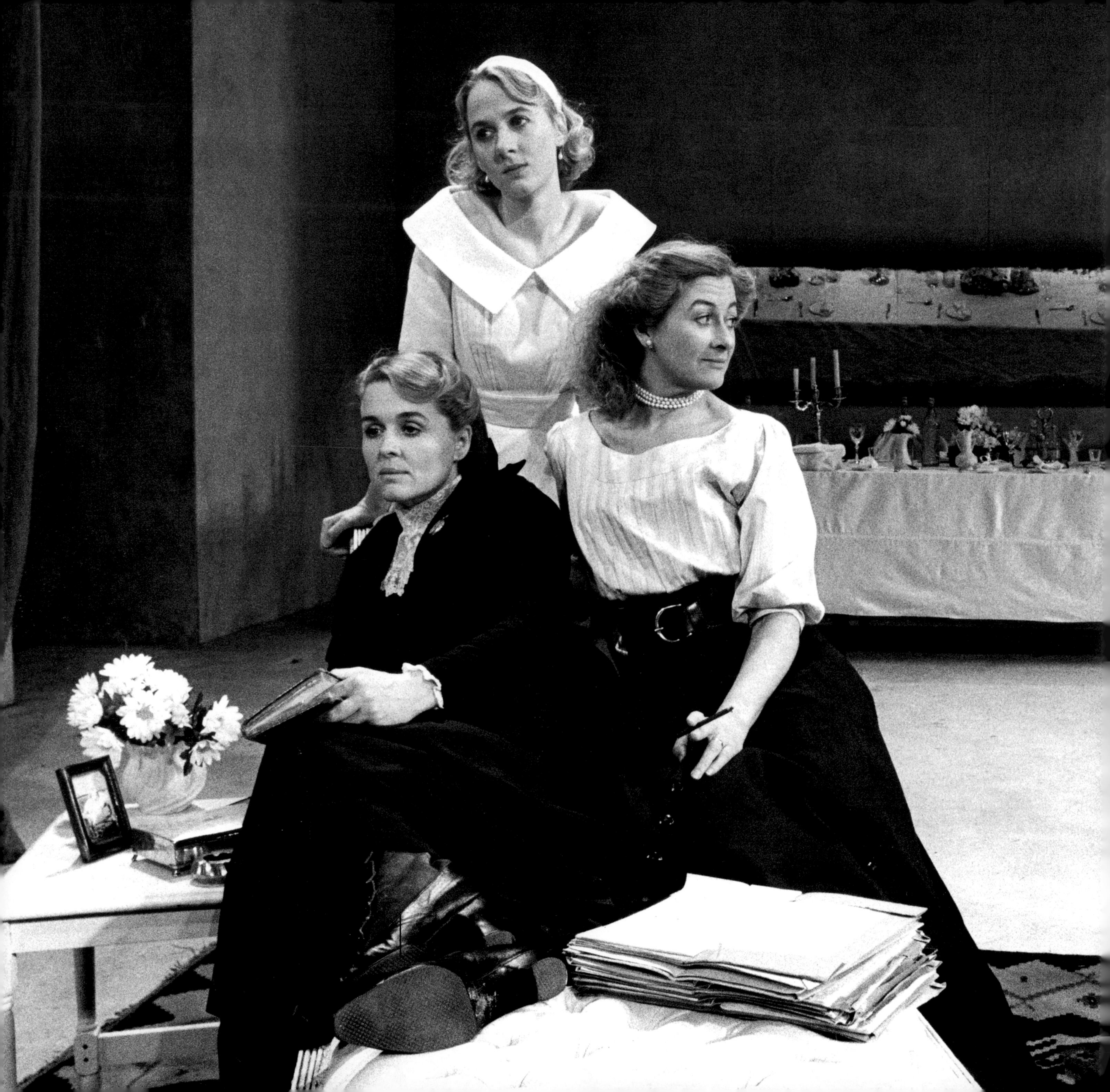

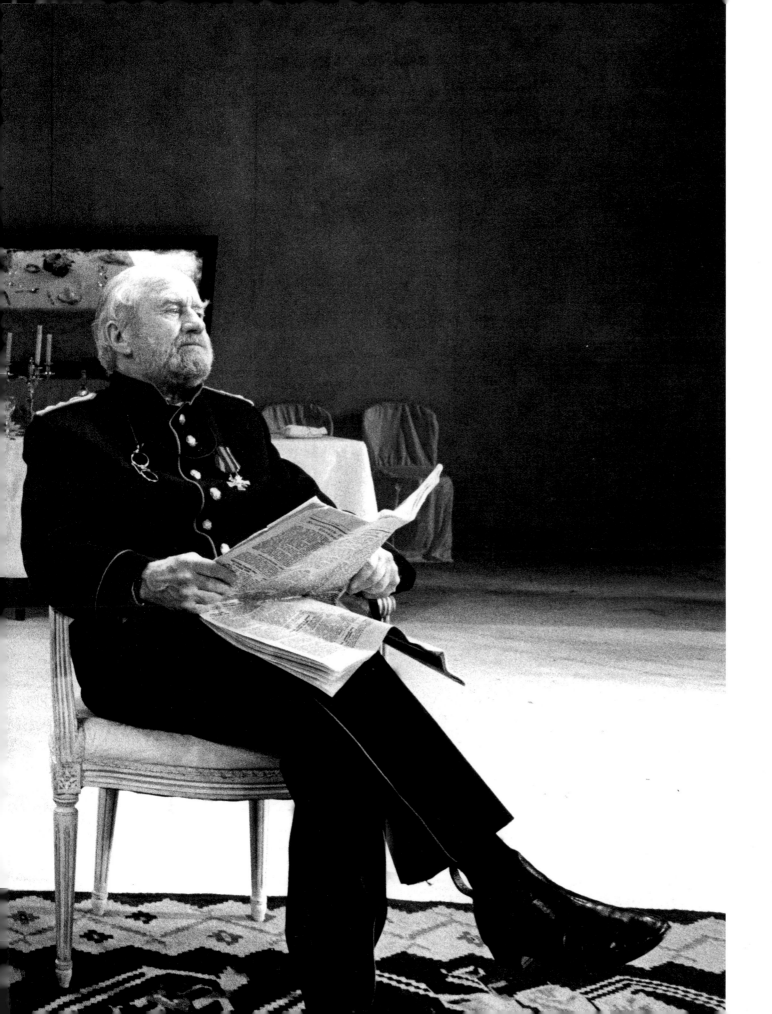

Sinéad Cusack as **Masha**, Niamh Cusack as **Irina**, Sorcha Cusack as **Olga**, Cyril Cusack as **Chebutykin** in *Three Sisters* by **Anton Chekhov** in a version by **Frank McGuinness**

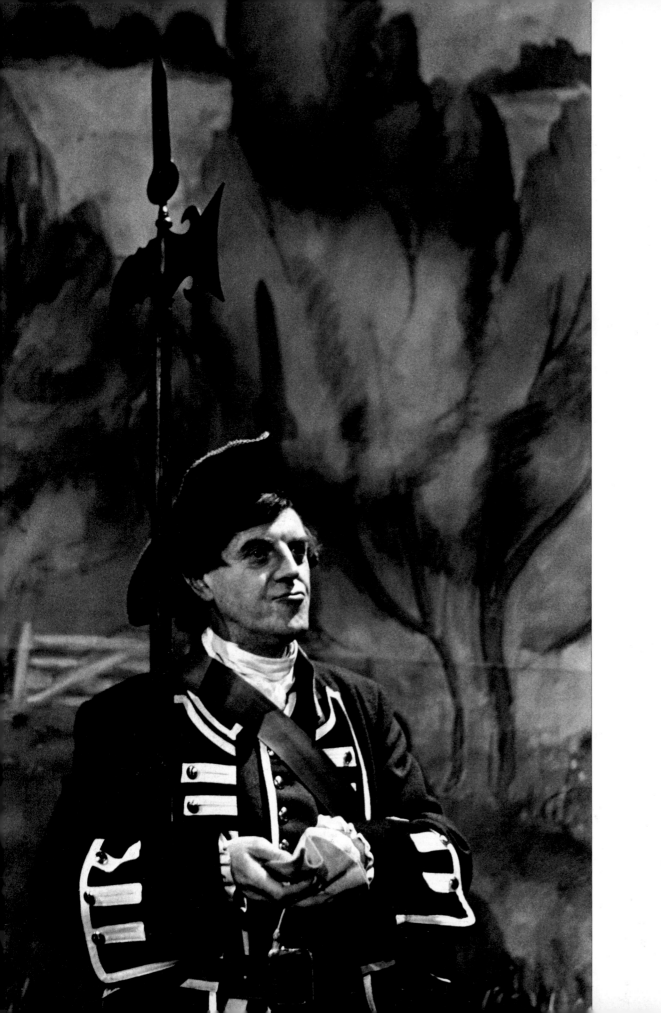

Eamon Morrissey as **Kite** in *The Recruiting Officer* by George Farquhar

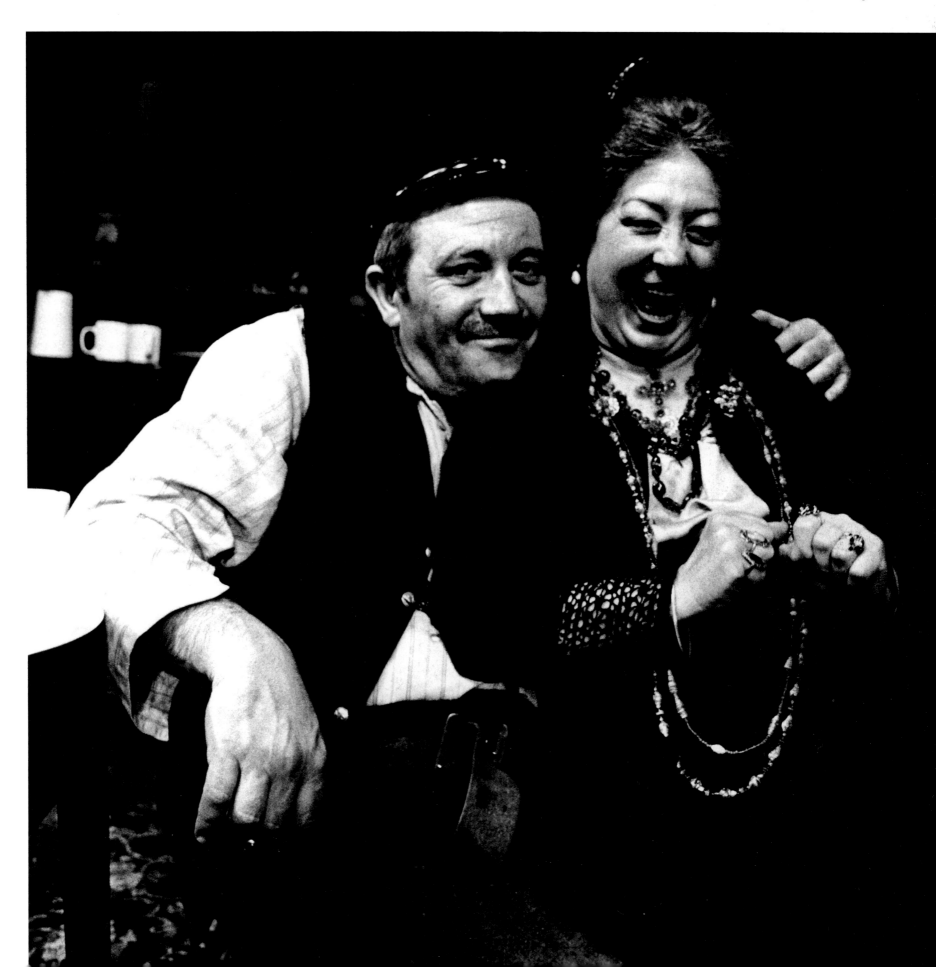

Donal McCann as **Captain Jack Boyle**, Maureen Potter as **Maisie Madigan** in *Juno and the Paycock* by **Sean O'Casey**

John Kavanagh as *Joxer Daly* in *Juno and the Paycock* by **Sean O'Casey**

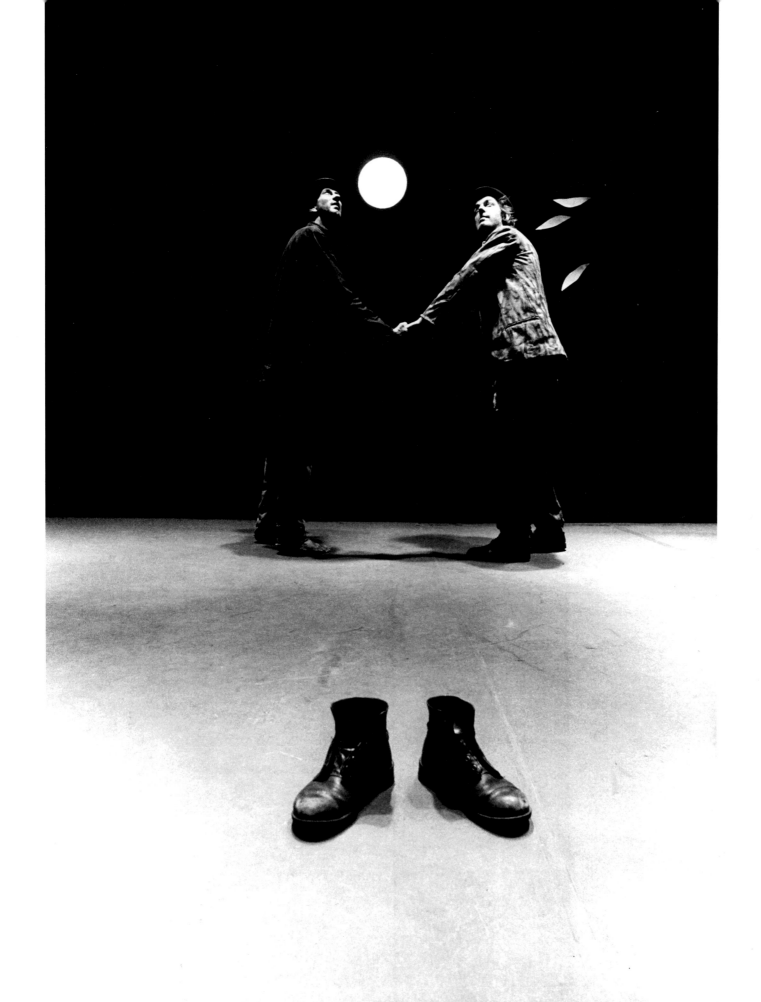

Barry McGovern as Estragon, Tom Hickey as Vladimir in *Waiting for Godot* by Samuel Beckett

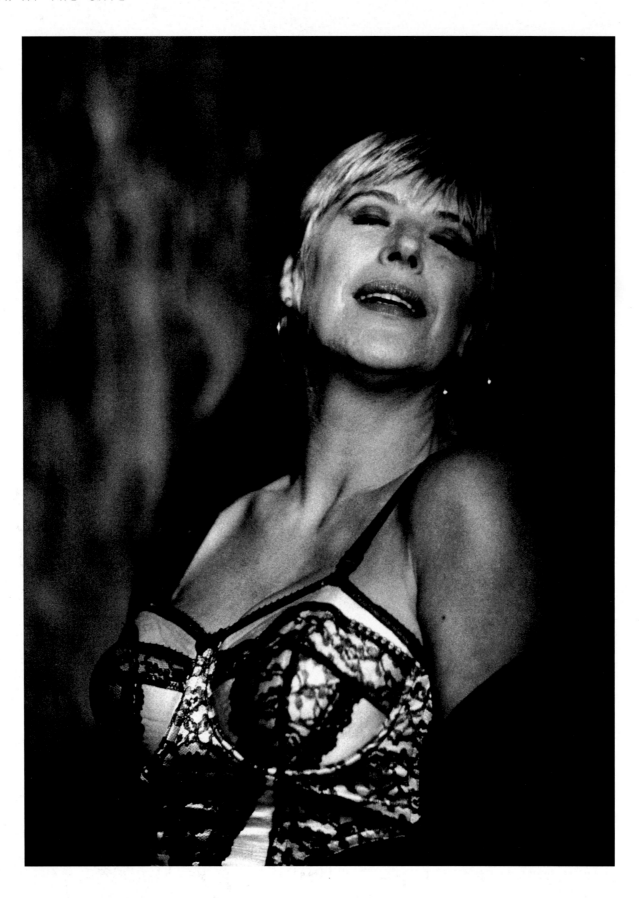

Marianne Faithfull as **Pirate Jenny** in *The Threepenny Opera* by **Bertolt Brecht** and **Kurt Weill** in a version by **Frank McGuinness**

Peter Holmes as **Antonio** in *Innocence, The Life of Caravaggio* by **Frank McGuinness**

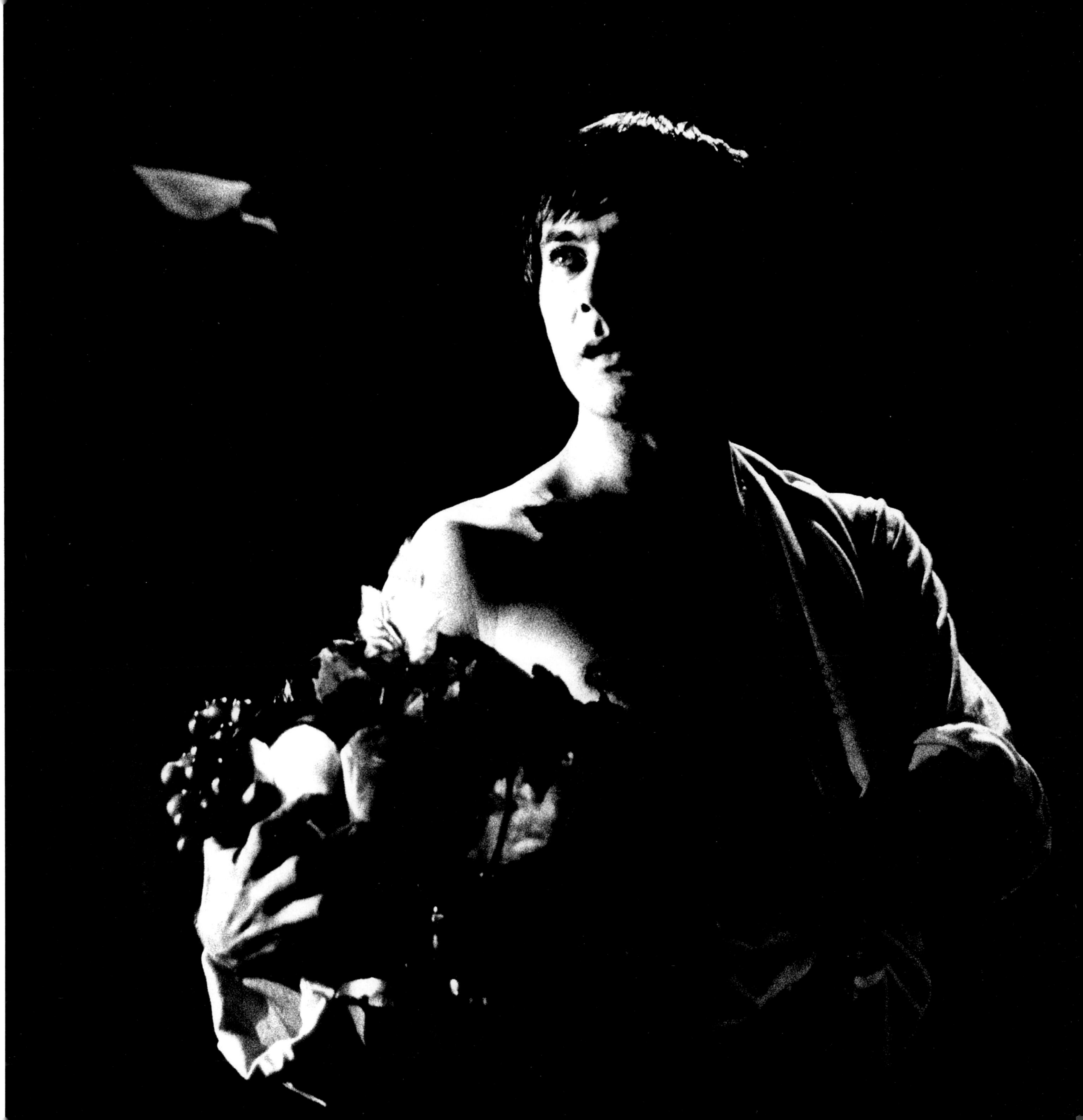

David Kelly as Al Lewis, Milo O'Shea as Willie Clark in *The Sunshine Boys* by Neil Simon

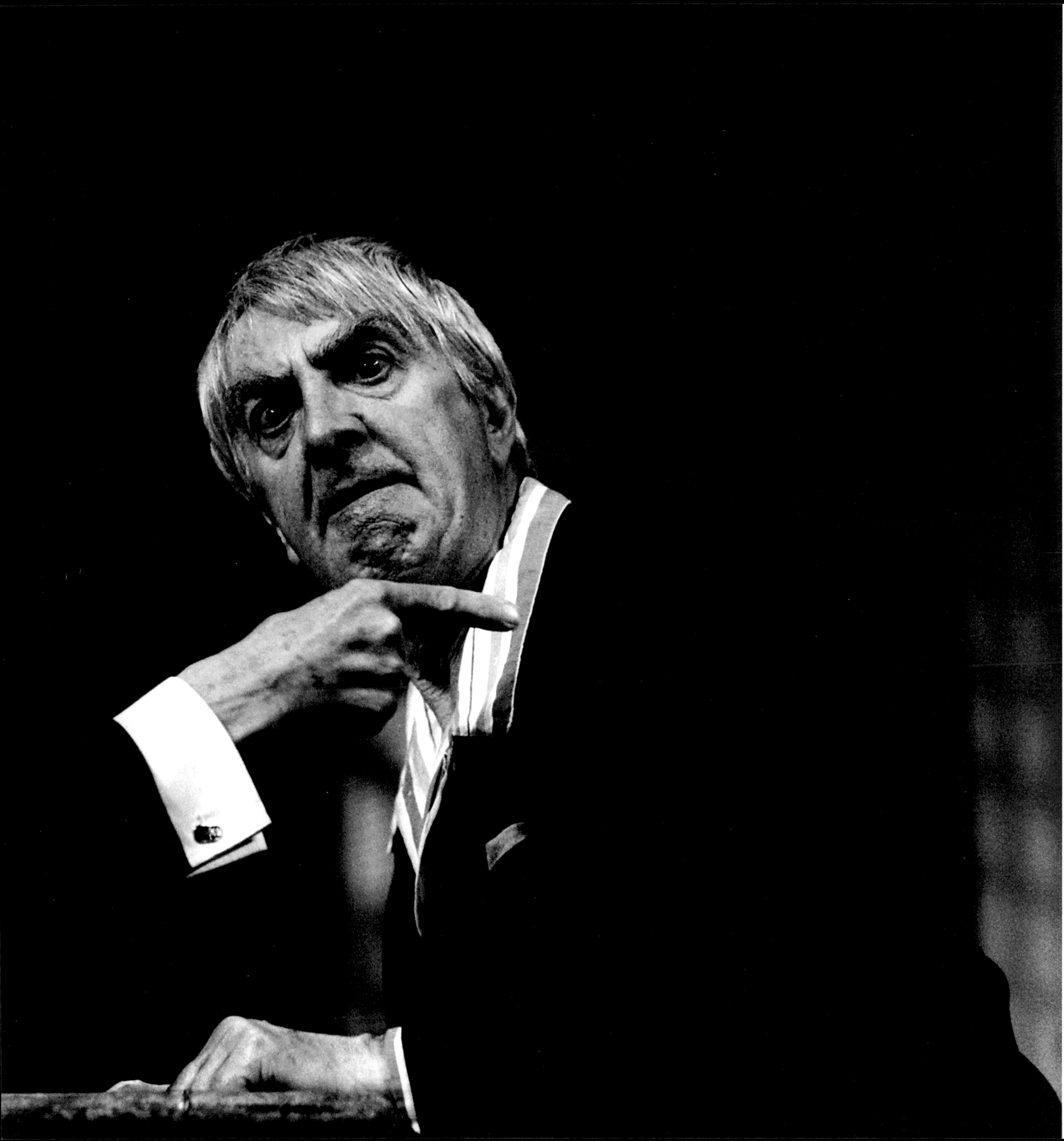

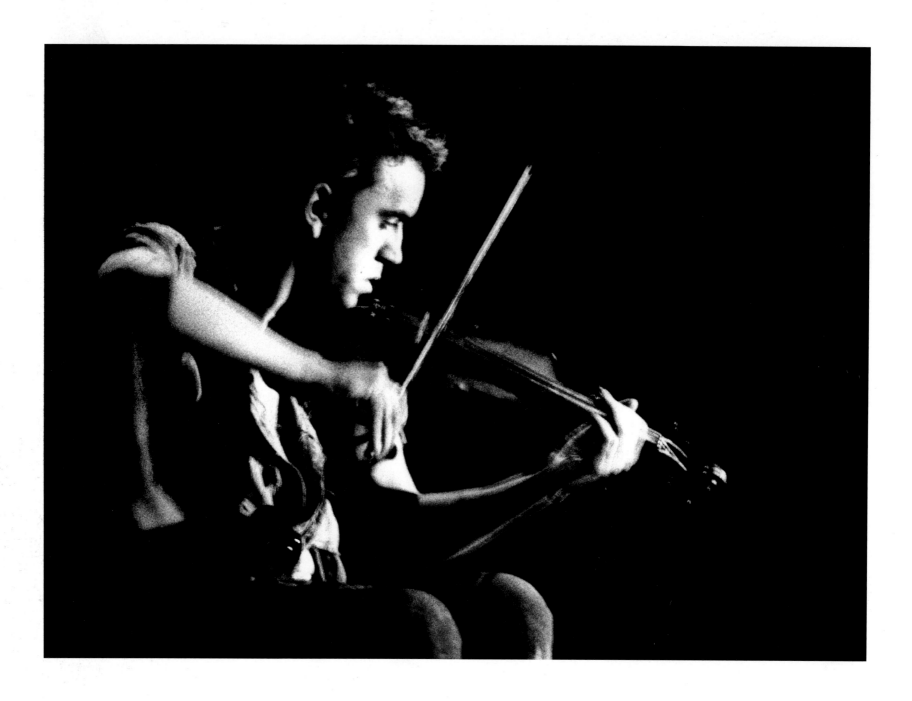

Phelim Drew as **A** in *Rough for Theatre I* by **Samuel Beckett**

Olwen Fouéré as **Salomé** in *Salomé* by **Oscar Wilde**

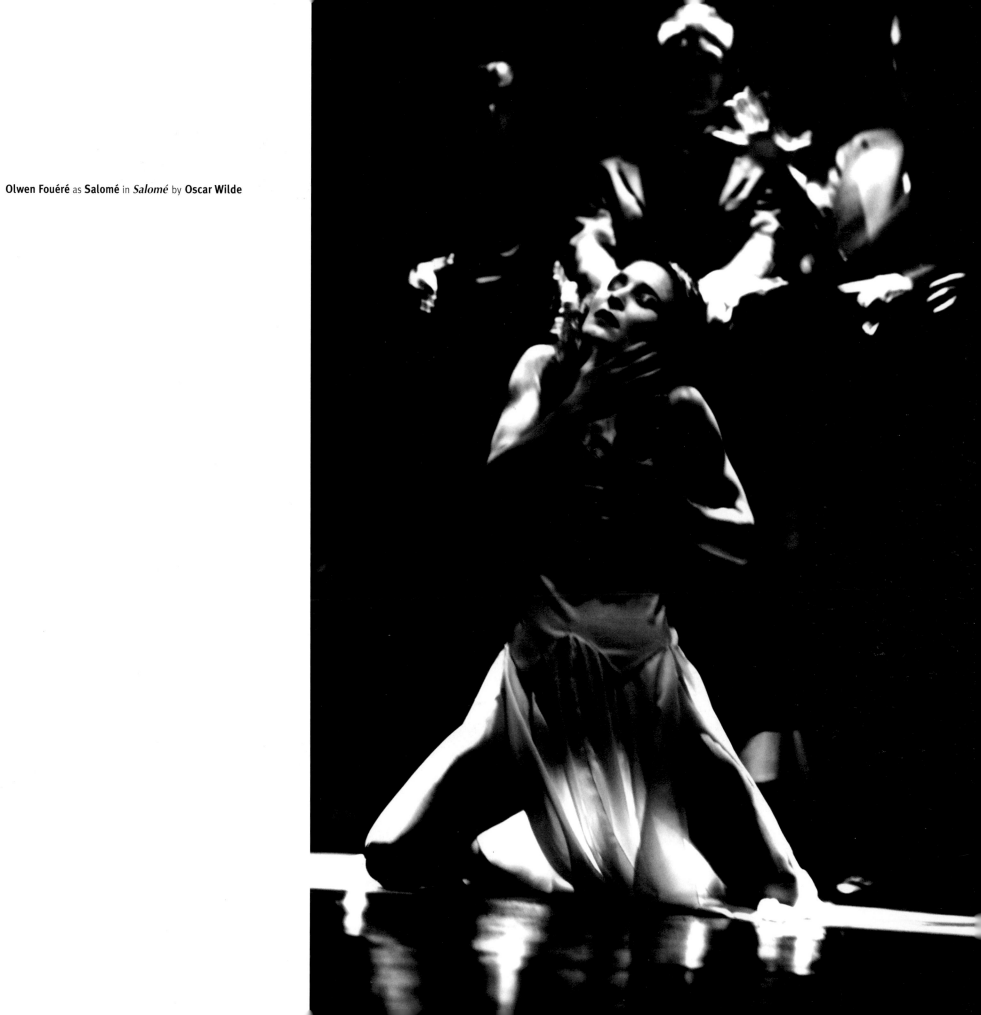

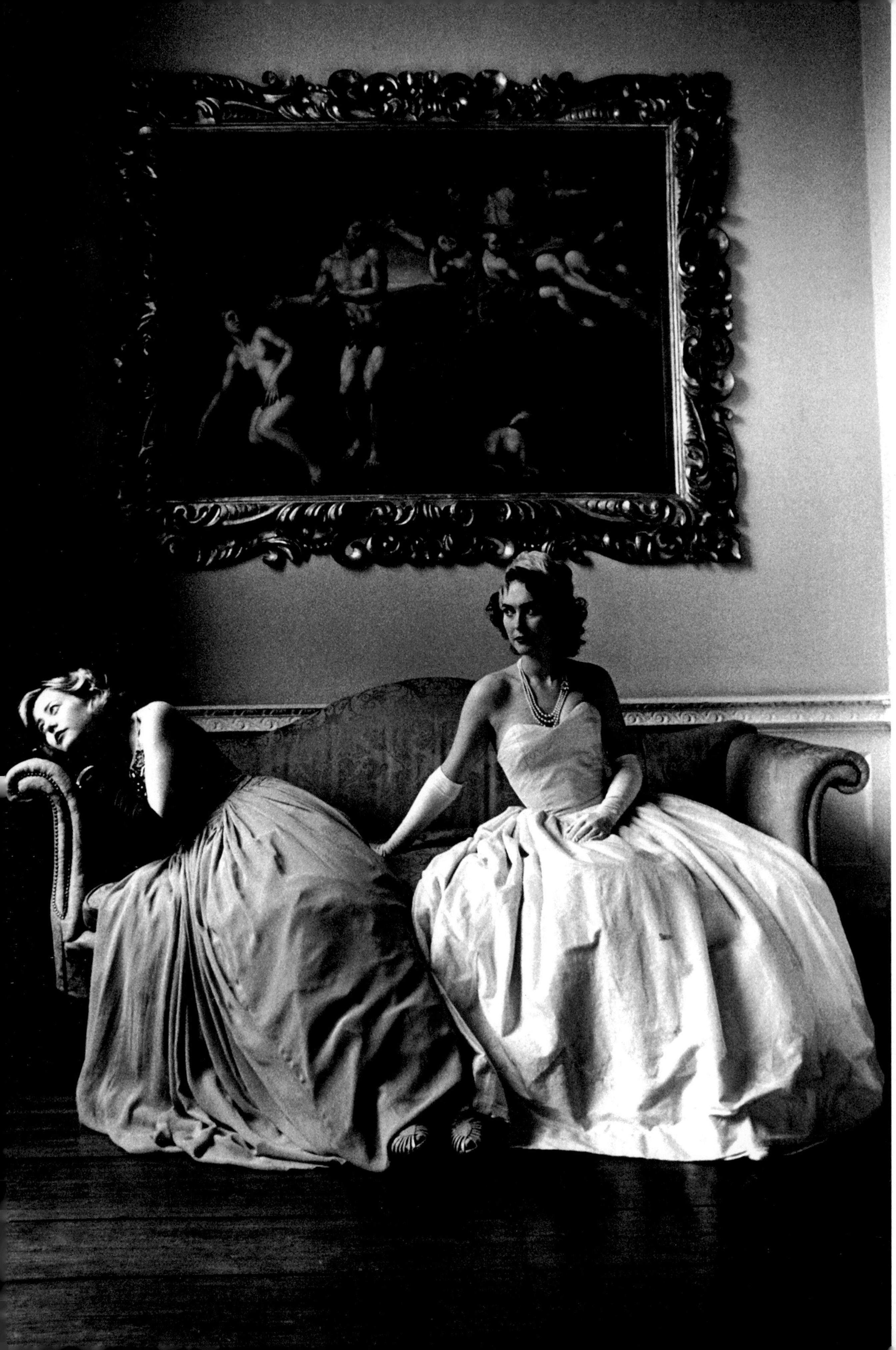

Angela Crowe as **Miss Graham, Sharon Devlin** as **Lady Stutfield** in ***Lady Windermere's Fan*** by **Oscar Wilde**

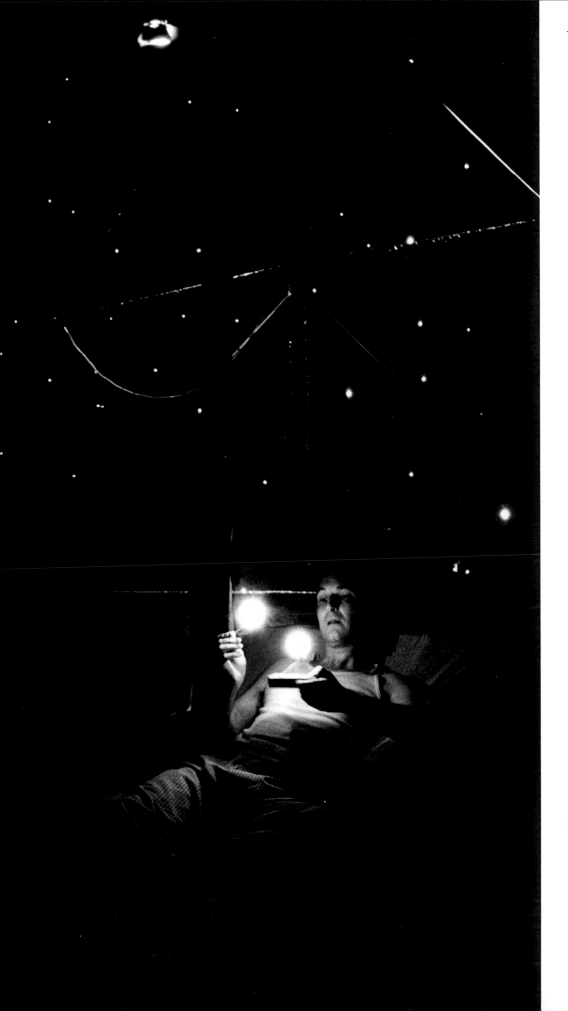

Donal O'Kelly in *Catalpa* by **Donal O'Kelly**

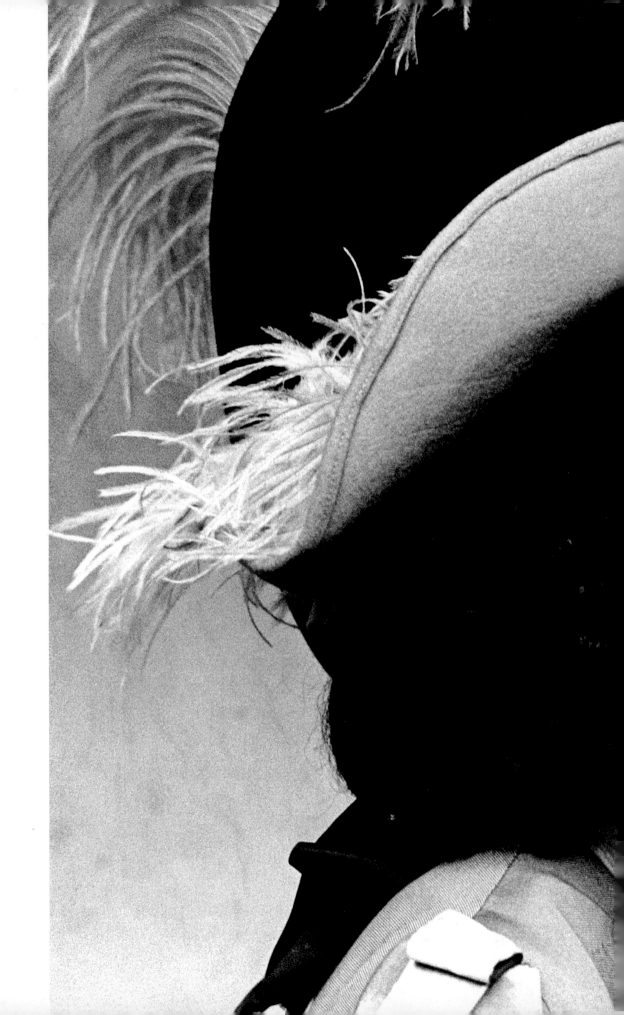

Barbara Brennan as **Silvia**, **Ian McElhinney** as **Captain Plume** in *The Recruiting Officer* by **George Farquhar**

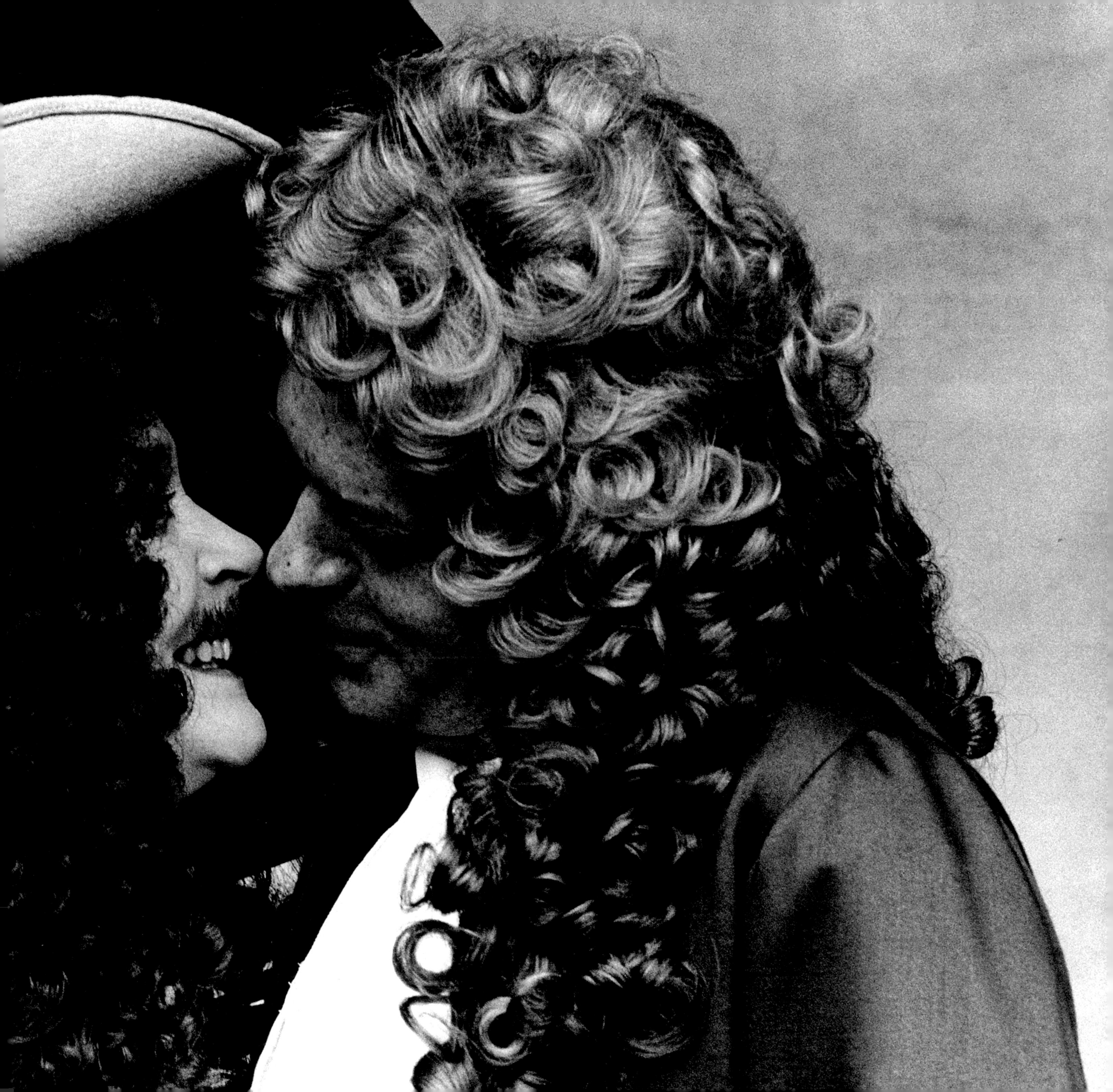

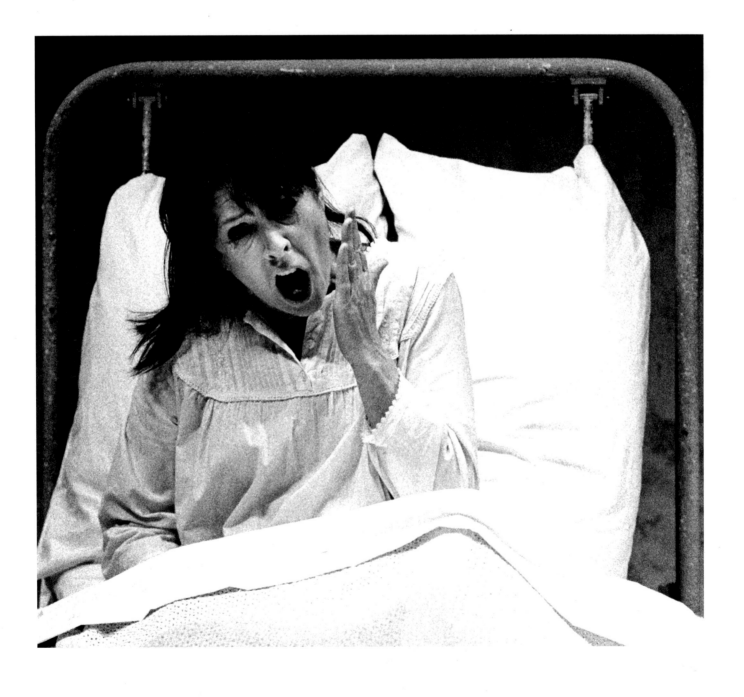

Penelope Wilton as **Deborah** in *A Kind of Alaska* by **Harold Pinter**

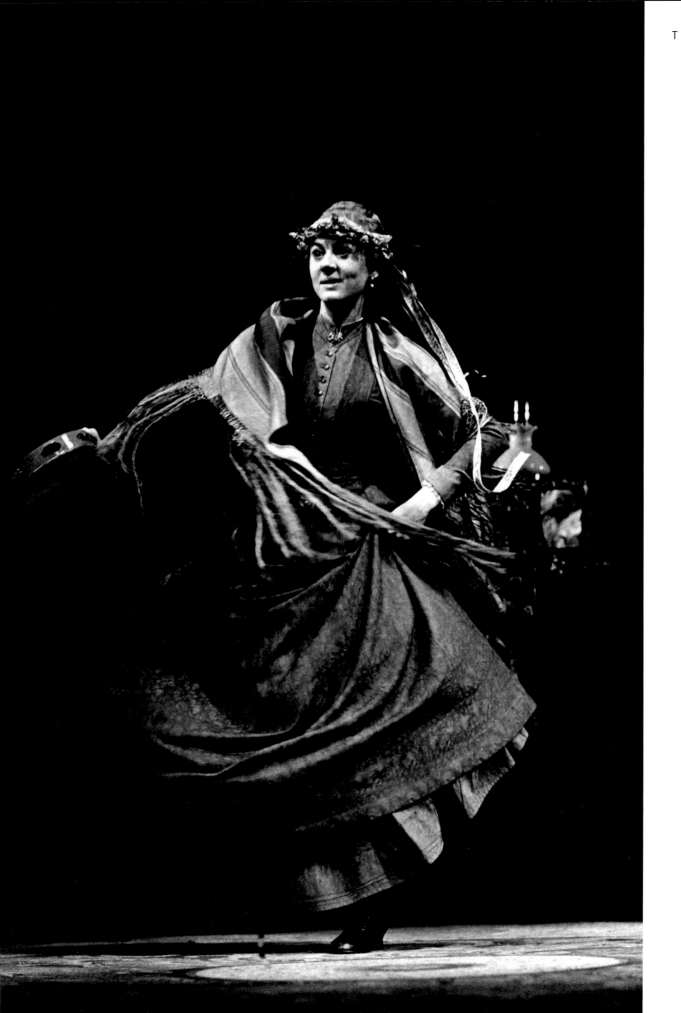

Niamh Cusack as **Nora** in *A Doll's House* by **Henrik Ibsen** based on the translation by **Joan Tindale**

Lindsay Duncan as Rebecca, Stephen Rea as Devlin in *Ashes to Ashes* by Harold Pinter

Pat Kinevane as **Cecil Graham** in ***Lady Windermere's Fan*** by **Oscar Wilde**

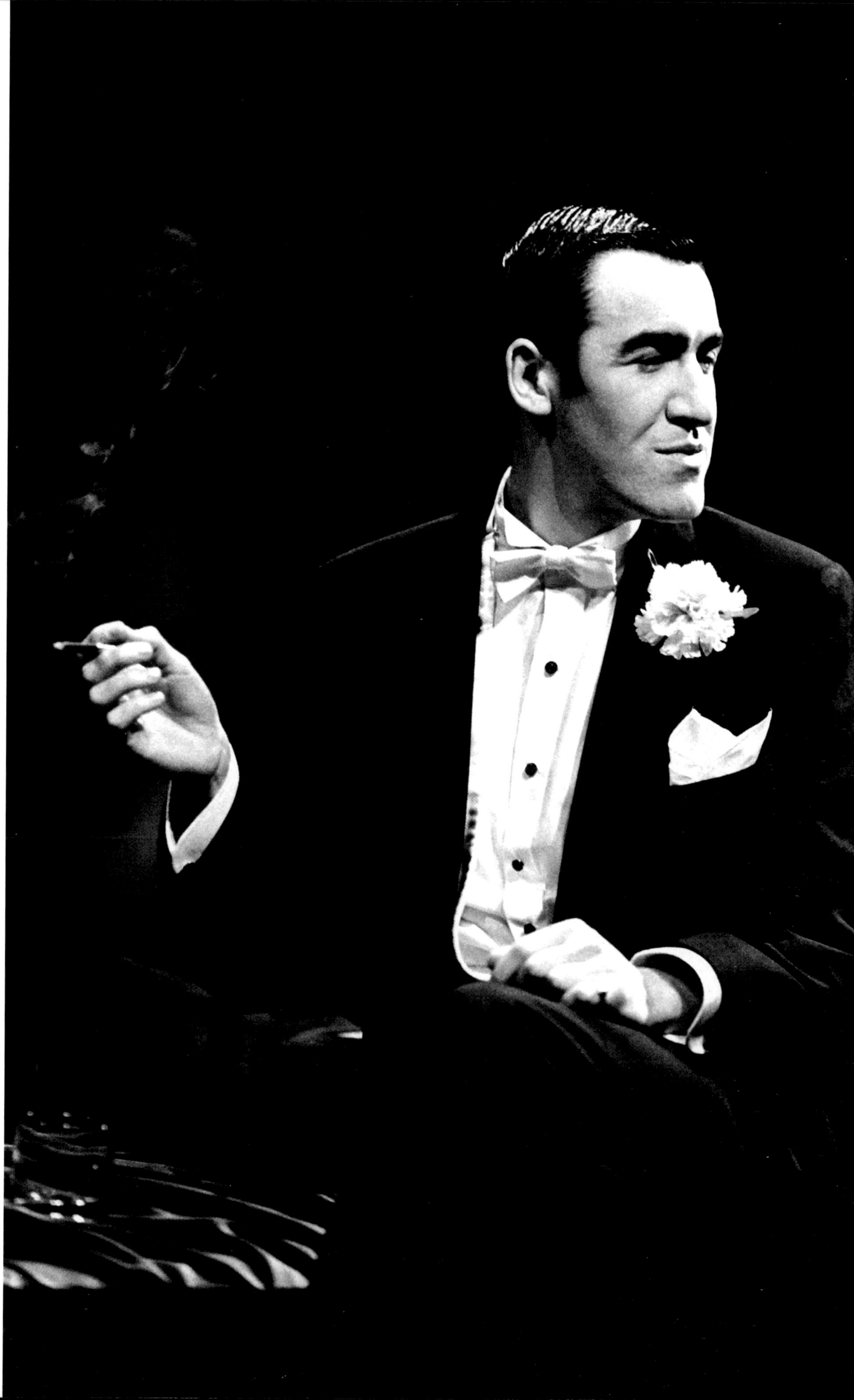

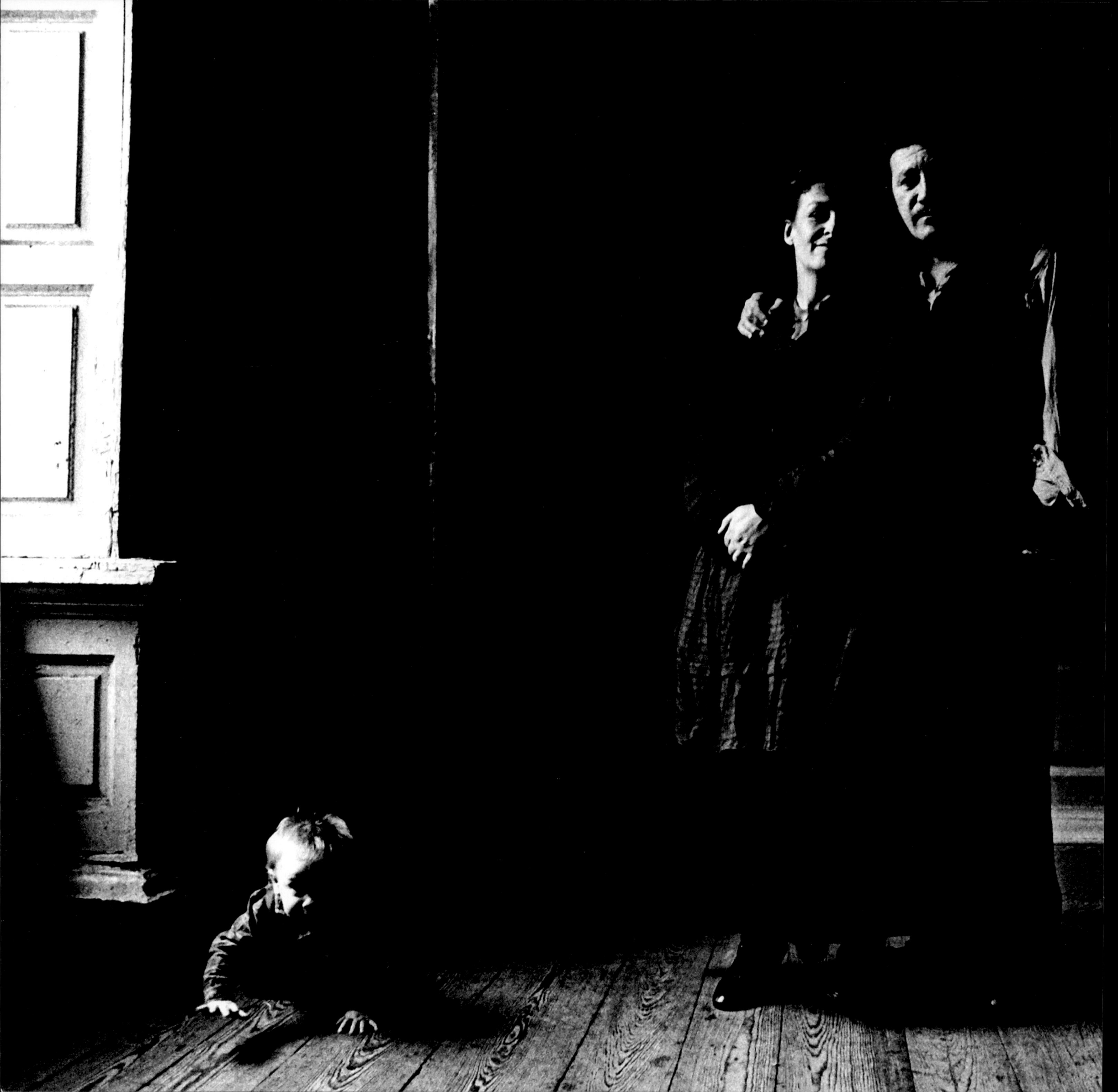

Geraldine Plunkett as **Juno Boyle**, Donal McCann as **Captain Jack Boyle** in *Juno and the Paycock* by **Sean O'Casey**

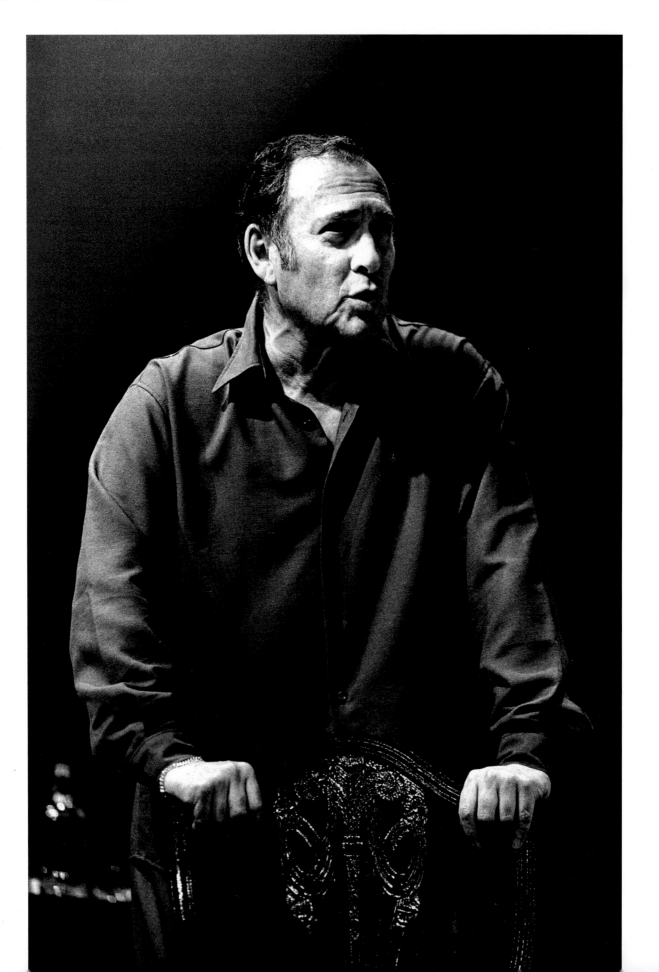

Harold Pinter as **Harry** in *The Collection* by **Harold Pinter**

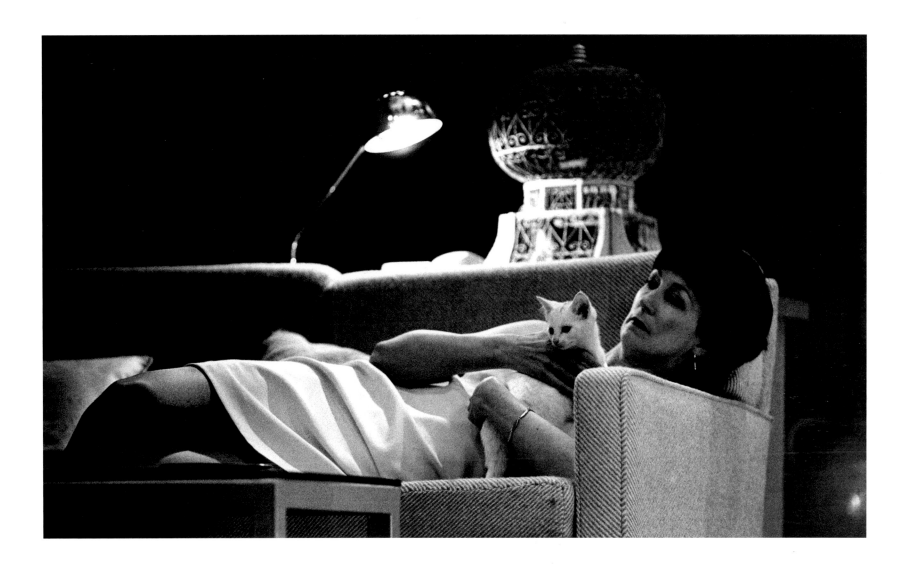

Ingrid Craigie as **Stella** in *The Collection* by **Harold Pinter**

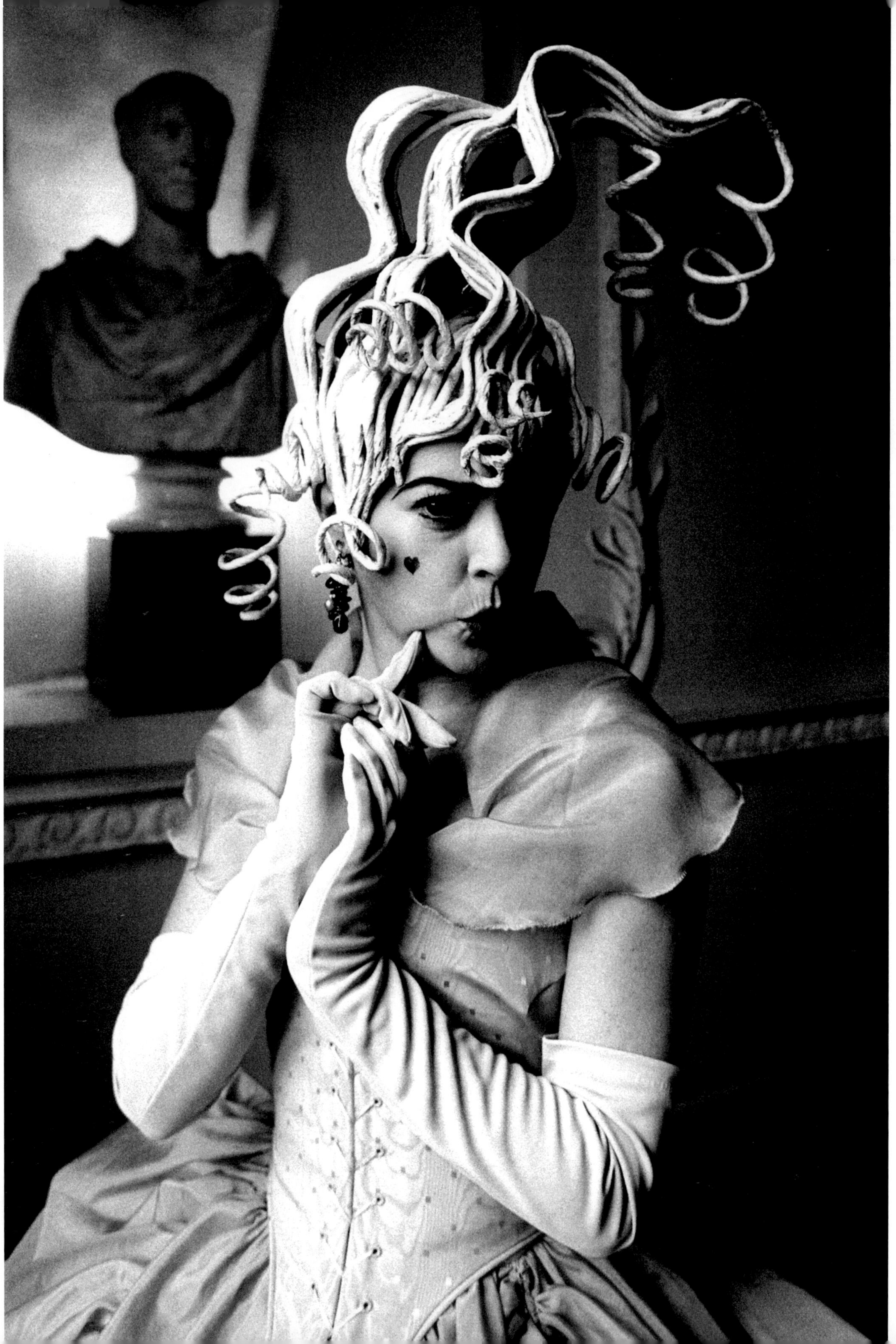

Gemma Craven as **Mrs Diggerty** in ***The London Vertigo*** by **Brian Friel** based on a play by **Charles Macklin**

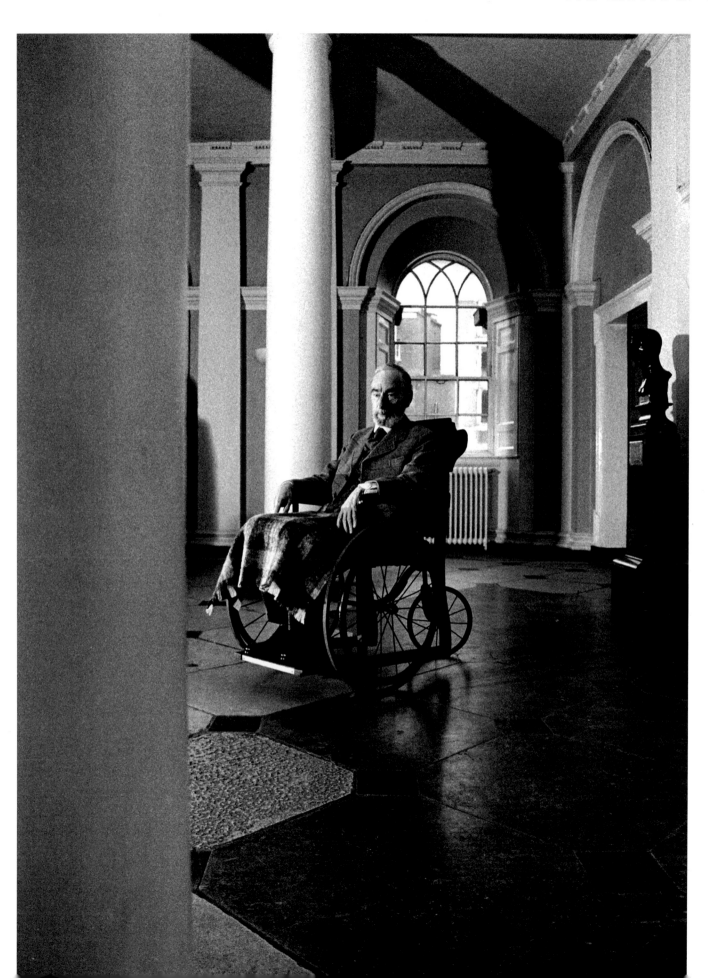

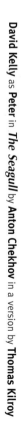

David Kelly as **Peter** in *The Seagull* by **Anton Chekhov** in a version by **Thomas Kilroy**

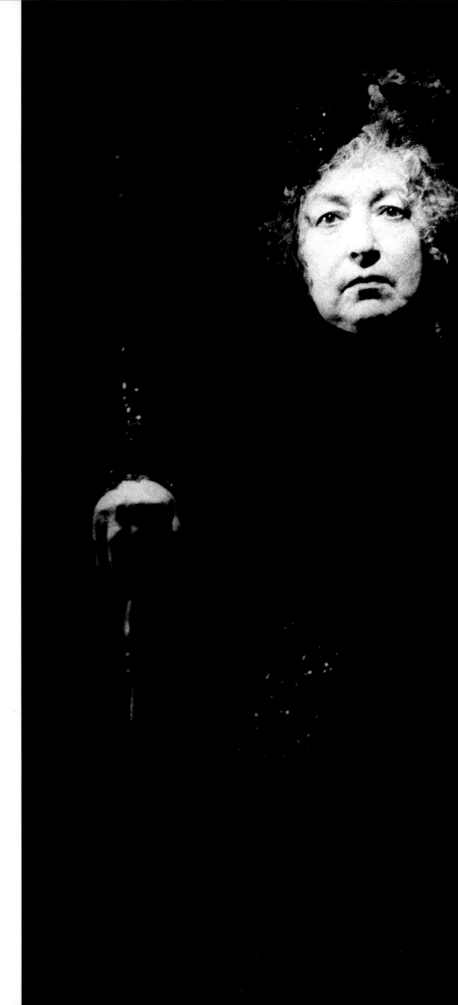

Maureen Potter as **Woman** in *Rockaby* by **Samuel Beckett**

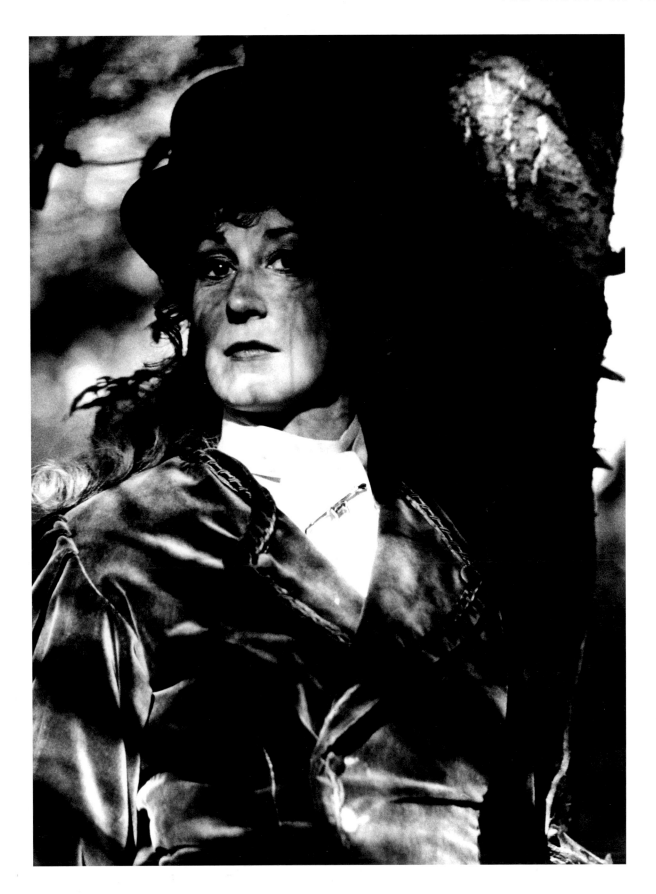

Ingrid Craigie as Gwen Mellors in The Mask of Moriarty by Hugh Leonard

Alan Stanford as **Hamm**, **Barry McGovern** as **Clov** in *Endgame* by **Samuel Beckett**

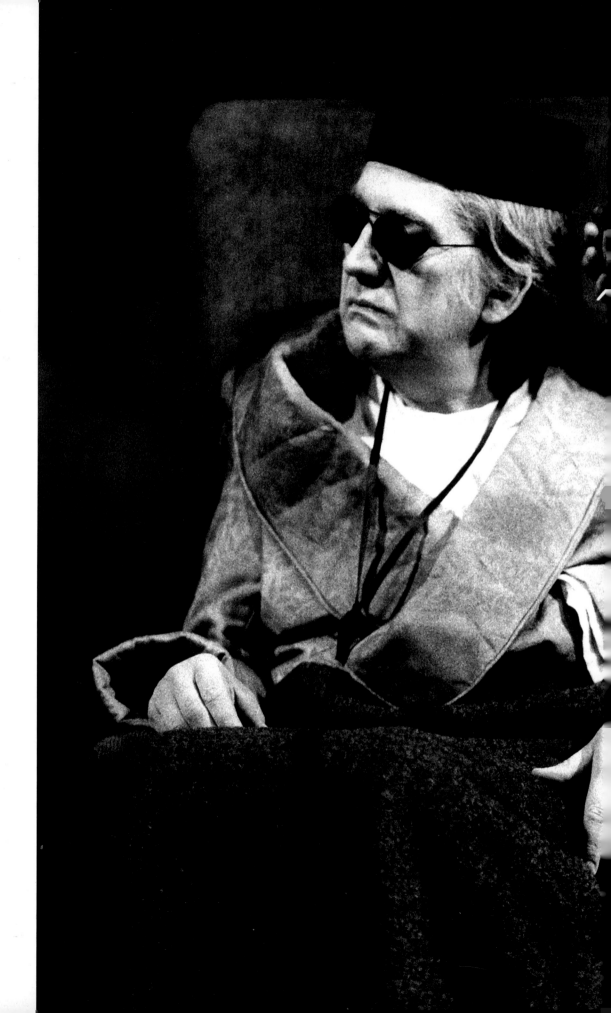

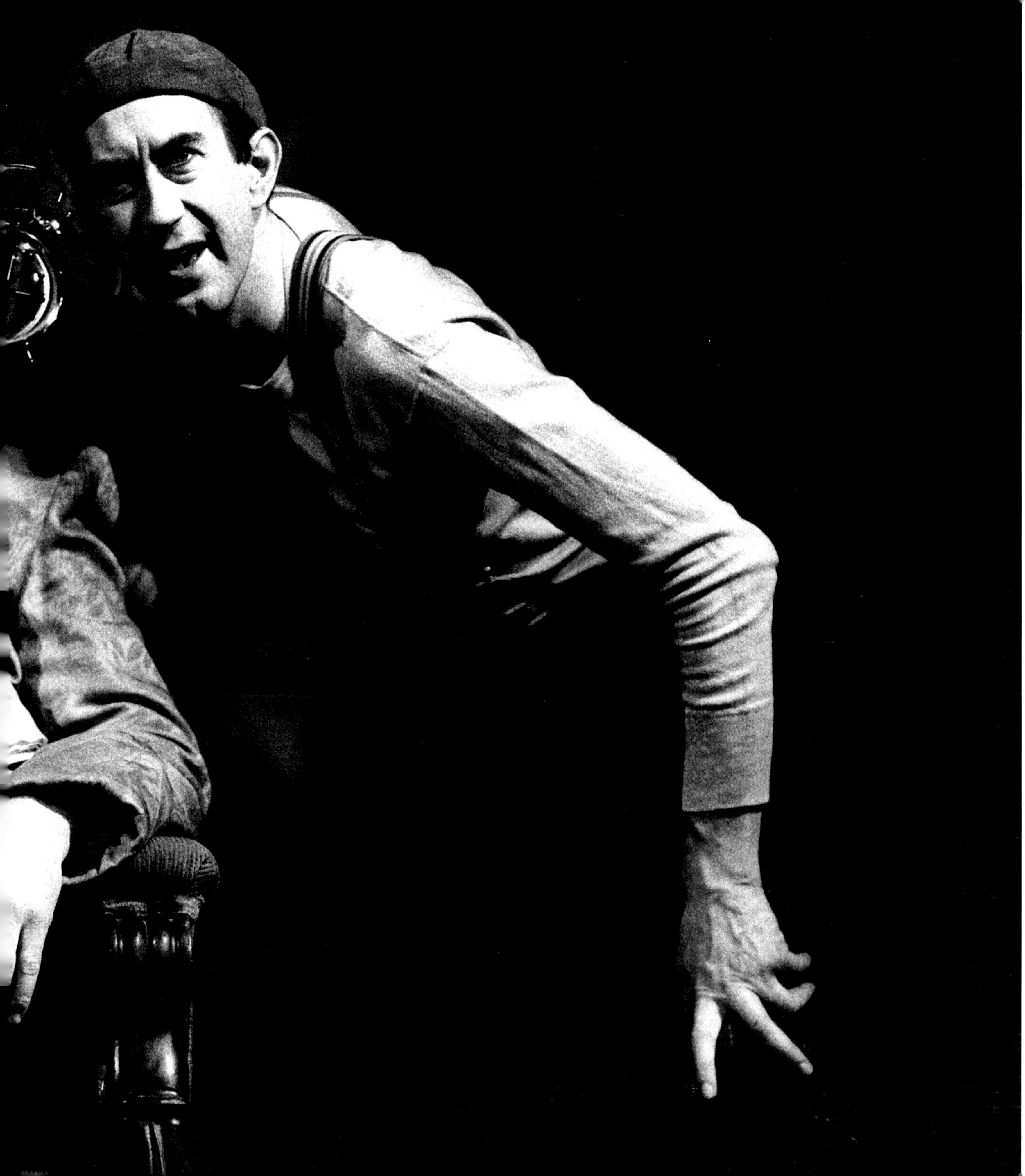

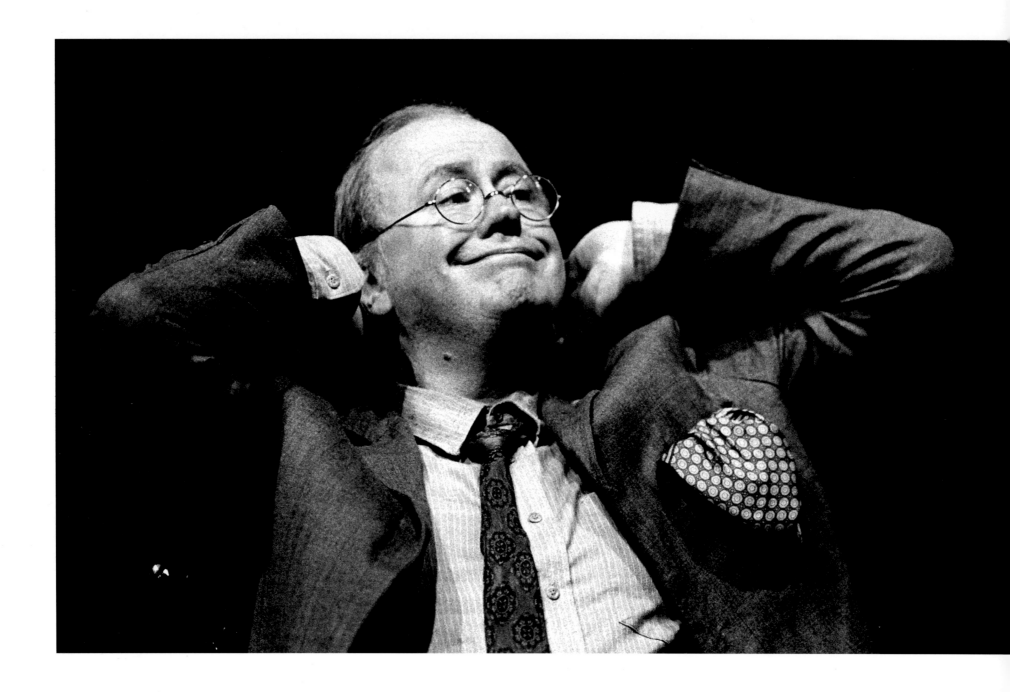

Niall Buggy as **Spooner** in *No Man's Land* by **Harold Pinter**

Jane Brennan as **Gila** in *One for the Road* by Harold Pinter

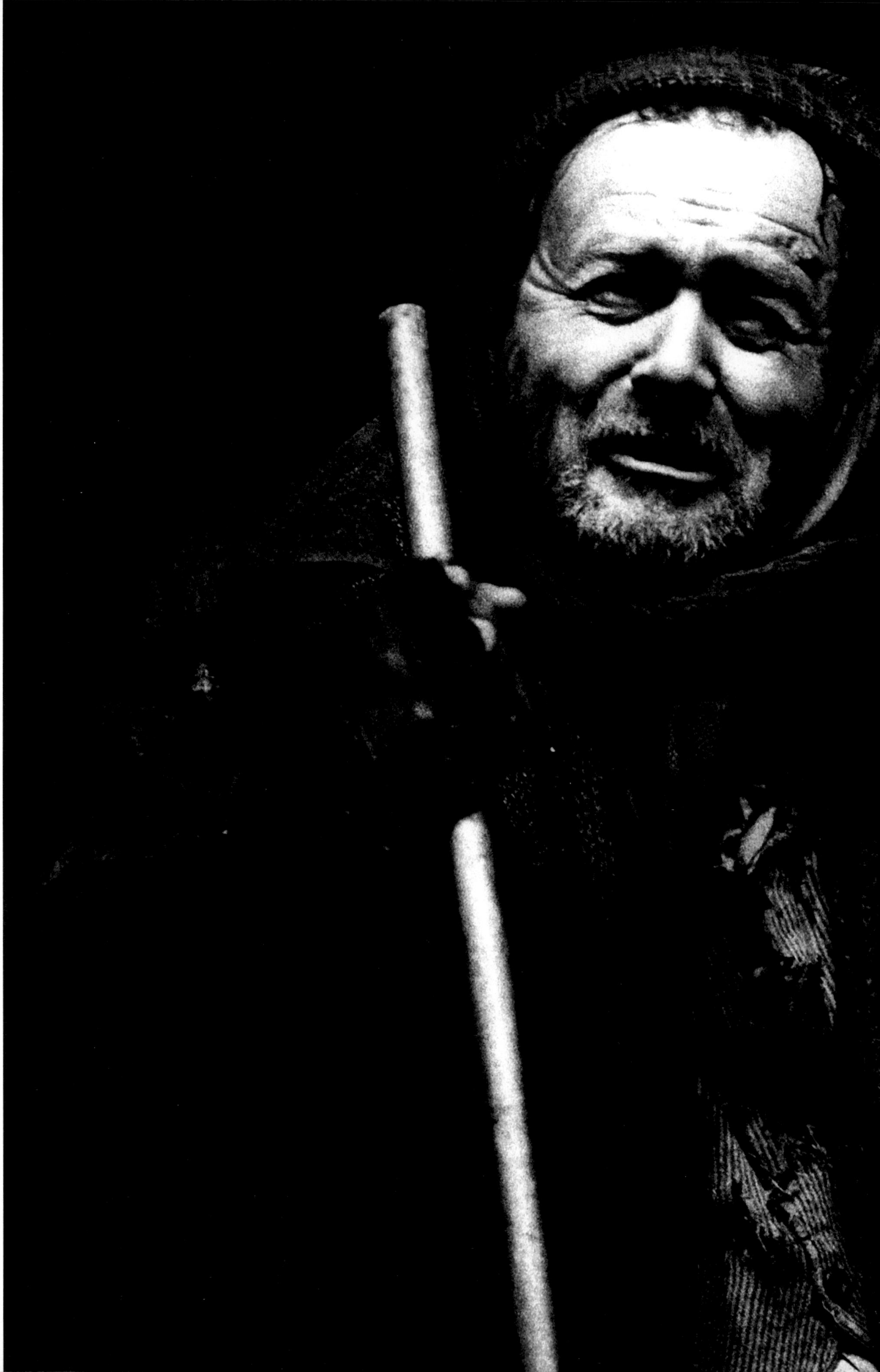

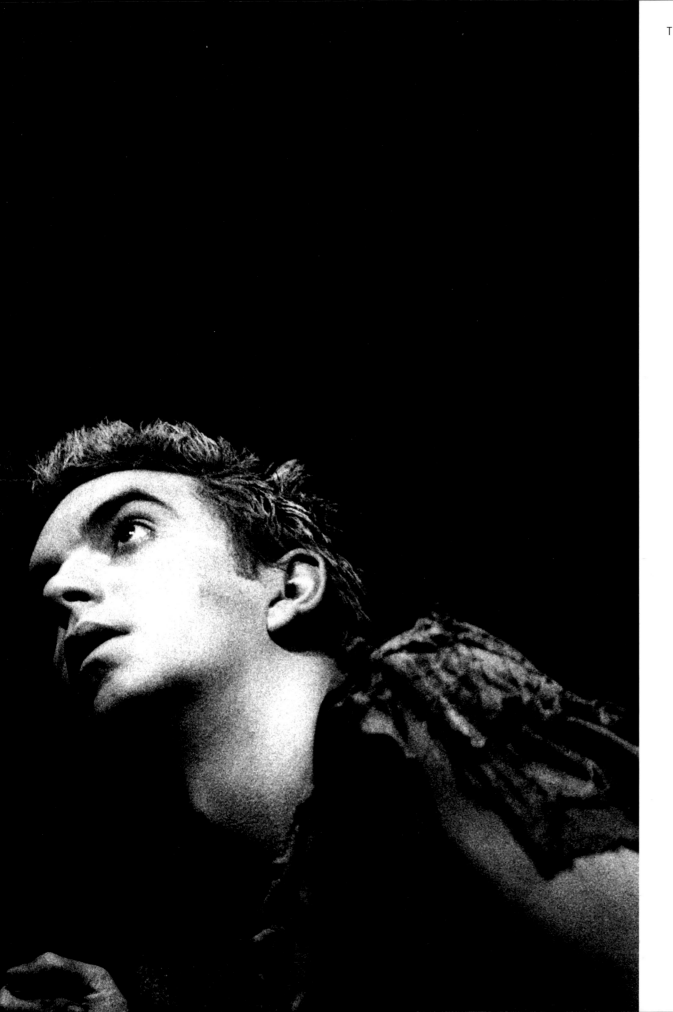

John Olohan as **B**, Phelim Drew as **A** in *Rough for Theatre 1* by **Samuel Beckett**

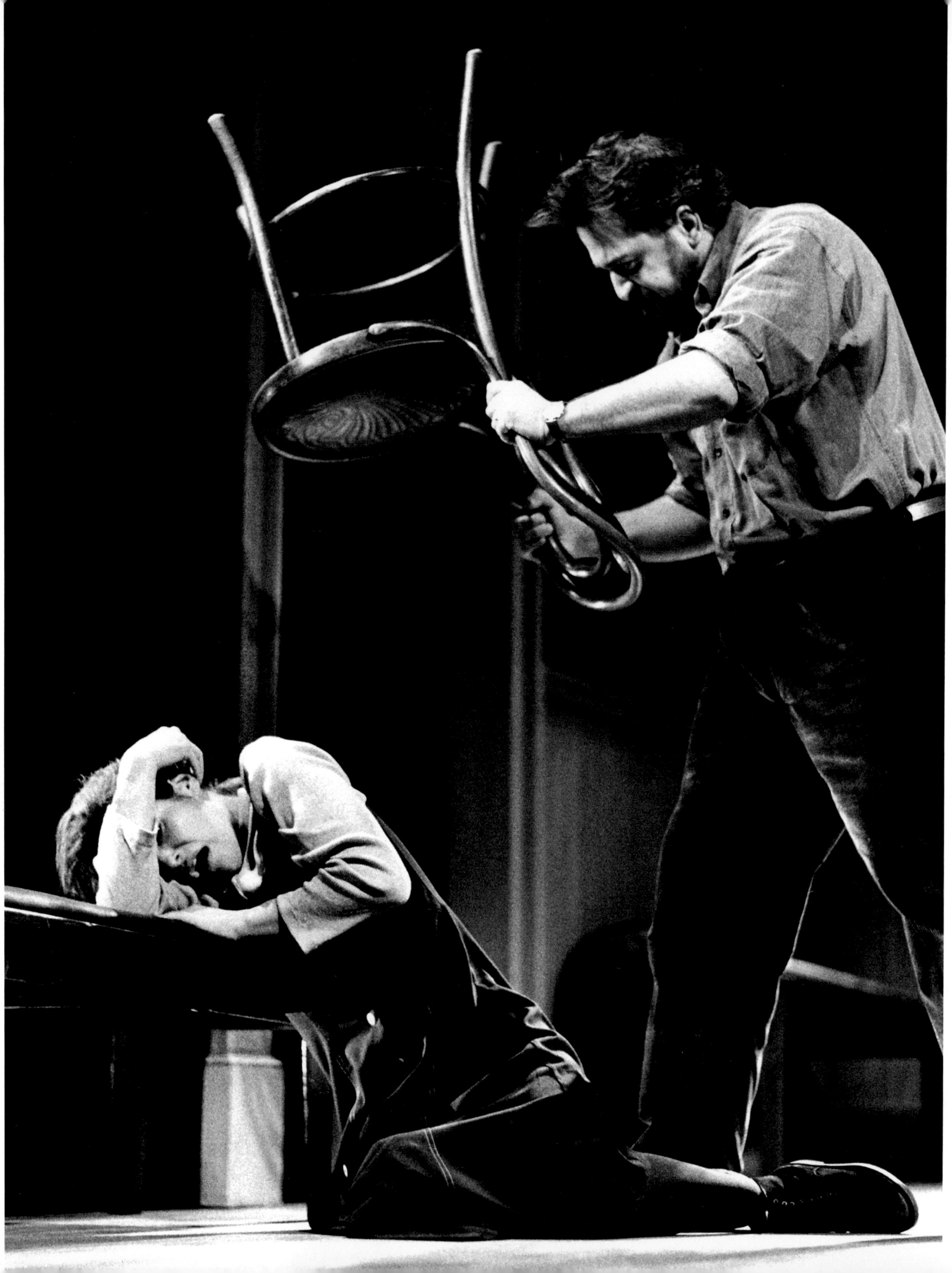

Dana Bledsoe as **Carol, Stanley Townsend** as **John** in *Oleanna* by **David Mamet**

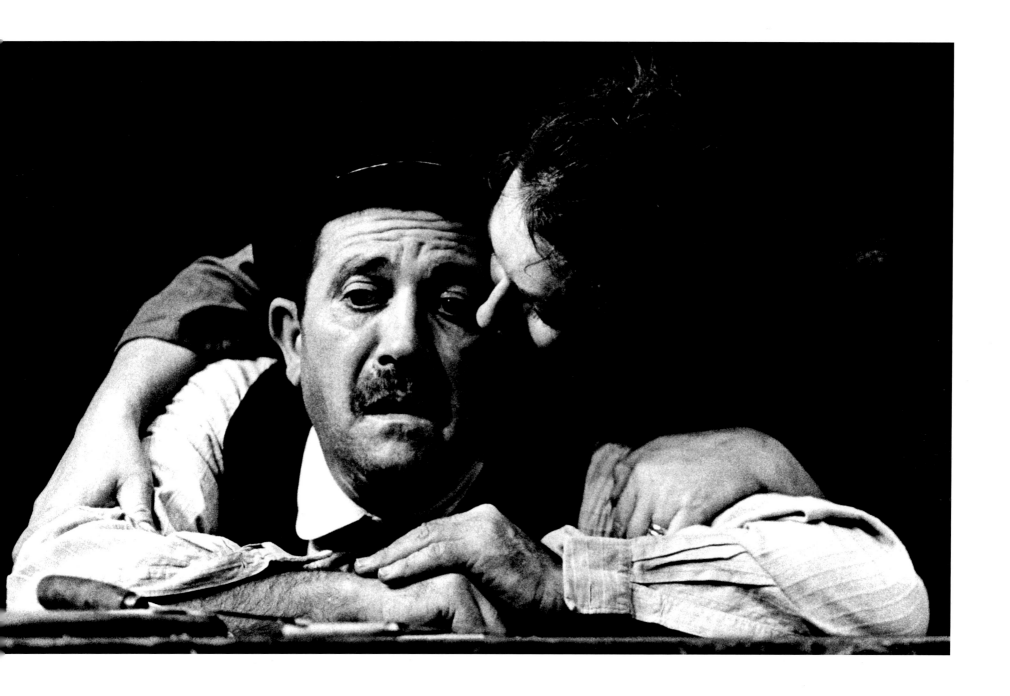

Donal McCann as Captain Jack Boyle, Geraldine Plunkett as Juno Boyle in *Juno and the Paycock* by Sean O'Casey

Seamus Forde as **Nagg** in *Endgame* by **Samuel Beckett**

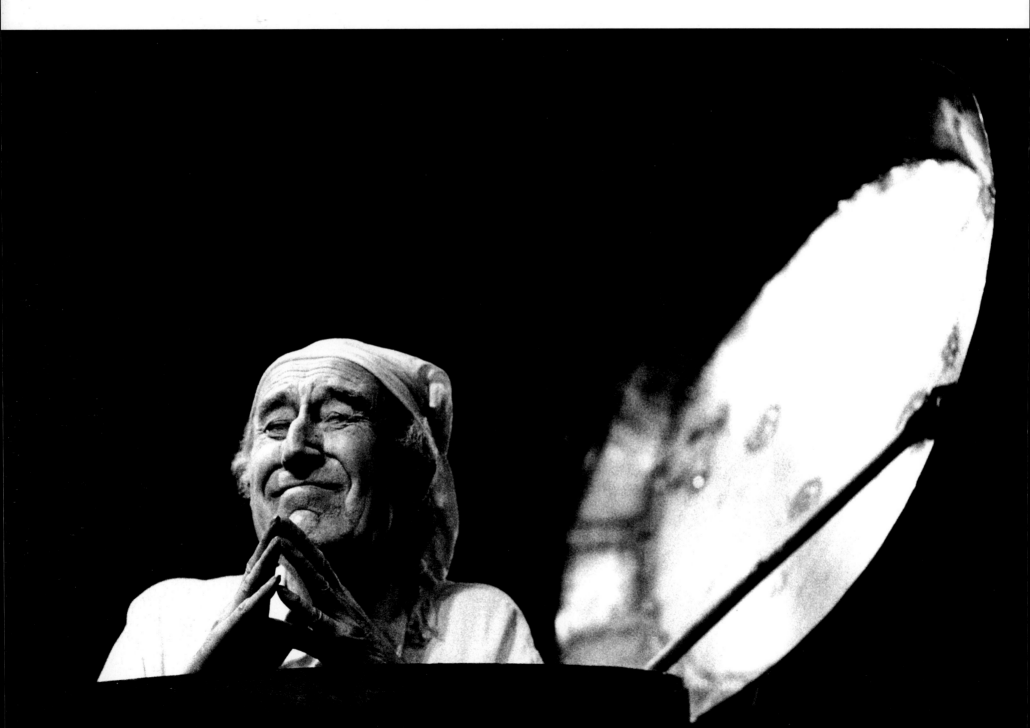

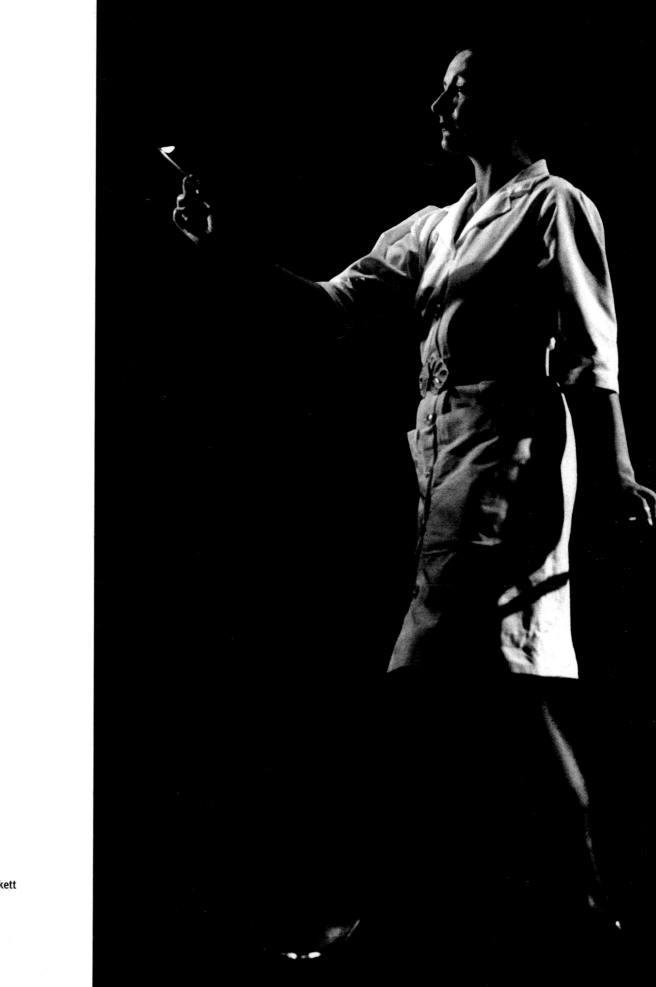

Helene Montague as **Assistant** in *Catastrophe* by **Samuel Beckett**

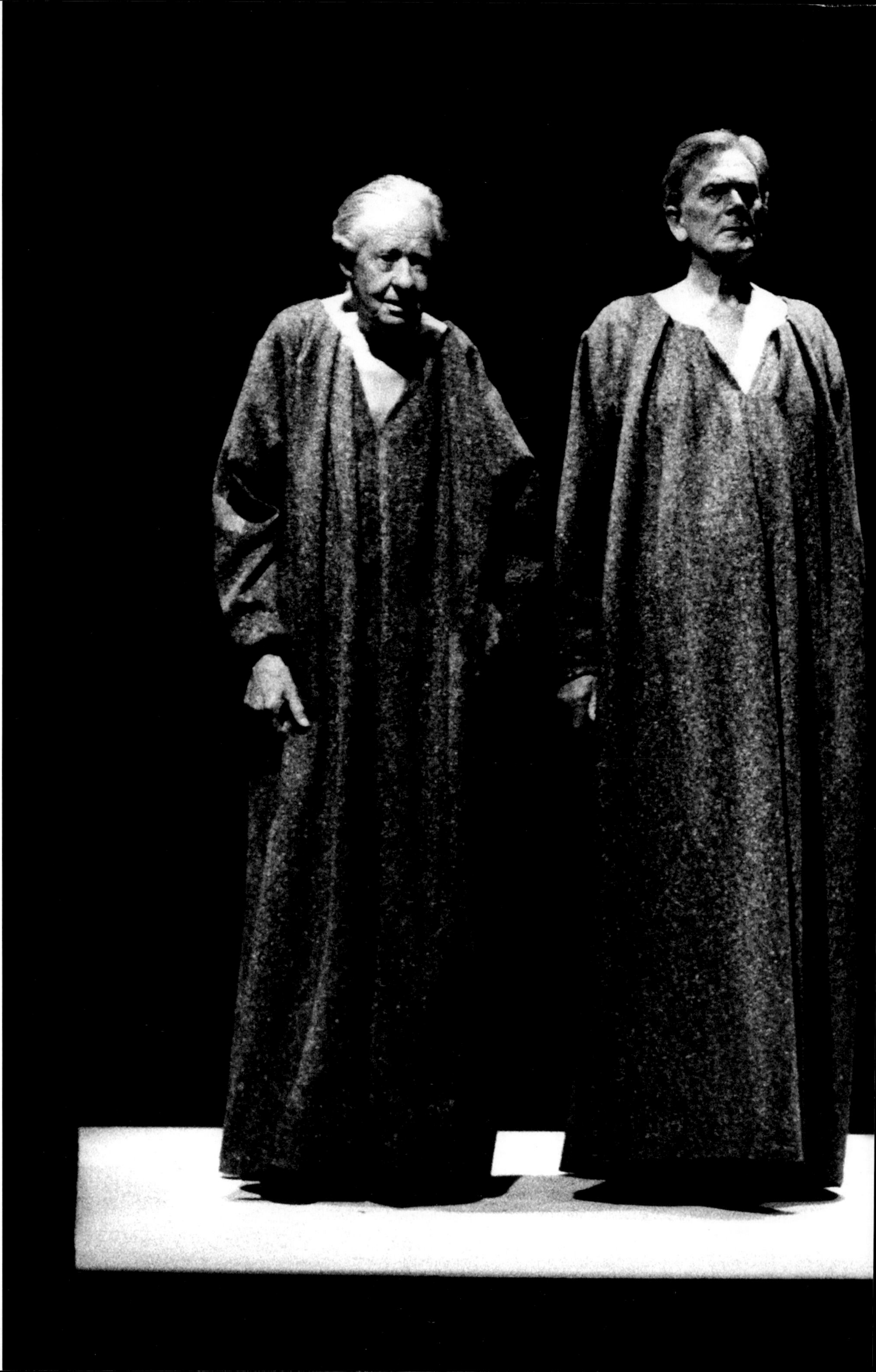

O Z Whitehead as **Bem, Barry Cassin** as **Bam, Seamus Forde** as **Bim, Micheál Ó Briain** as **Bom** in *What Where* by **Samuel Beckett**

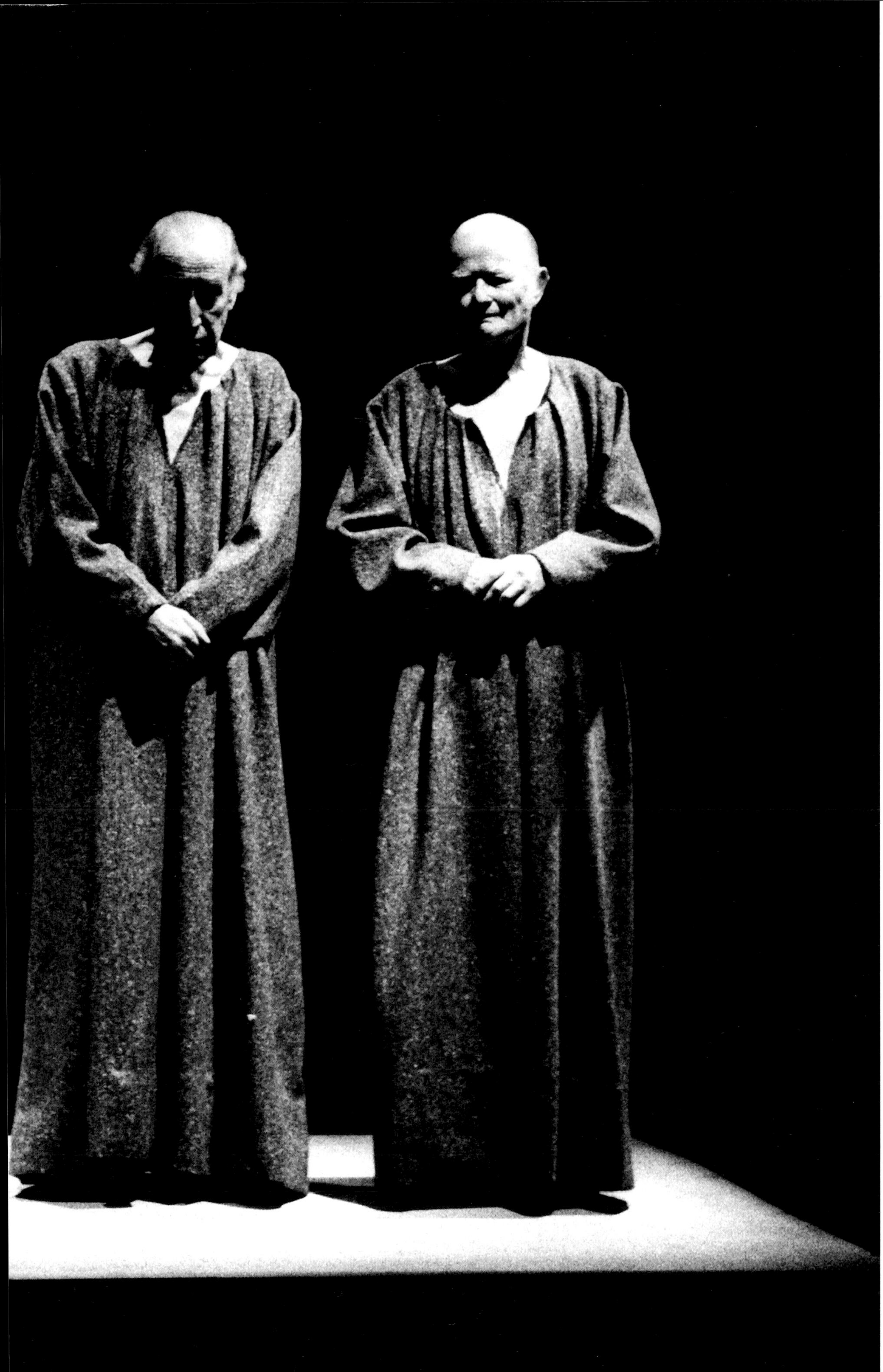

Michael Pennington as **Nicolas**, Nicholas Grennell as **Victor** in *One for the Road* by **Harold Pinter**

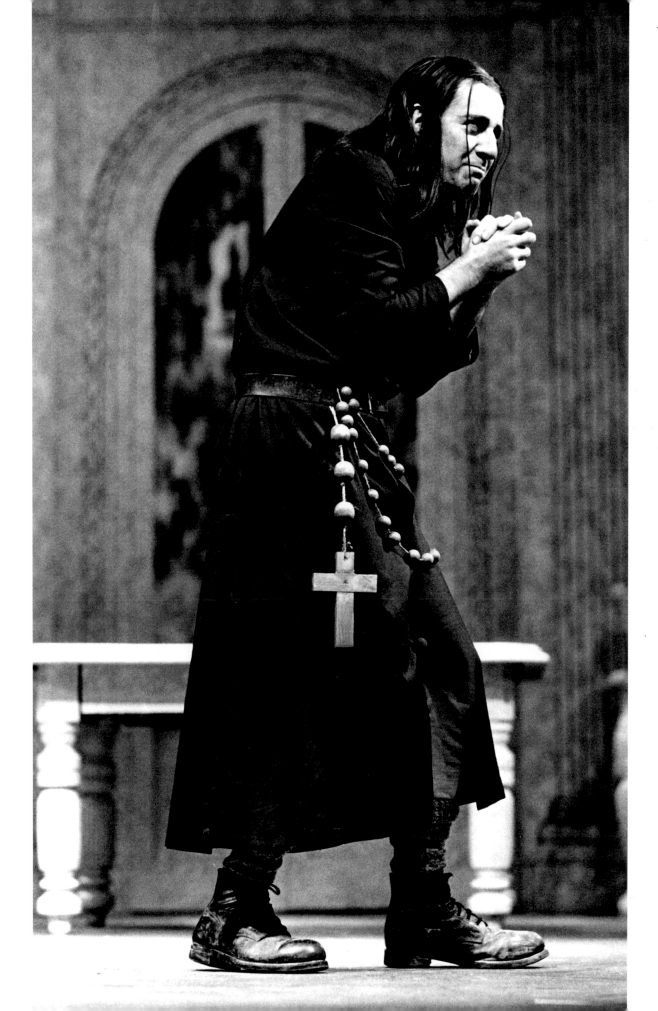

Stephen Brennan as **Tartuffe** in **Molière's *Tartuffe*** in a version by **Michael West**

Flo McSweeney as Titania, Stephen Brennan as Oberon in *A Midsummer Night's Dream* by William Shakespeare

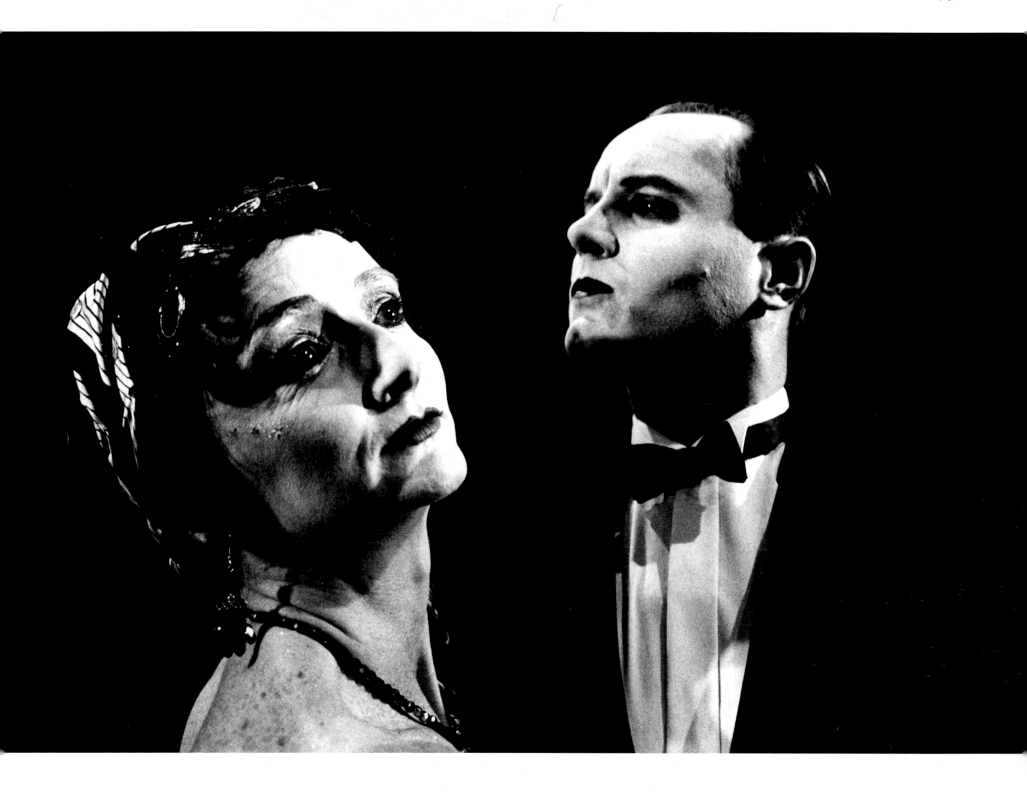

Bairbre Ní Chaoimh as **a guest at the dinner, Michael James Ford** as **the page of Herodias** in *Salomé* by **Oscar Wilde**

David Kelly as **Krapp** in *Krapp's Last Tape* by **Samuel Beckett**

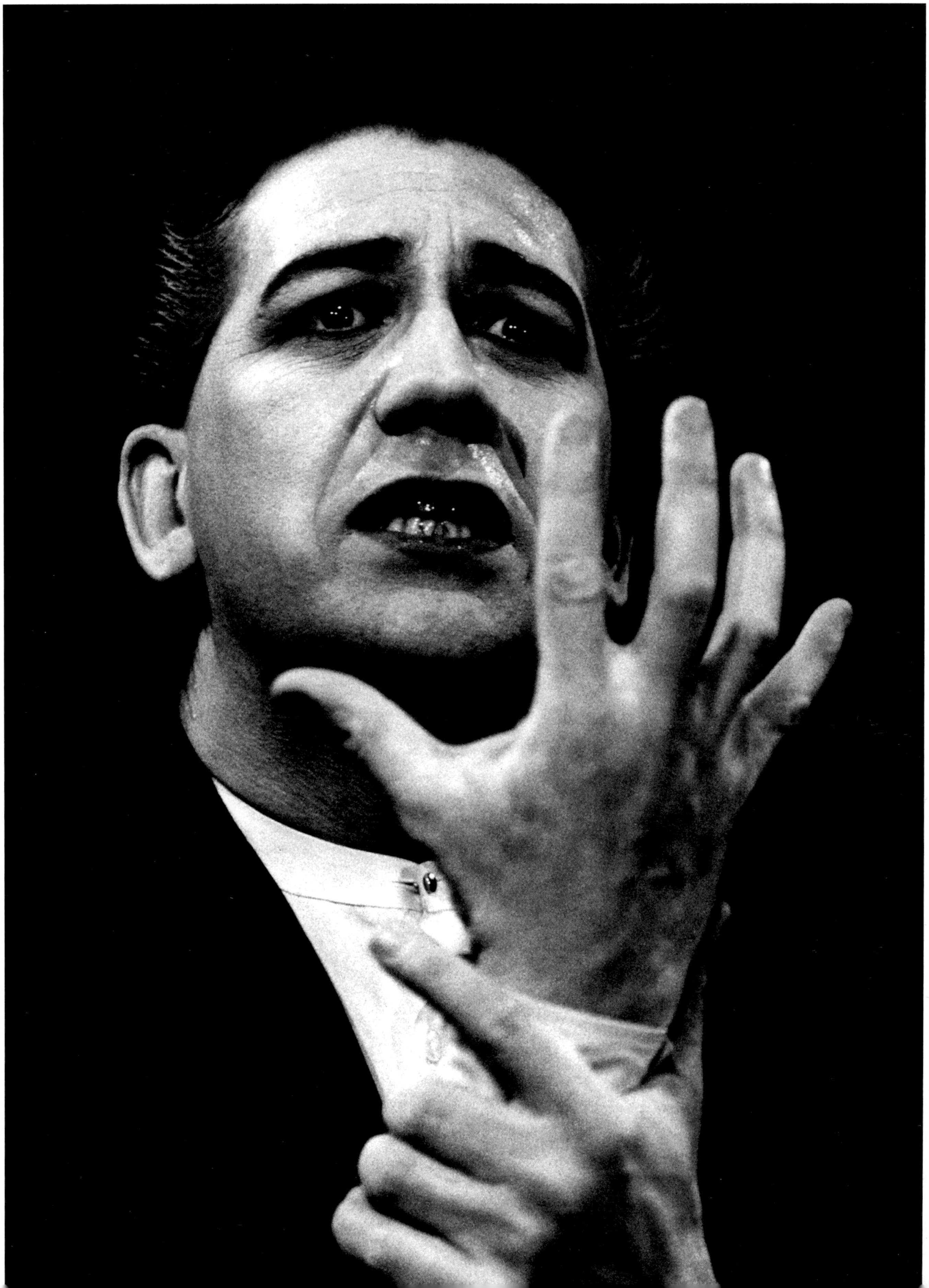

Alan Stanford as **Herod** in ***Salomé*** by **Oscar Wilde**

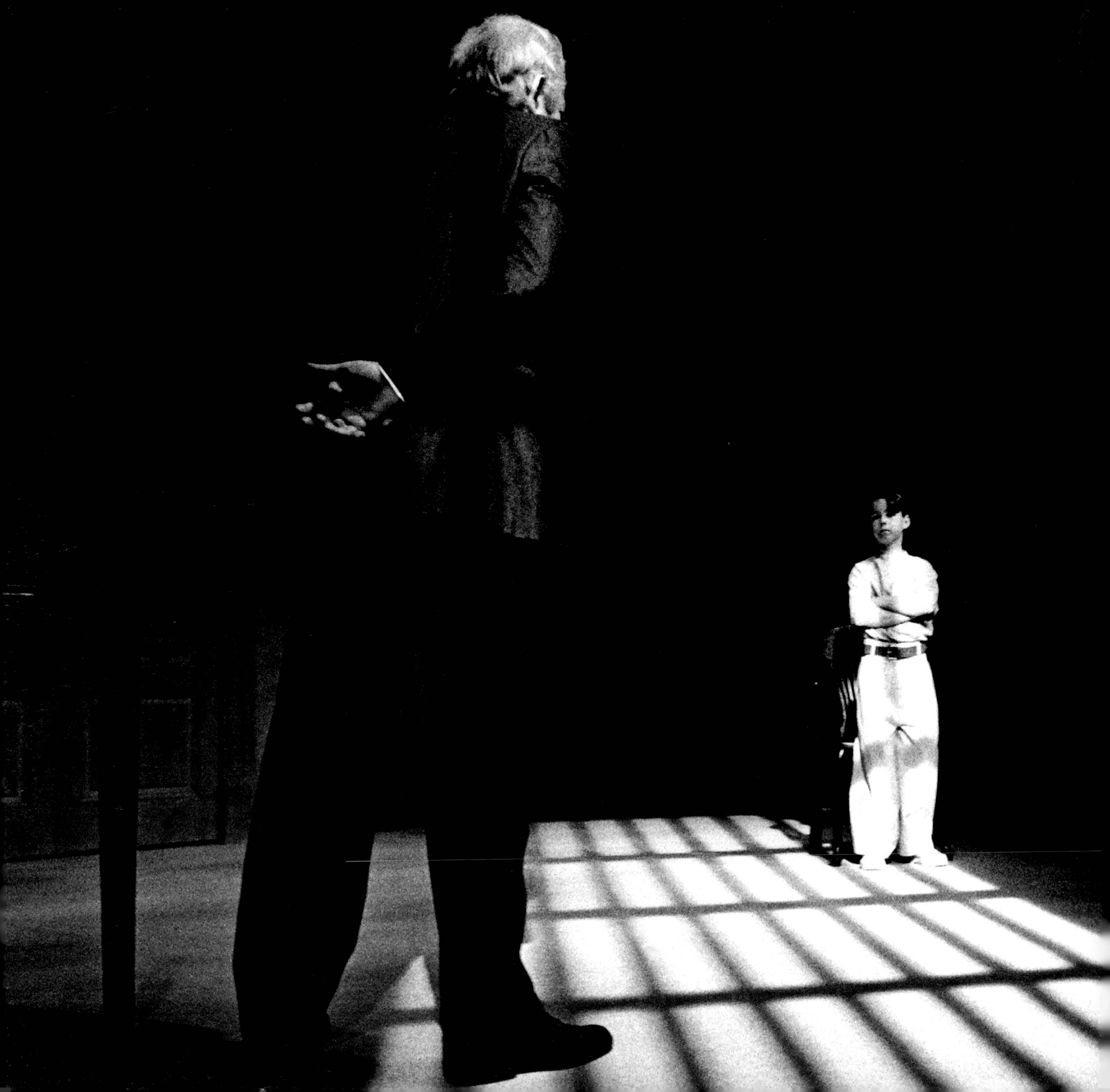

Michael Pennington as **Nicolas**, Ciarán Fitzgerald as **Nicky** in *One for the Road* by Harold Pinter

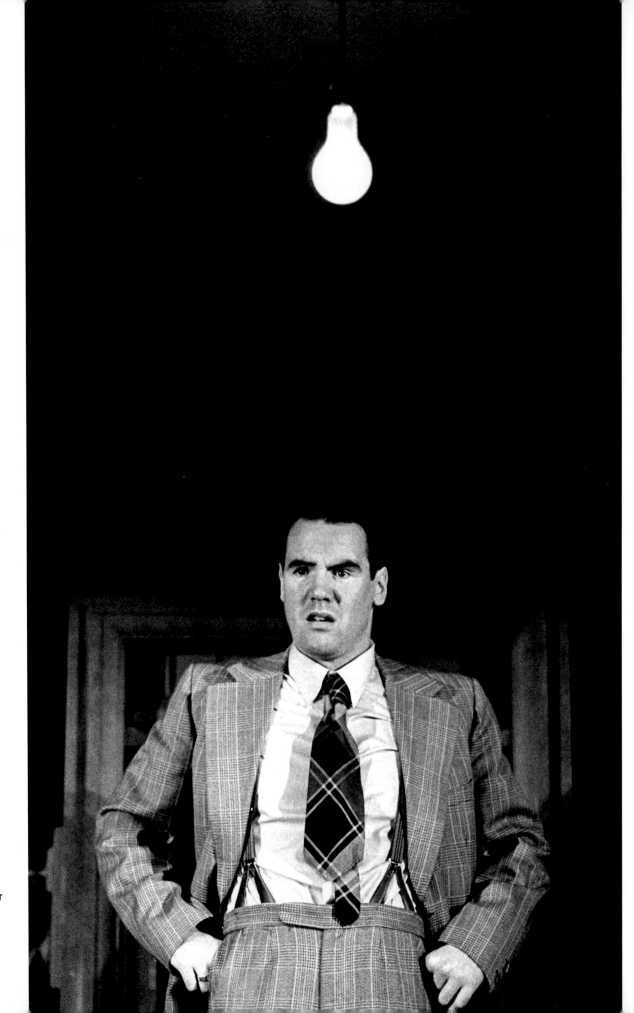

David Herlihy as **Gus** in *The Dumb Waiter* by **Harold Pinter**

Ian McElhinney as **Ben** in *The Dumb Waiter* by **Harold Pinter**

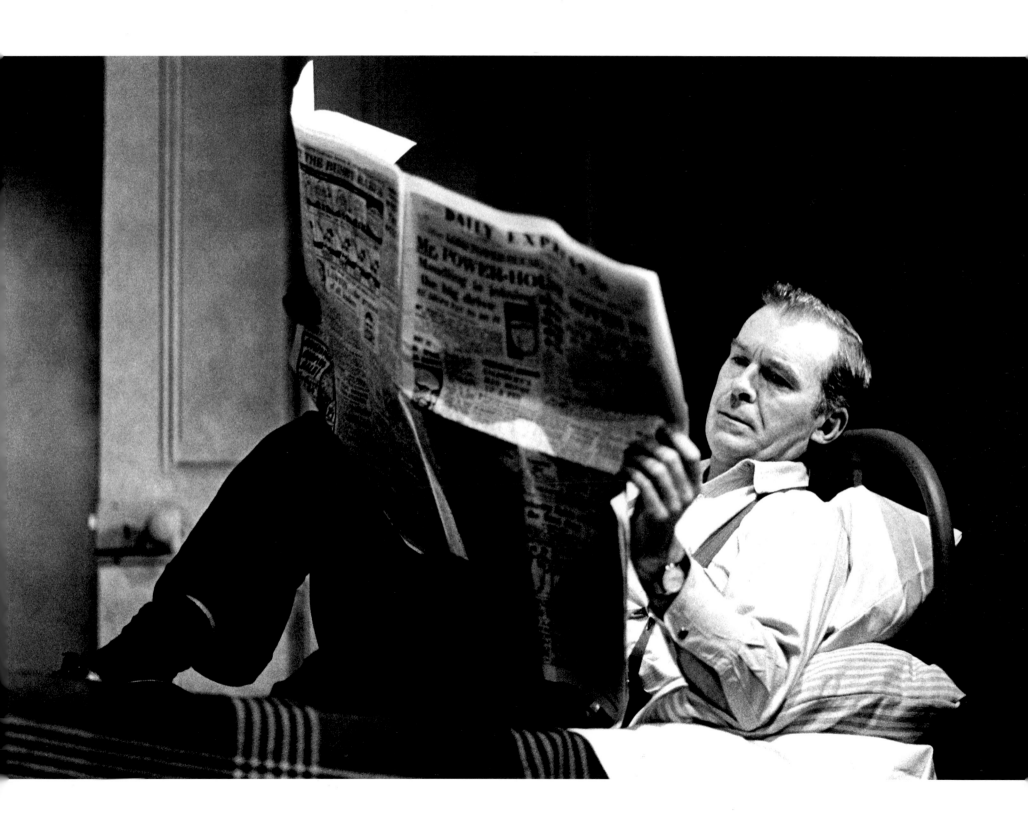

Jeananne Crowley as **Lady Touchwood** in *The Double Dealer* by **William Congreve**

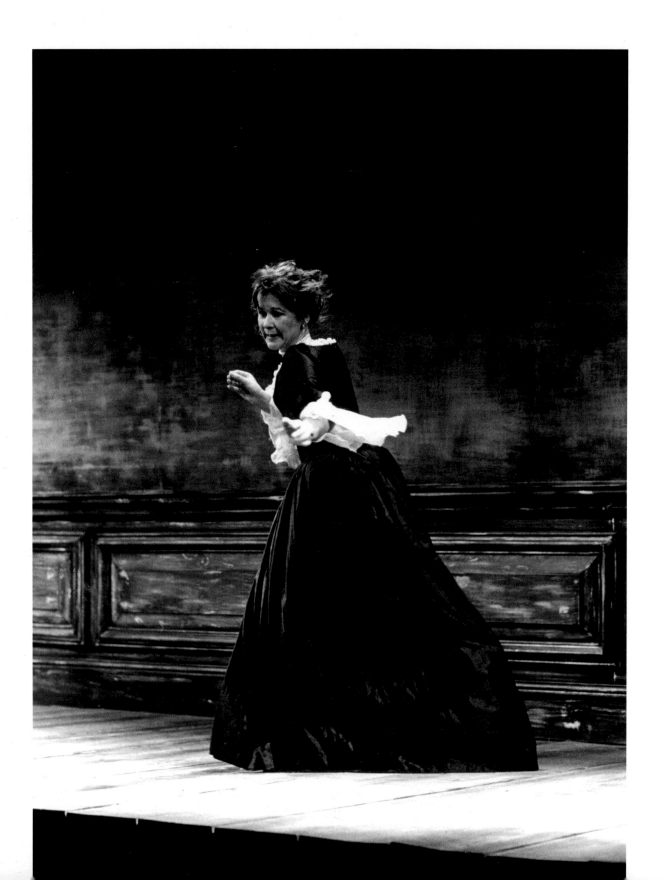

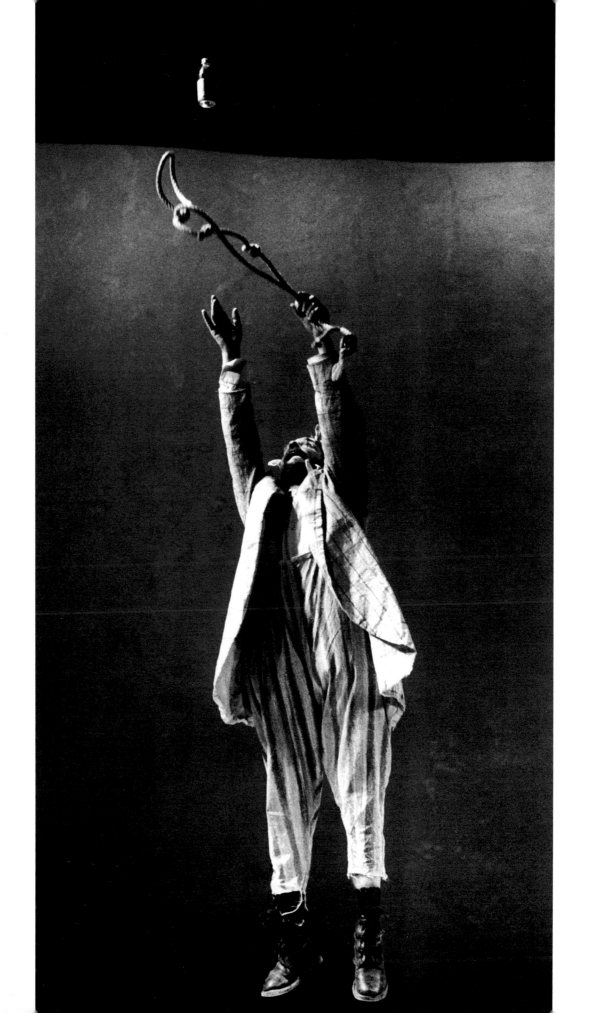

Derek Chapman as Man in *Act Without Words I* by Samuel Beckett

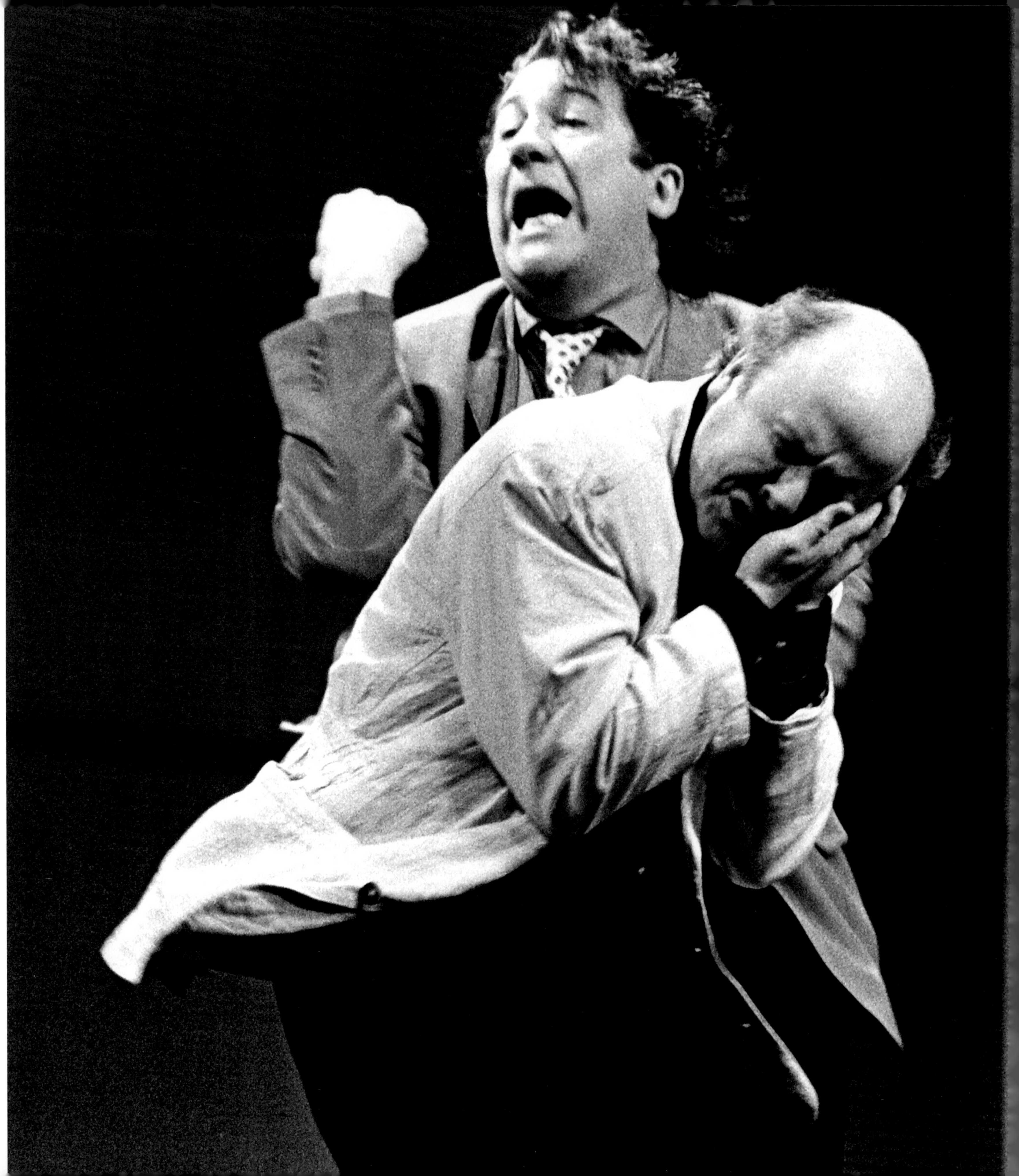

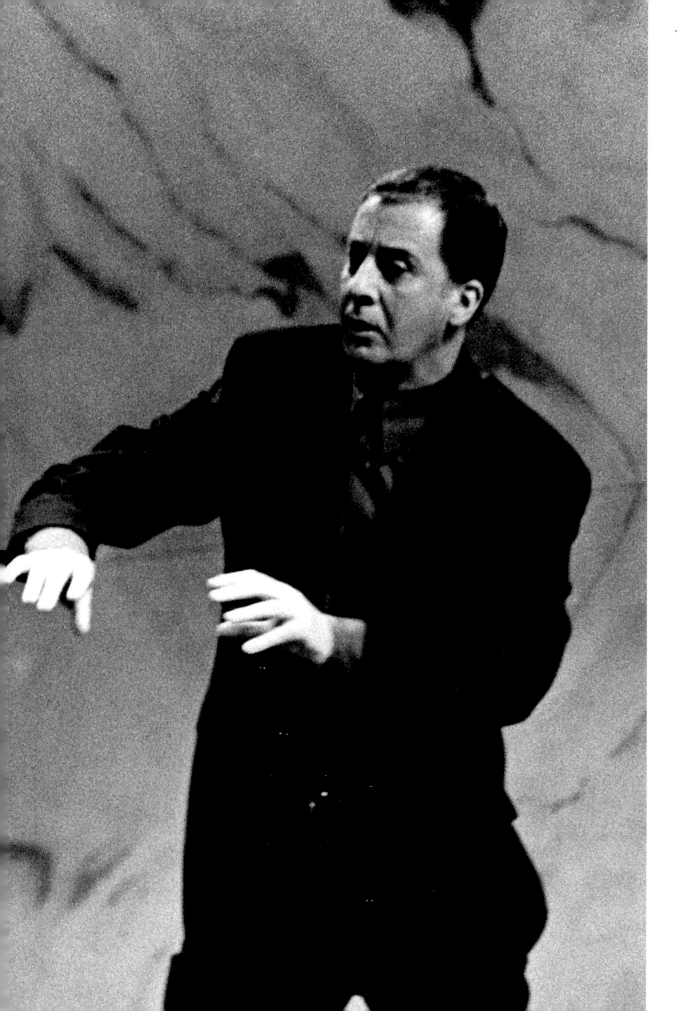

Alan Stanford as **Marc**, **Mark Lambert** as **Yvan**, **Stephen Brennan** as **Serge** in **Art** by **Yasmina Reza** translated by **Christopher Hampton**

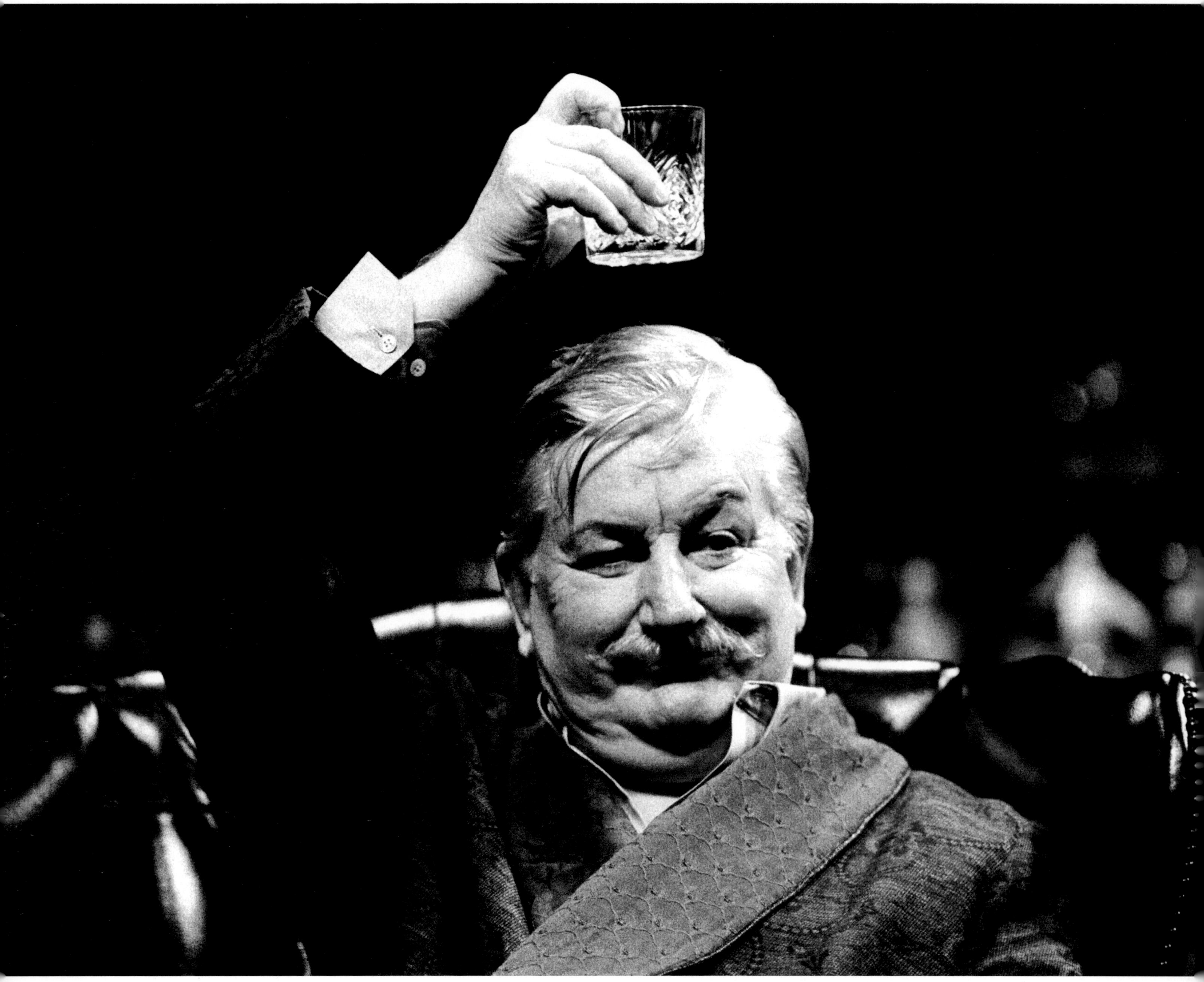

T P McKenna as **Hirst** in *No Man's Land* by **Harold Pinter**

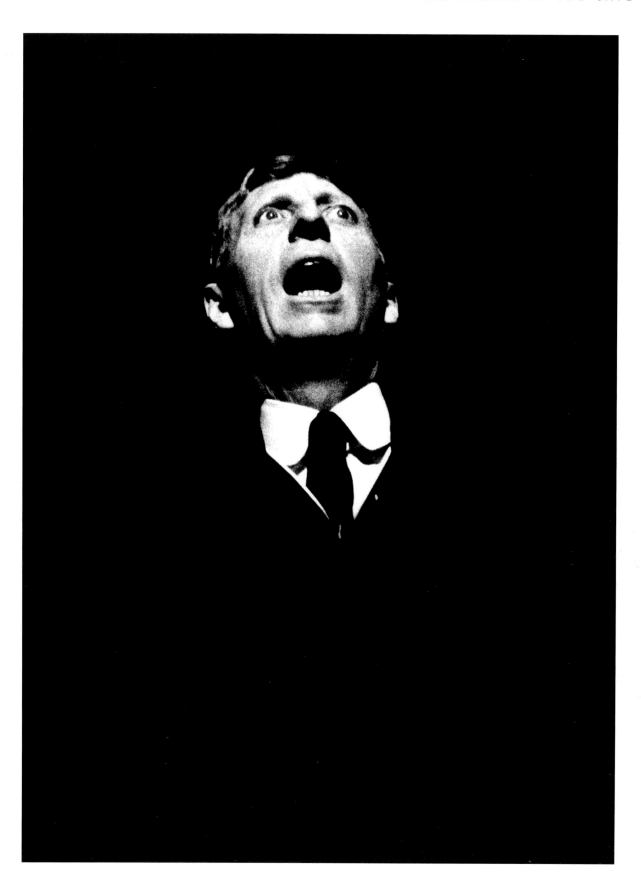

Tom Baker as **Sherlock Holmes** in *The Mask of Moriarty* by **Hugh Leonard**

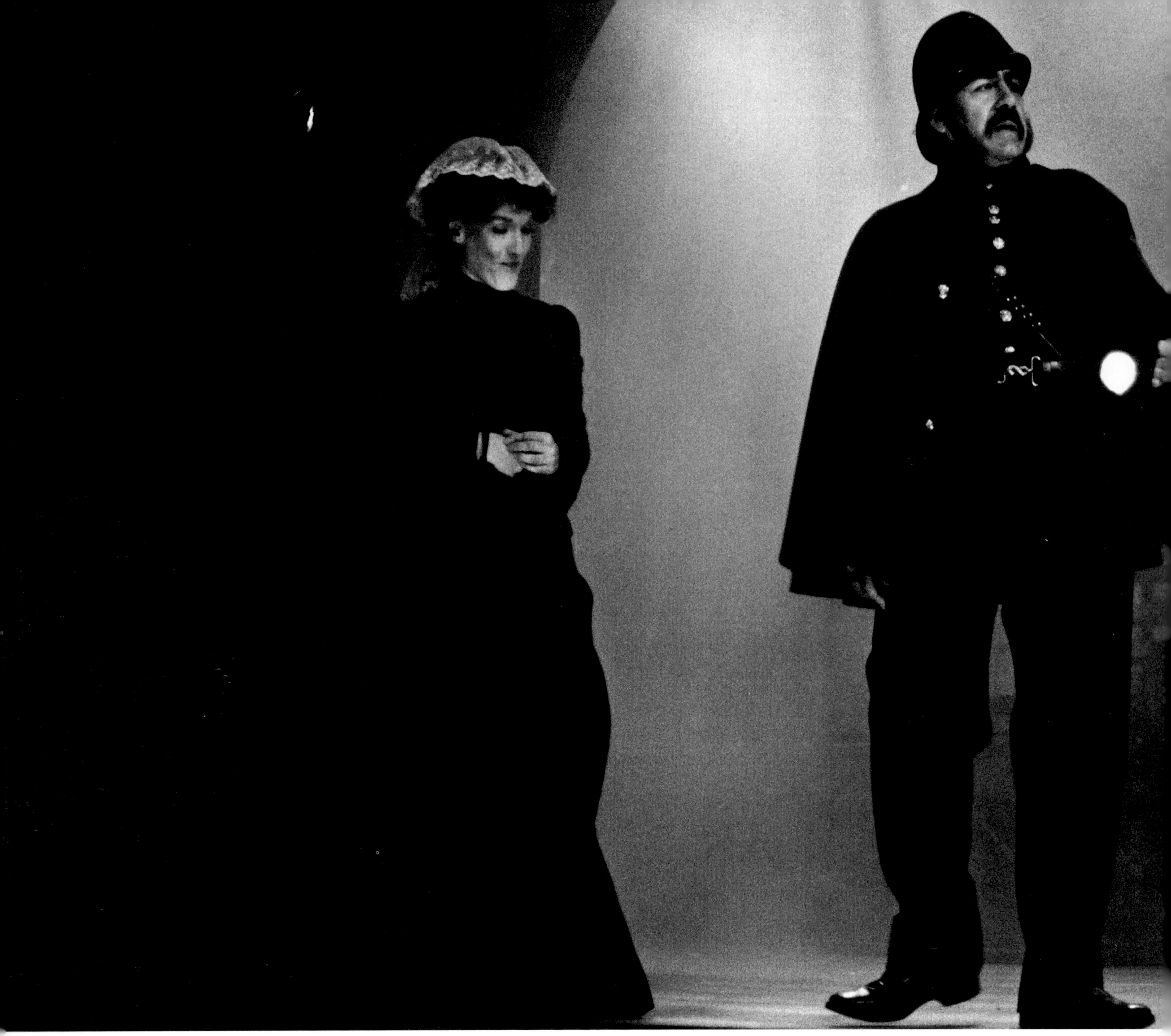

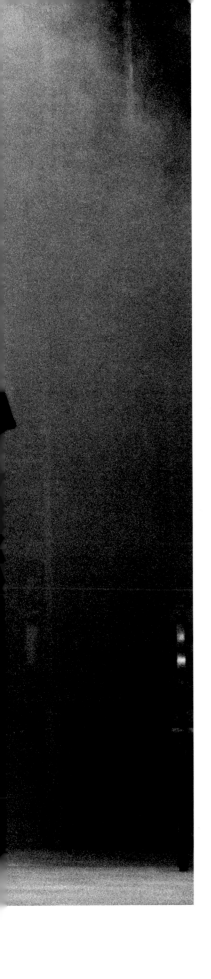

Cinzia Hardy as **Methylated Mary, David Henry** as **Herbert Travesty** in *The Mask of Moriarty* by **Hugh Leonard**

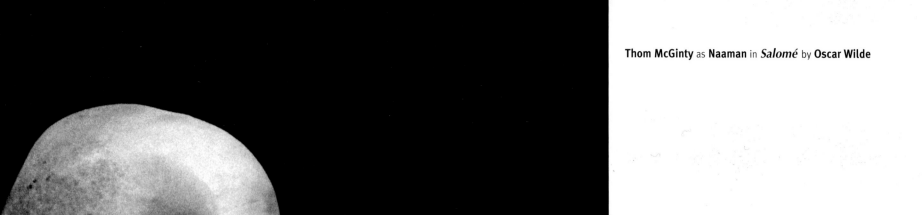

Thom McGinty as Naaman in *Salomé* by Oscar Wilde

Catherine Byrne as **Molly Sweeney, Mark Lambert** as **Frank Sweeney** in *Molly Sweeney* by **Brian Friel**

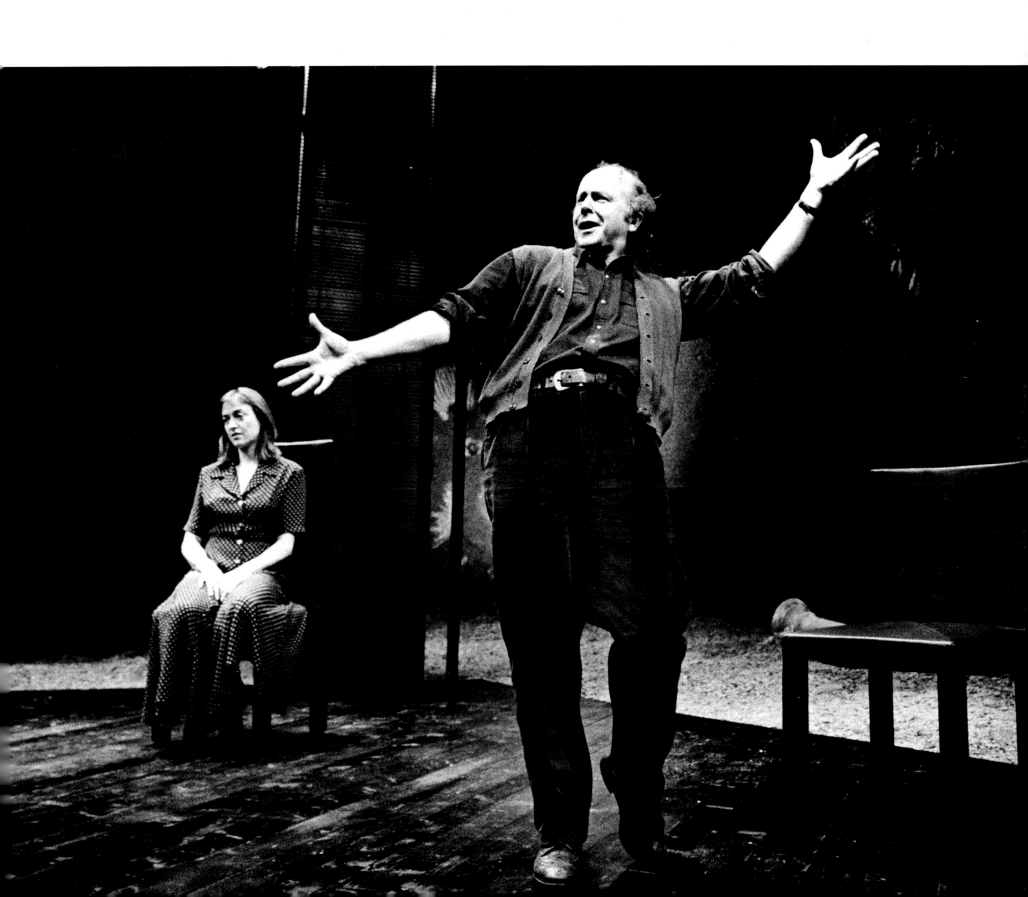

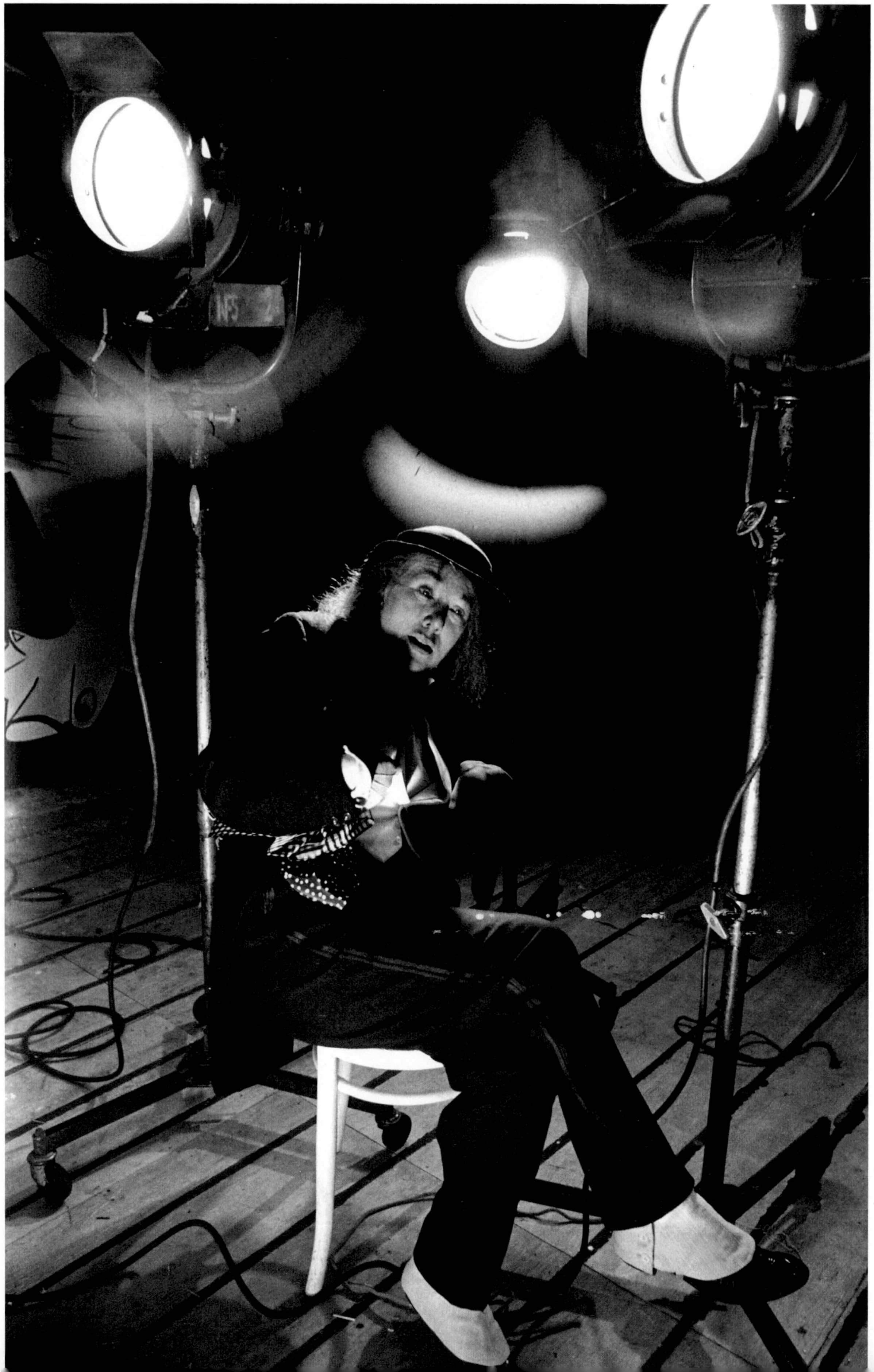

Rosaleen Linehan as **Feste** in ***Twelfth Night*** by **William Shakespeare**

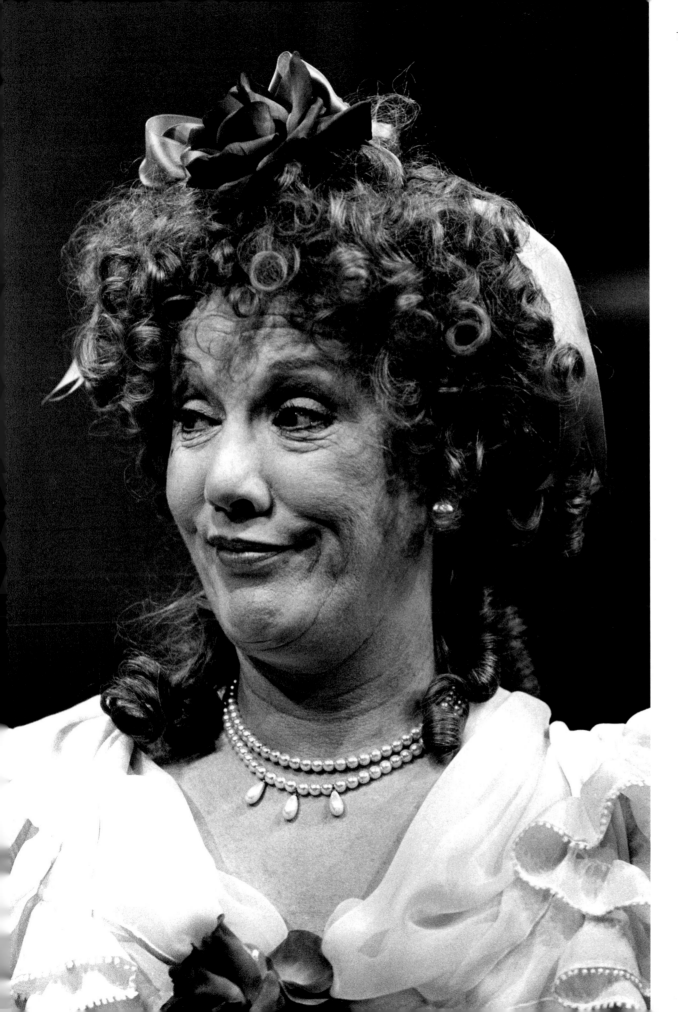

Rosaleen Linehan *as* **Mrs Malaprop** *in The Rivals* by **Richard Brinsley Sheridan**

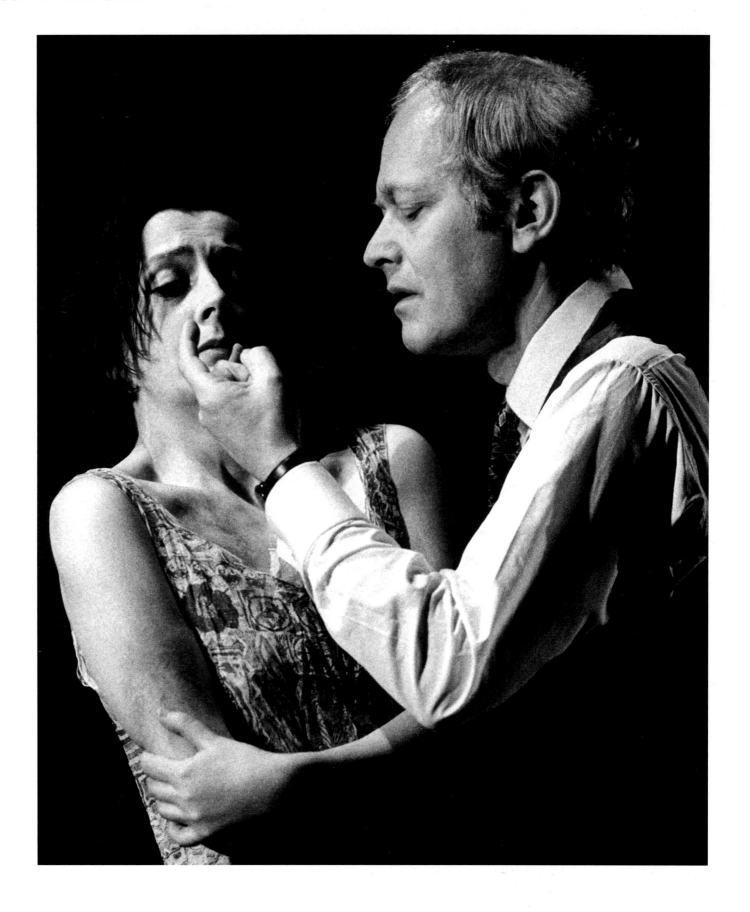

Jane Brennan AS **Gila**, Michael Pennington AS **Nicolas** IN *One for the Road* BY **Harold Pinter**

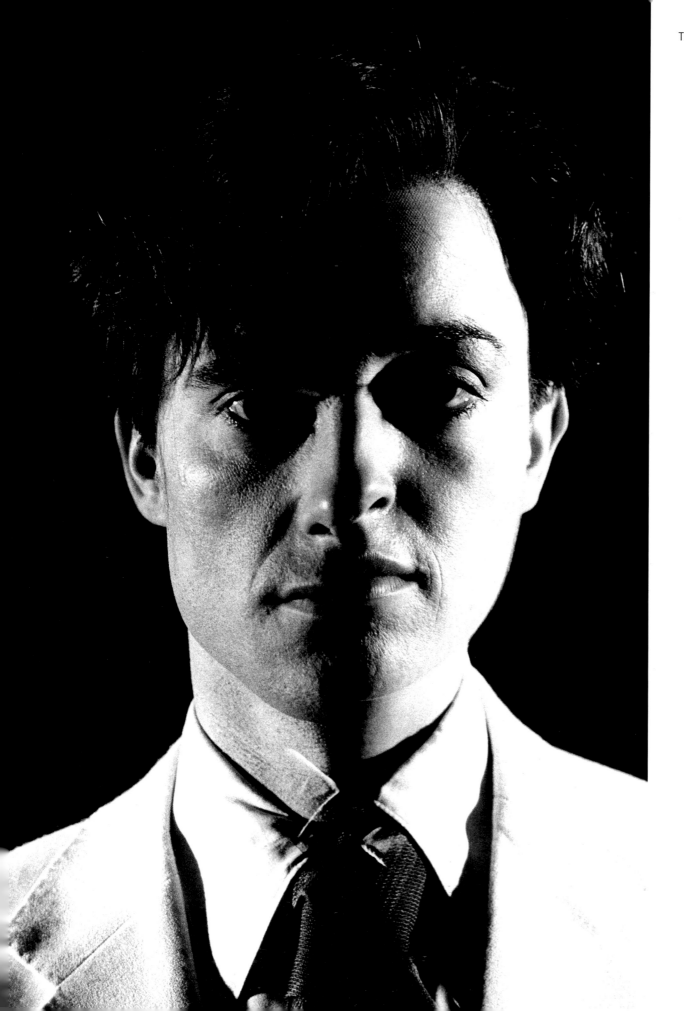

Barry Lynch as **Sebastian**, Catherine Byrne as **Cesario** in *Twelfth Night* by **William Shakespeare**

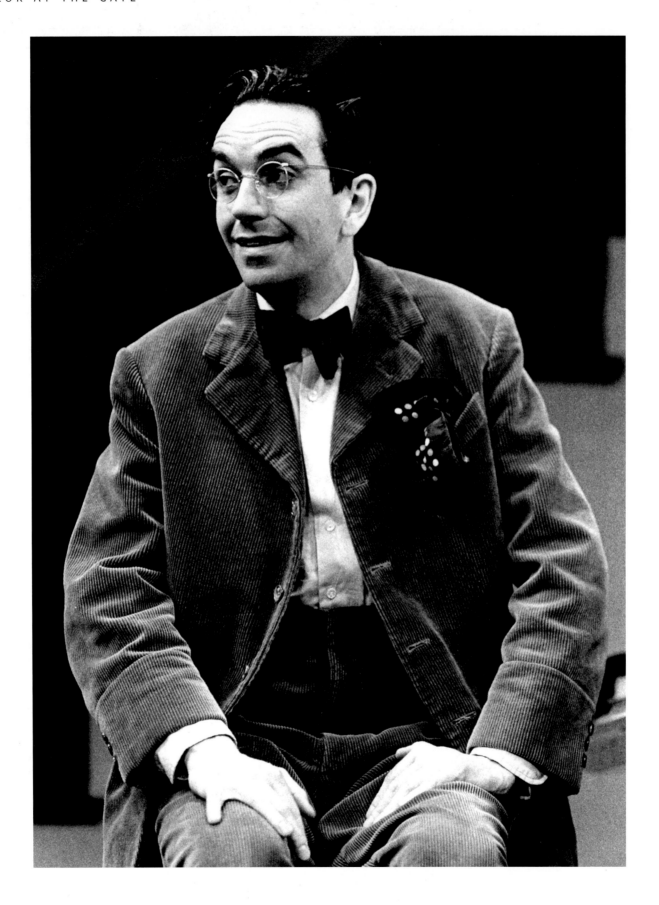

Phelim Drew as **Roland Maule** in *Present Laughter* by Noël Coward

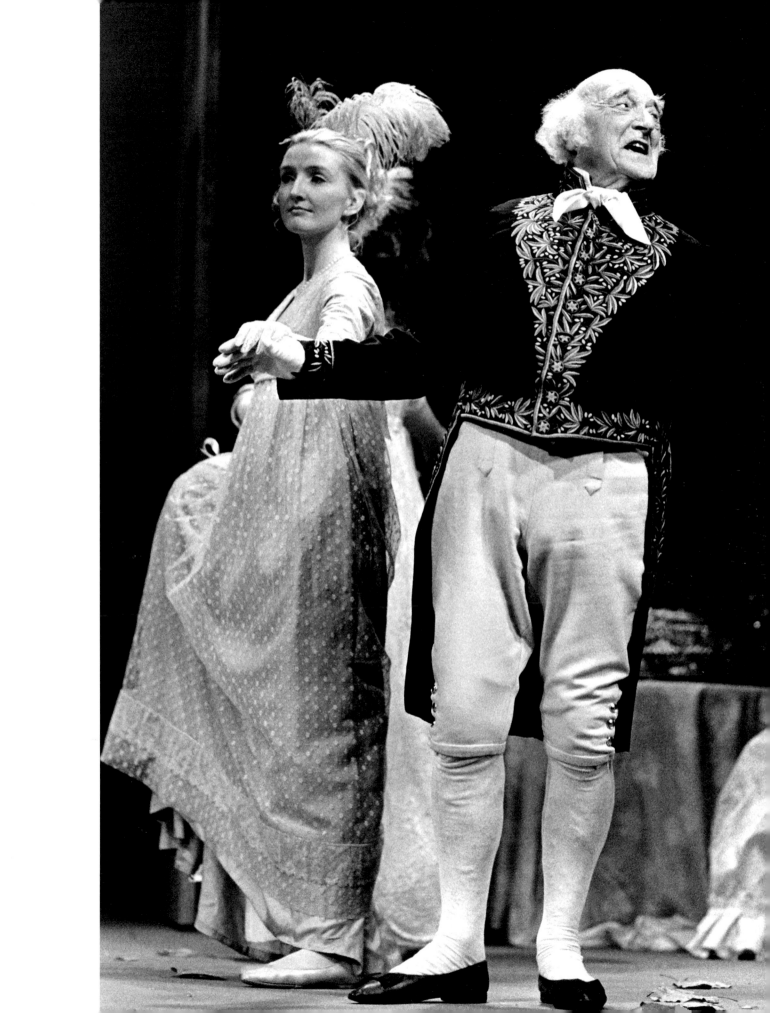

Claudia Carroll as **Caroline Bingley**, Christopher Casson as **Sir William Lucas** in *Pride and Prejudice* by Jane Austen

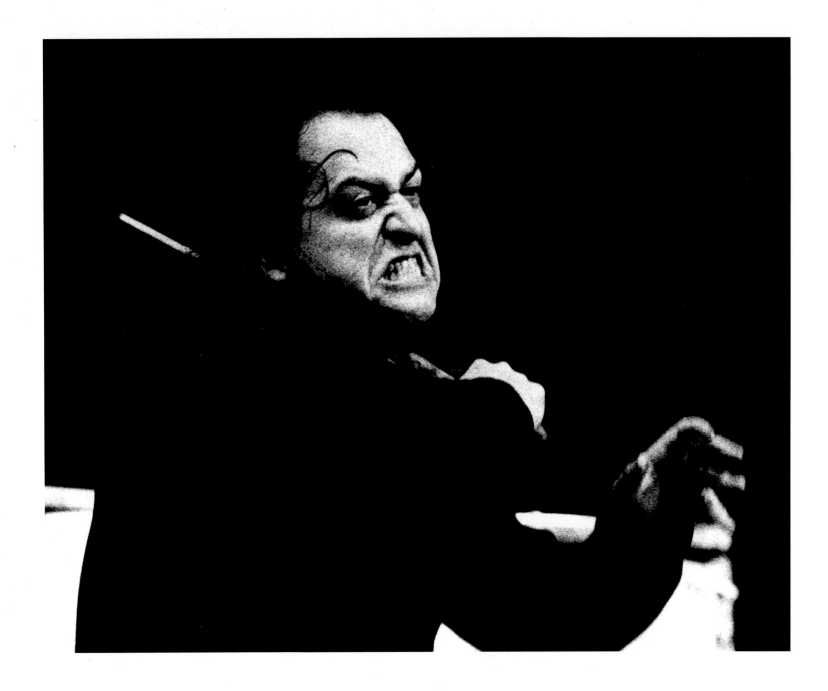

Overleaf: **Barry McGovern** as **Estragon** in *Waiting for Godot* by **Samuel Beckett**   **Stanley Townsend** as **Maskwell** in *The Double Dealer* by **William Congreve**

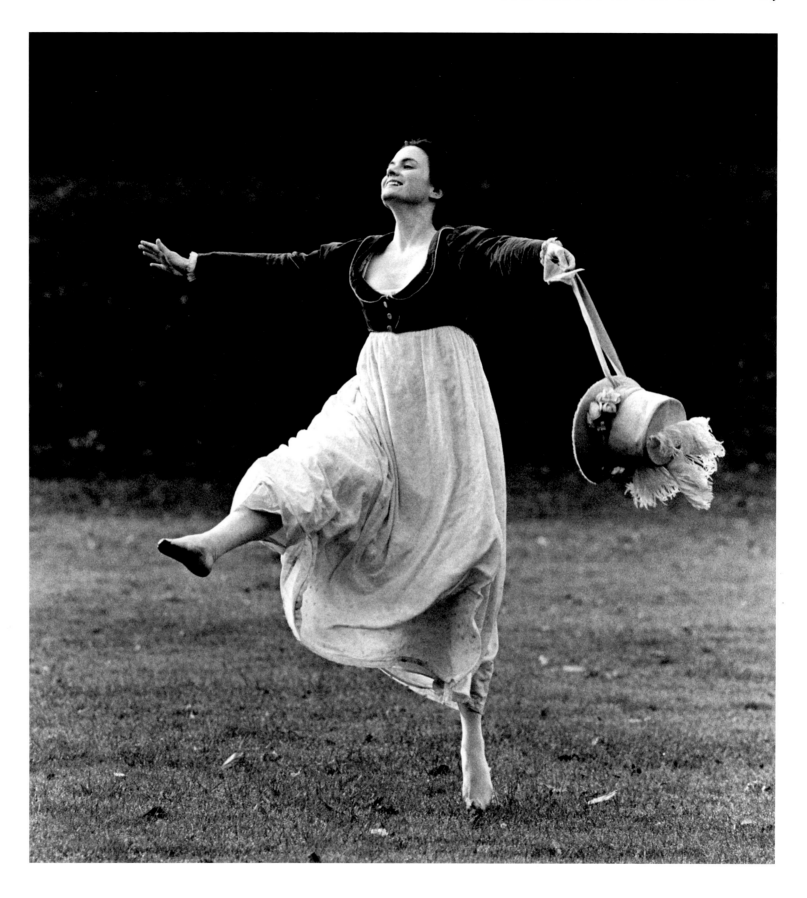

Alison McKenna as **Lydia Bennet** in *Pride and Prejudice* by **Jane Austen** adapted for the stage by **James Maxwell**

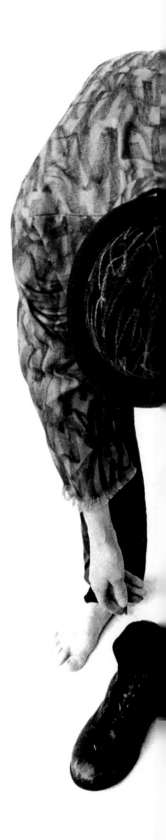

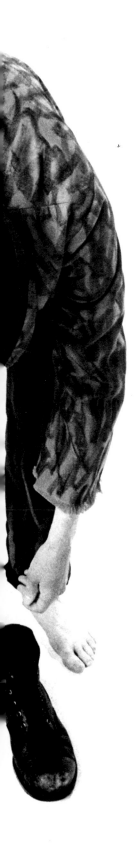

Garrett Keogh as Caravaggio in Innocence, The Life of Caravaggio by Frank McGuinness

Kate Flynn as Lena in *Innocence, The Life of Caravaggio* by Frank McGuinness

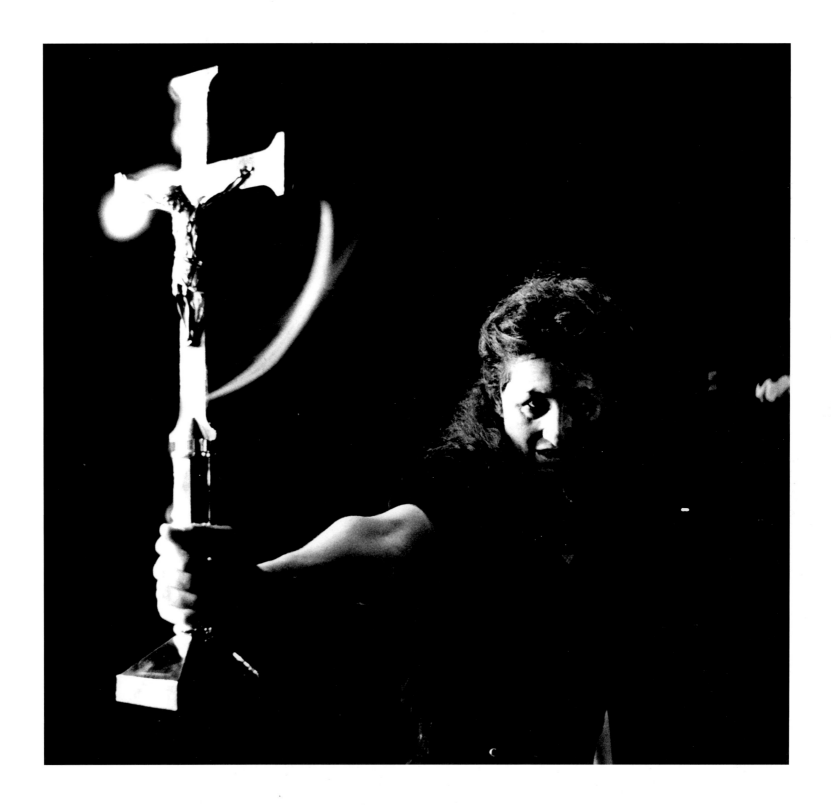

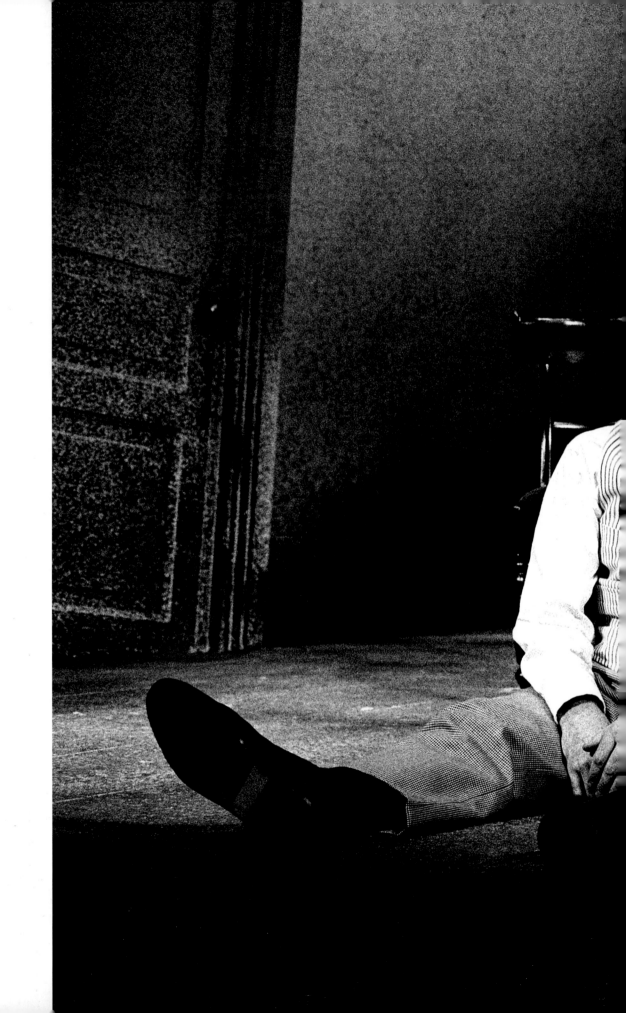

James Laurenson as **Mr Aston**, **Gillian Barge** as **Isobel Desmond** in *The Seagull* by **Anton Chekhov** in a version by **Thomas Kilroy**

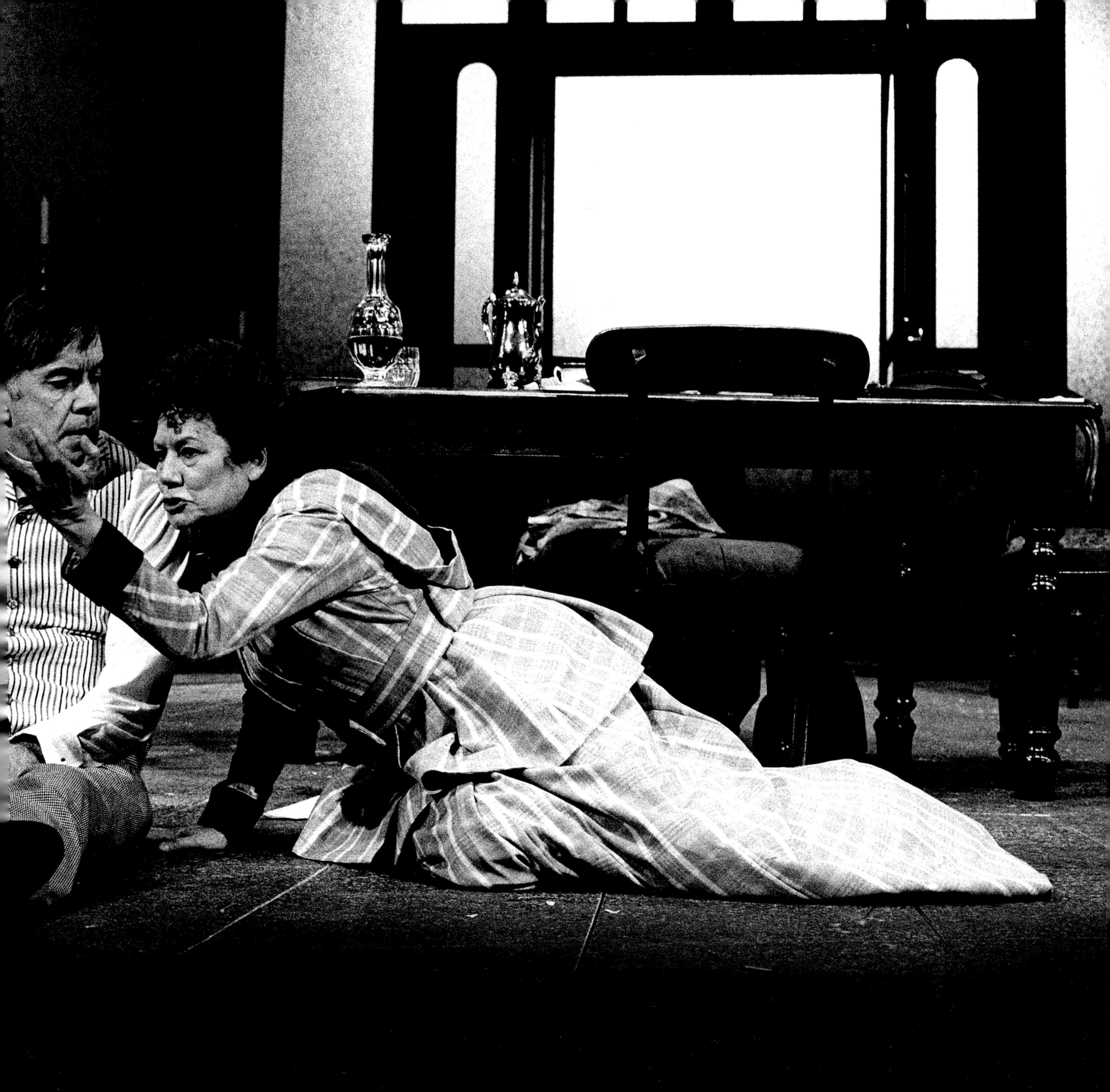

Brendan Gleeson as **Epikhodov** in *The Cherry Orchard* by **Anton Chekhov** in a version by **Michael Bogdanov**

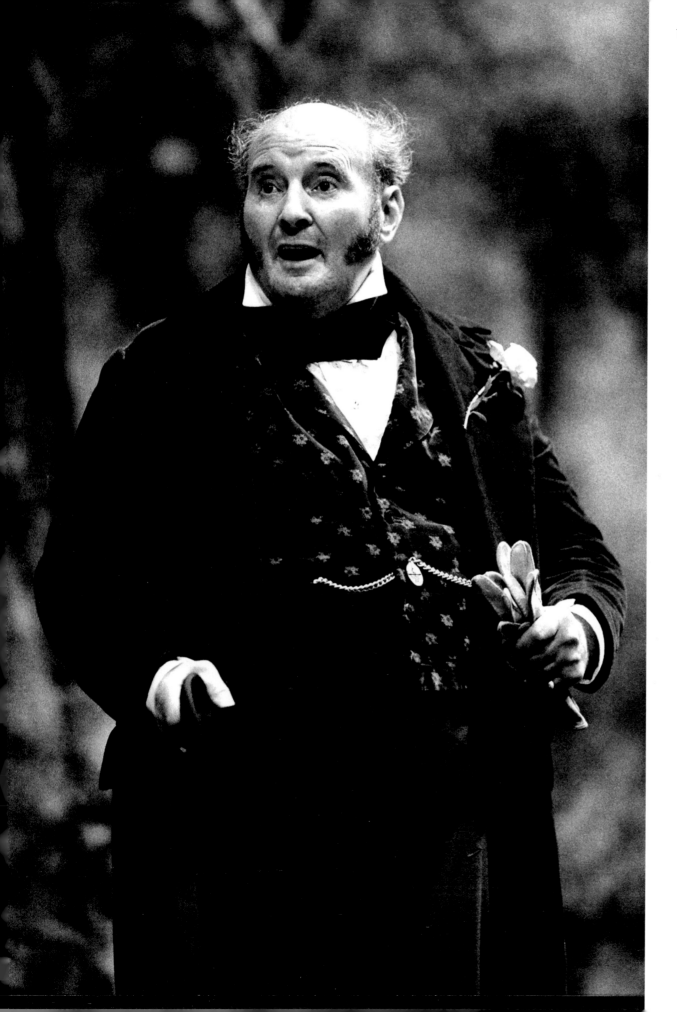

John Cowley as **Bolshintsov** in **Brian Friel's** version of **A Month in the Country** by **Ivan Turgenev**

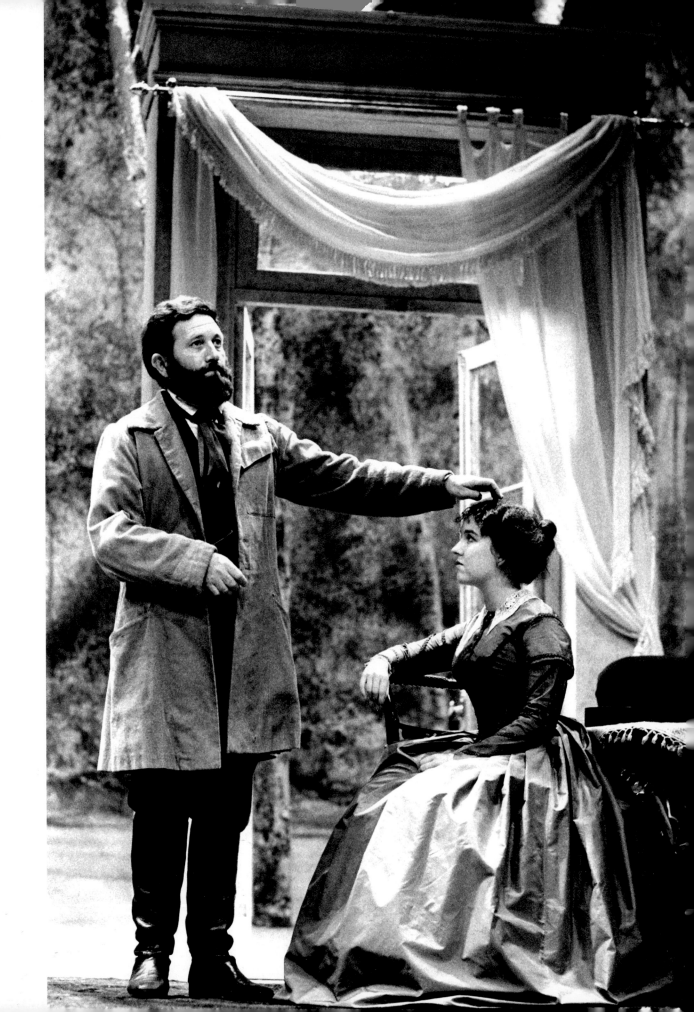

Donal McCann as **Shpigelsky**, Karen Ardiff as **Vera** in Brian Friel's version of *A Month in the Country* by Ivan Turgenev

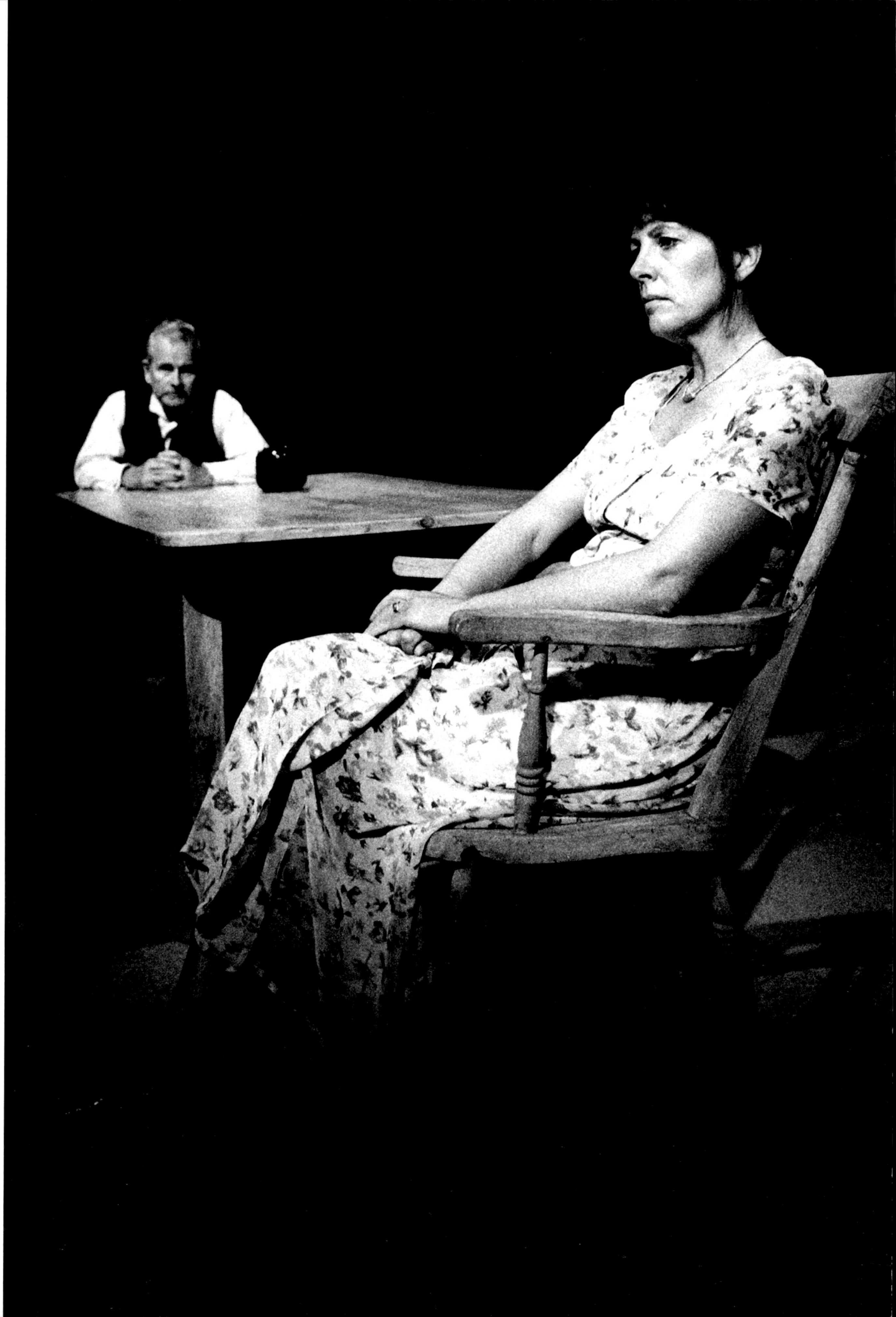

Ian Holm as **Duff**, **Penelope Wilton** as **Beth** in ***Landscape*** by **Harold Pinter**

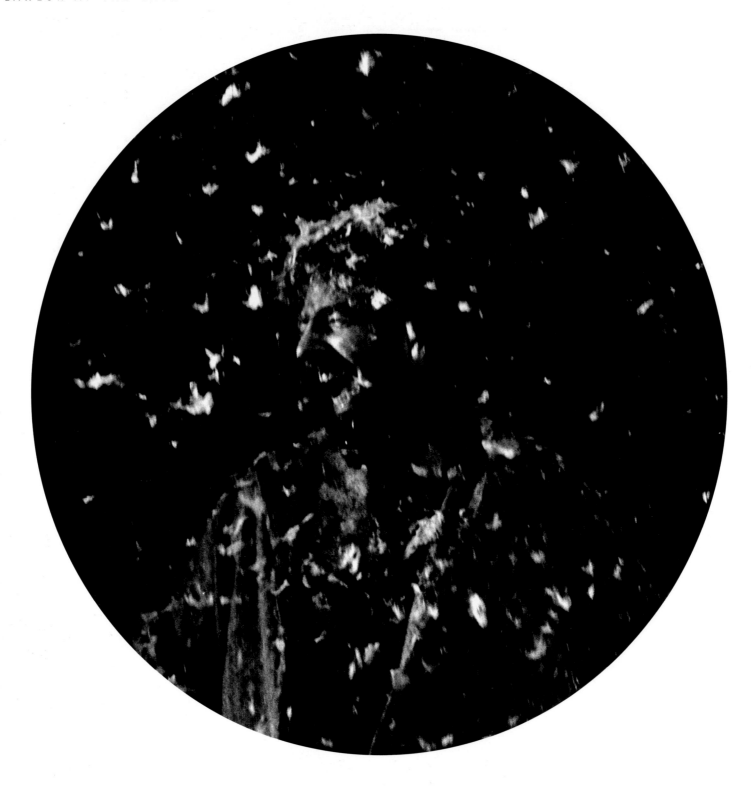

Garrett Keogh as **Caravaggio** in *Innocence, The Life of Caravaggio* by **Frank McGuinness**

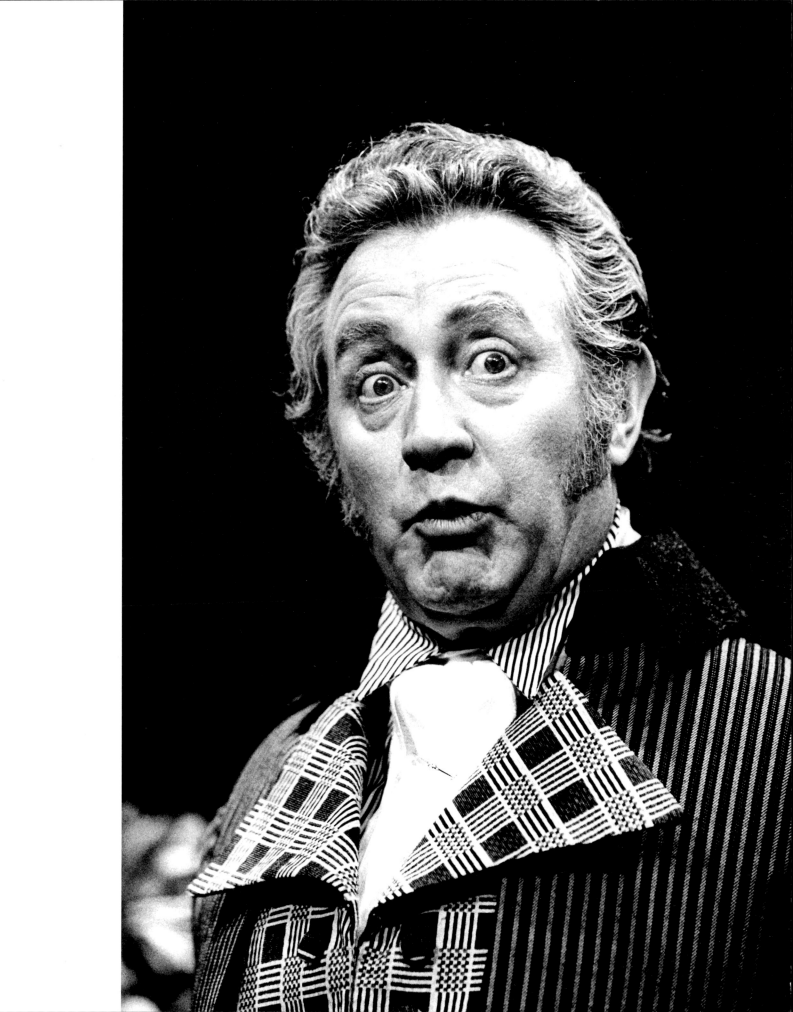

Bill Golding as **Sir Peter Teazle** in *The School for Scandal* by **Richard Brinsley Sheridan**

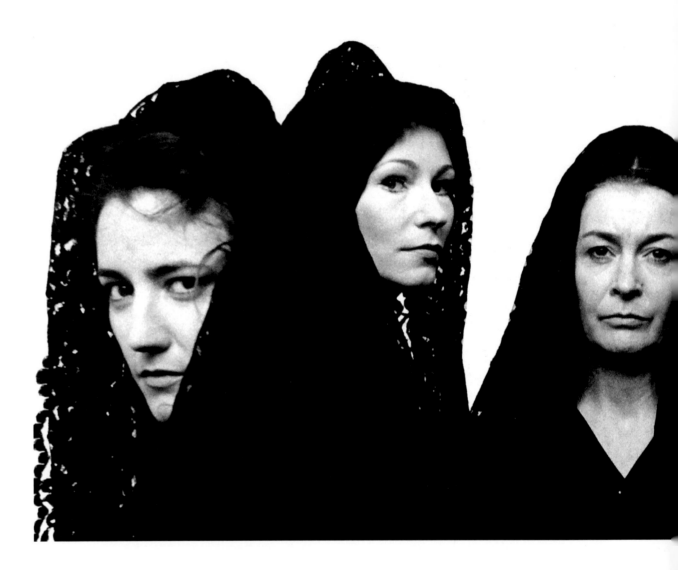

Orla Brady as **Adela**, Katherine O'Toole as **Martirio**, Barbara Brennan as **Magdalena**, Jane Brennan as **Amelia**, Bernadett

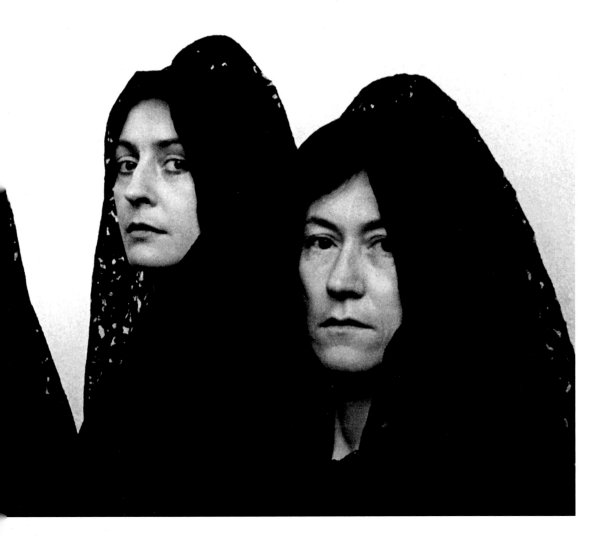

as **Angustias** in *The House of Bernarda Alba* by **Federico García Lorca** in a translation by **Aidan Mathews**

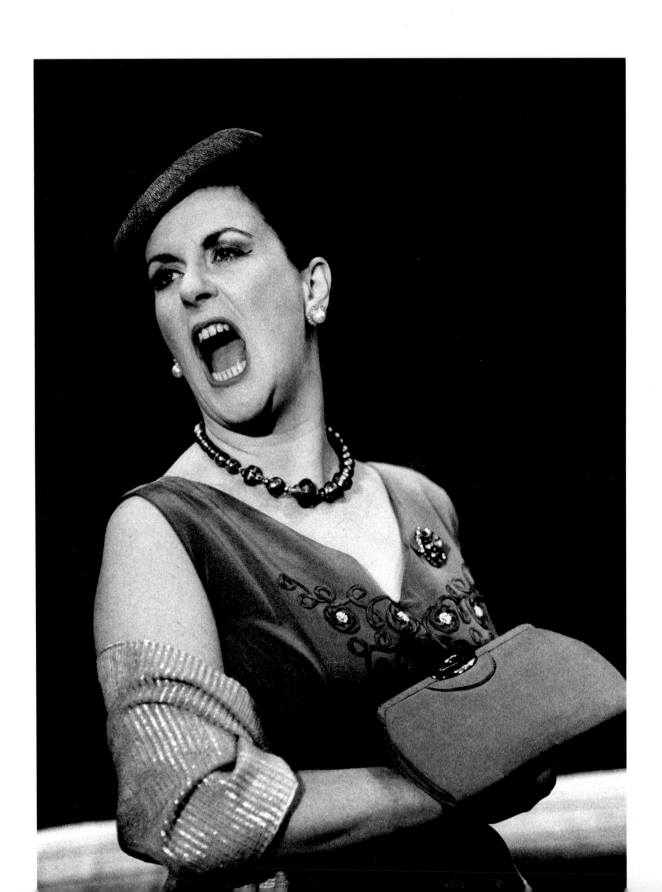

Marion O'Dwyer as **Lucy** in *The Threepenny Opera* by **Bertolt Brecht** and **Kurt Weill** in a version by **Frank McGuinness**

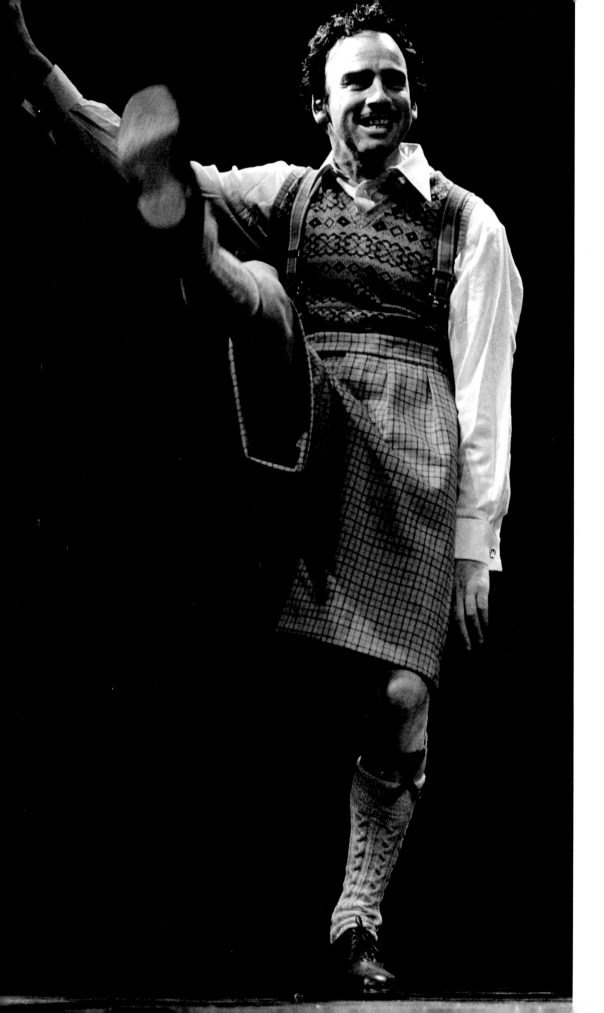

John Kavanagh as **Malvolio** in *Twelfth Night* by **William Shakespeare**

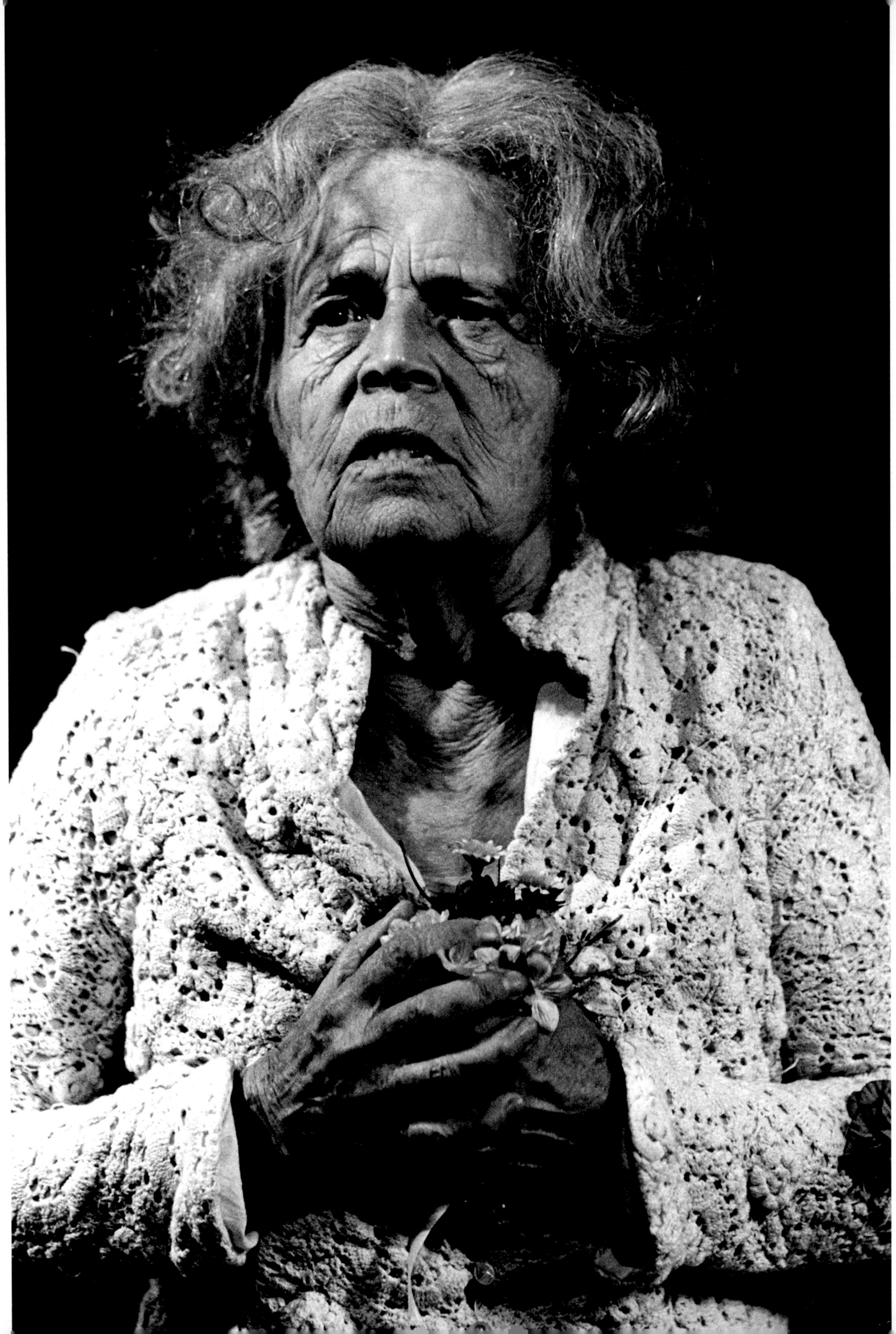

Patricia Hayes as **Maria Josefa** in ***The House of Bernarda Alba*** by **Federico García Lorca** in a translation by **Aidan Mathews**

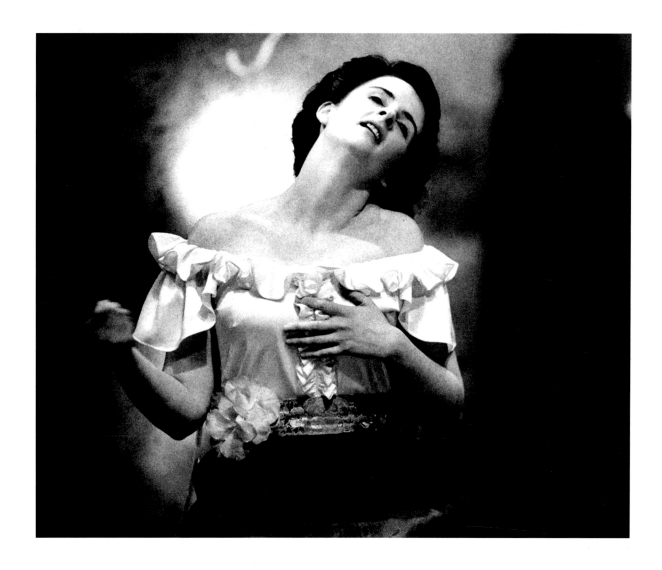

Anna Healy as **Dunyasha** in *The Cherry Orchard* by **Anton Chekhov** in a version by **Michael Bogdanov**

Susan FitzGerald as **La Marquise de Merteuil** in *Les Liaisons Dangereuses* by **Christopher Hampton** from the novel by **Choderlos de Laclos**

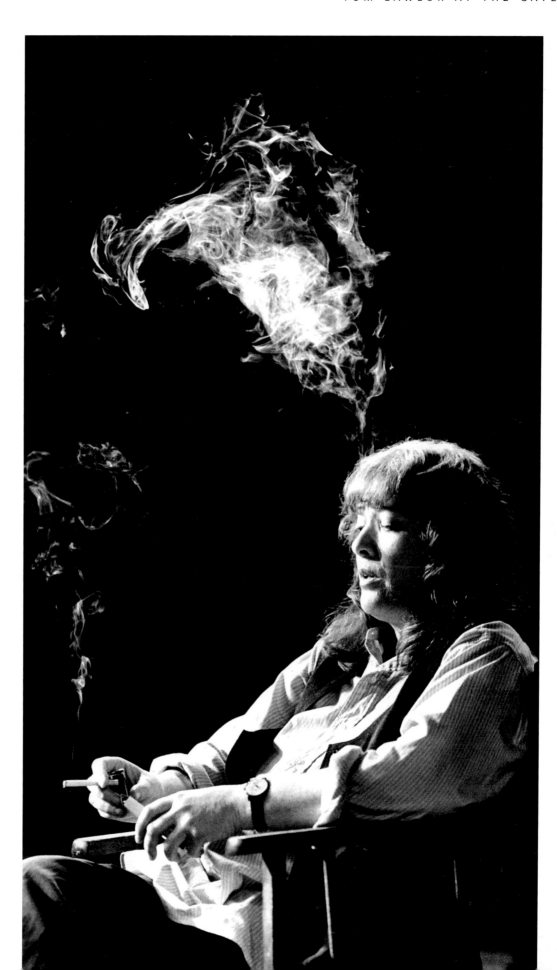

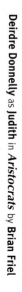
Deirdre Donnelly as **Judith** in *Aristocrats* by **Brian Friel**

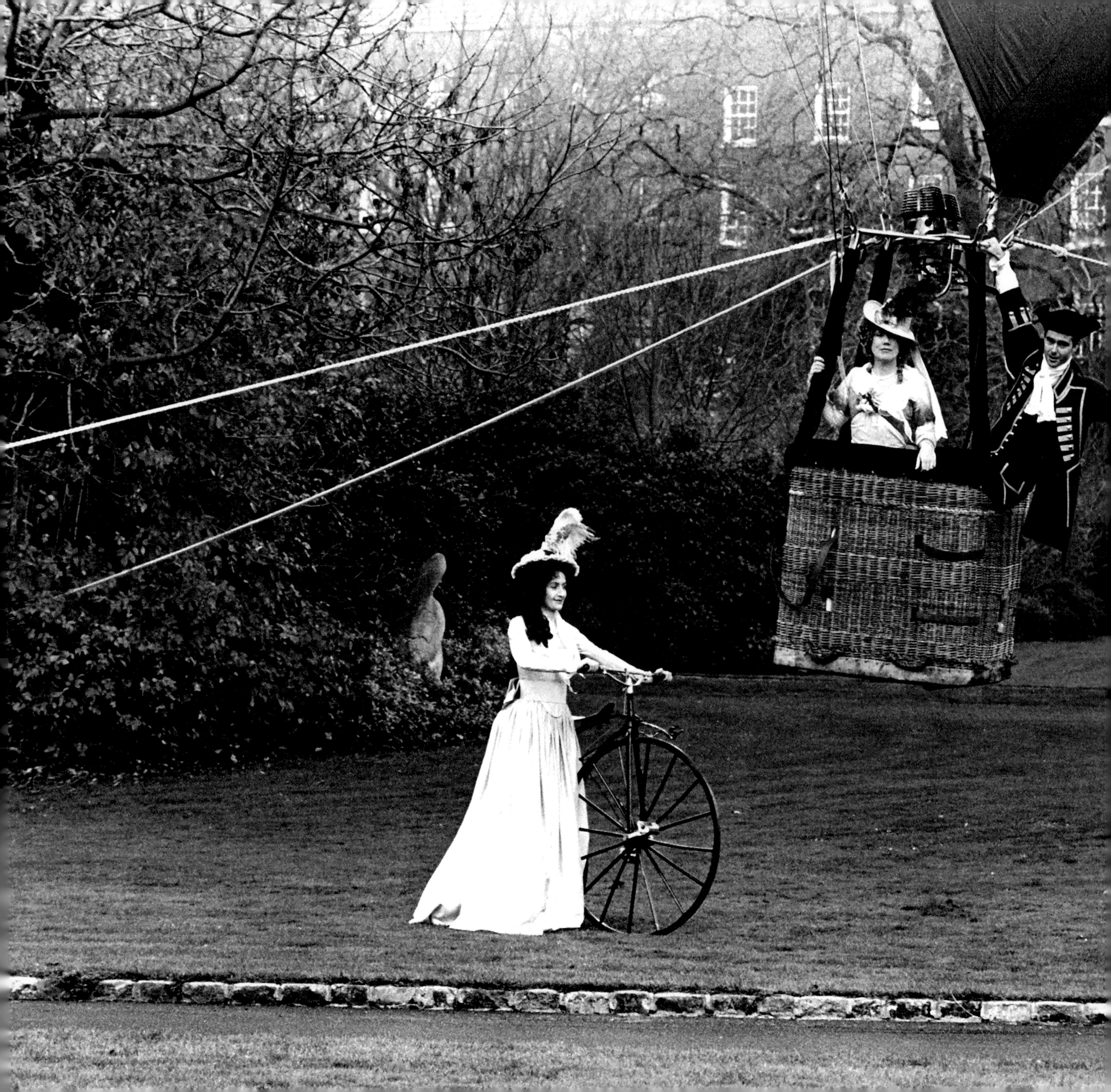

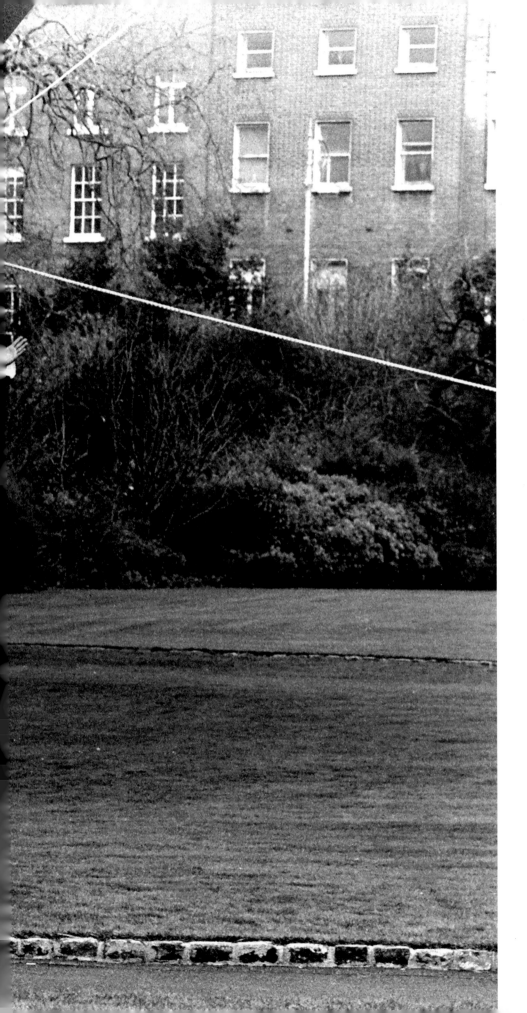

Jane Brennan as **Lydia Languish**, Rosaleen Linehan as **Mrs Malaprop**, Barry Lynch as **Captain Absolute** in *The Rivals* by **Richard Brinsley Sheridan**

Doreen Hepburn as **Ase, Joe Dowling** as **Peer Gynt** in *Peer Gynt* by **Henrik Ibsen** in a version by **Frank McGuinness**

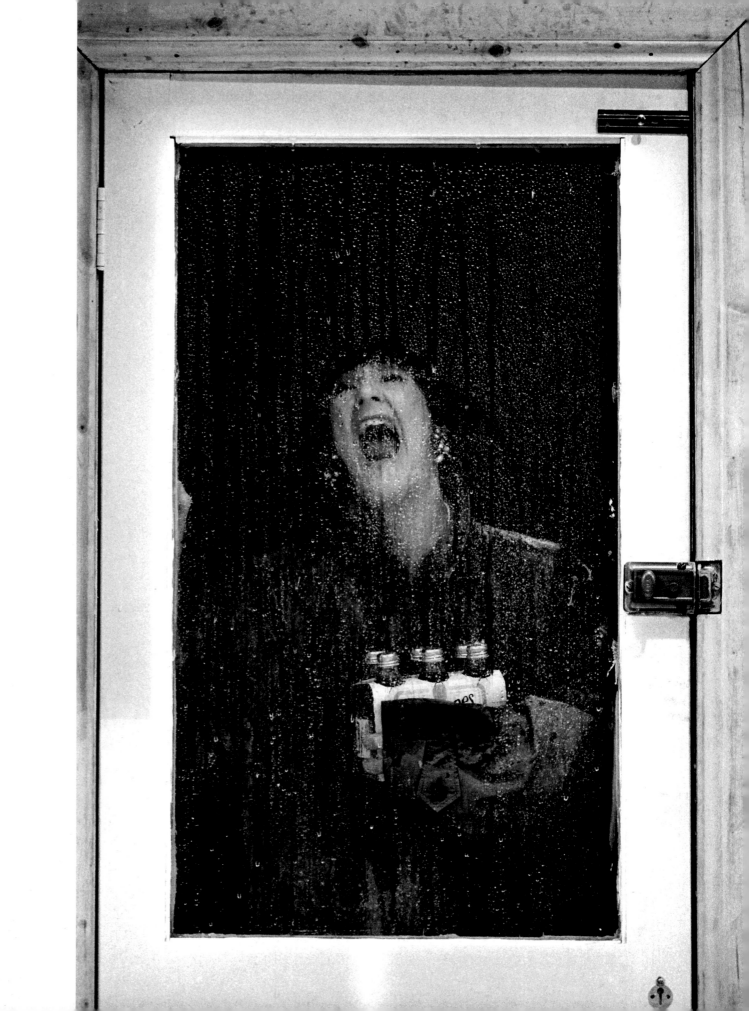

Pauline McLynn as **Jane** in *Absurd Person Singular* by **Alan Ayckbourn**

Corinne Jaber as **Woman**, Bruce Myers as **Man** in *Dybbuk* by **Bruce Myers** adapted from the play by **Anski**

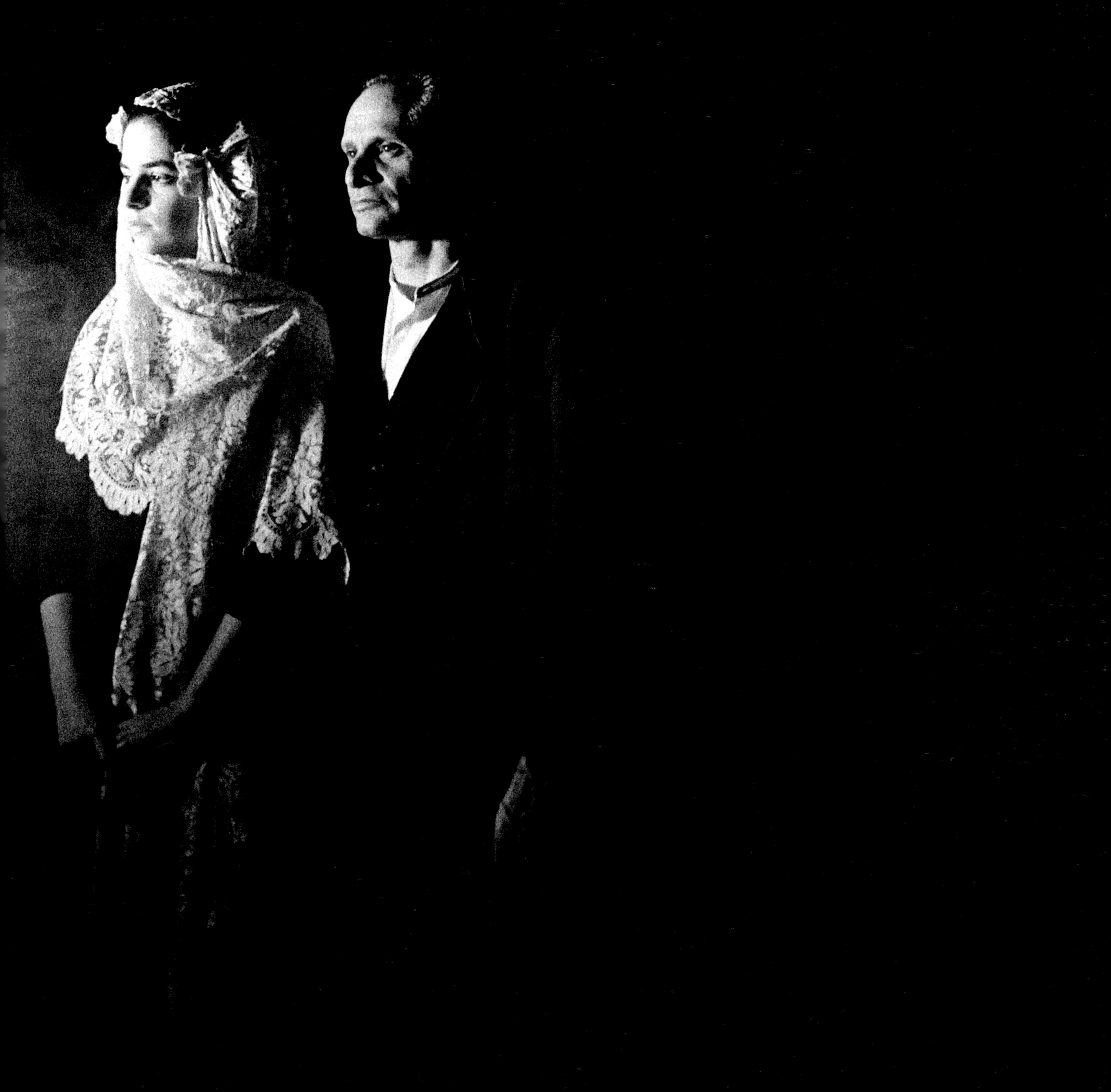

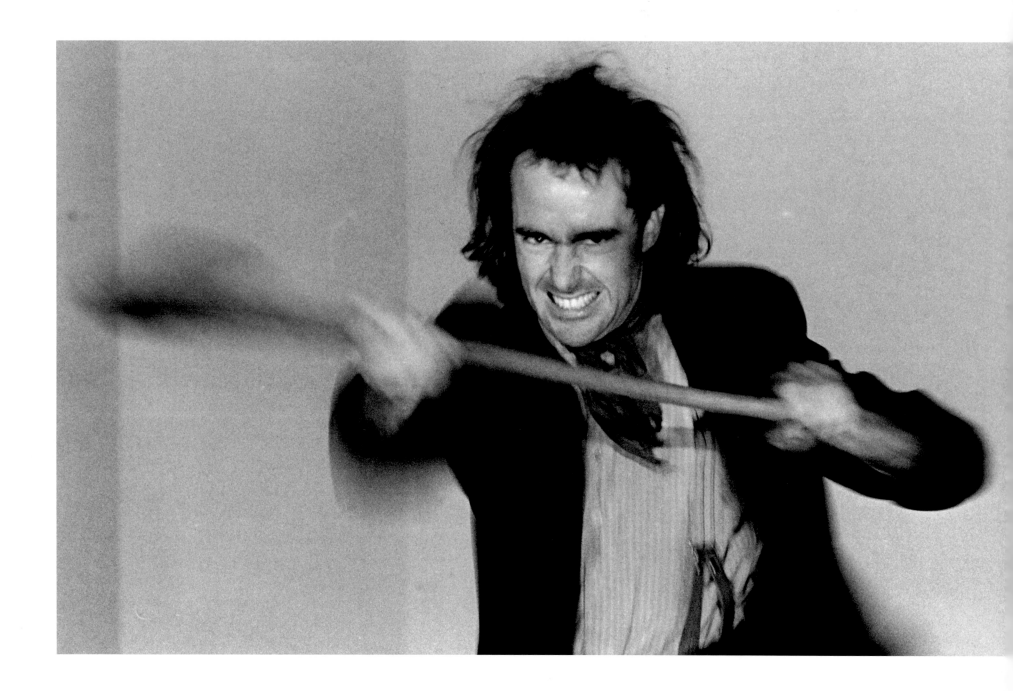

Barry Lynch as **Peer Gynt** in *Peer Gynt* by **Henrik Ibsen** in a version by **Frank McGuinness**

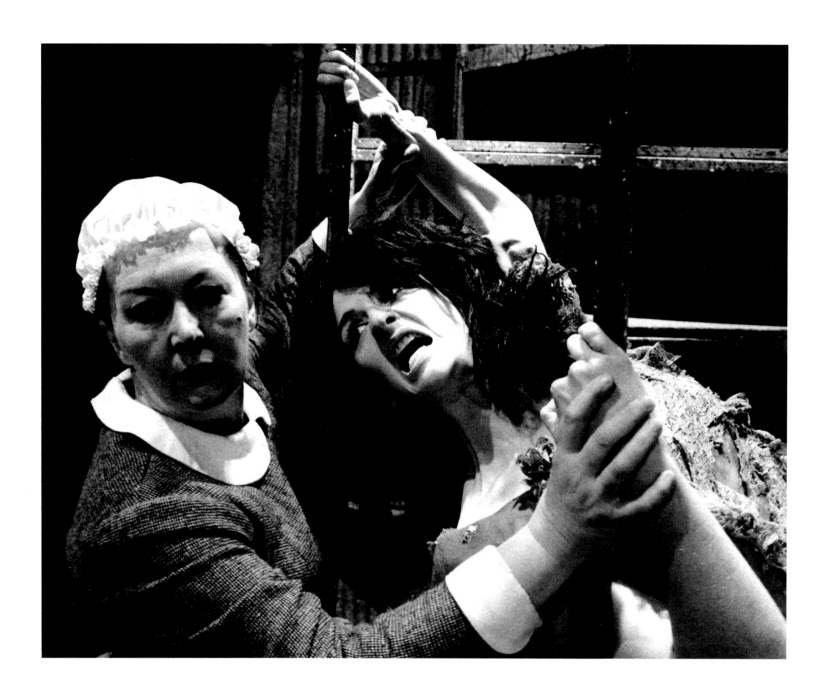

Máire Hastings as **Mrs Brocklehurst, Anna Healy** as **Mrs Rochester** in *Jane Eyre* by **Charlotte Brontë** adapted for the stage by **Fay Weldon**

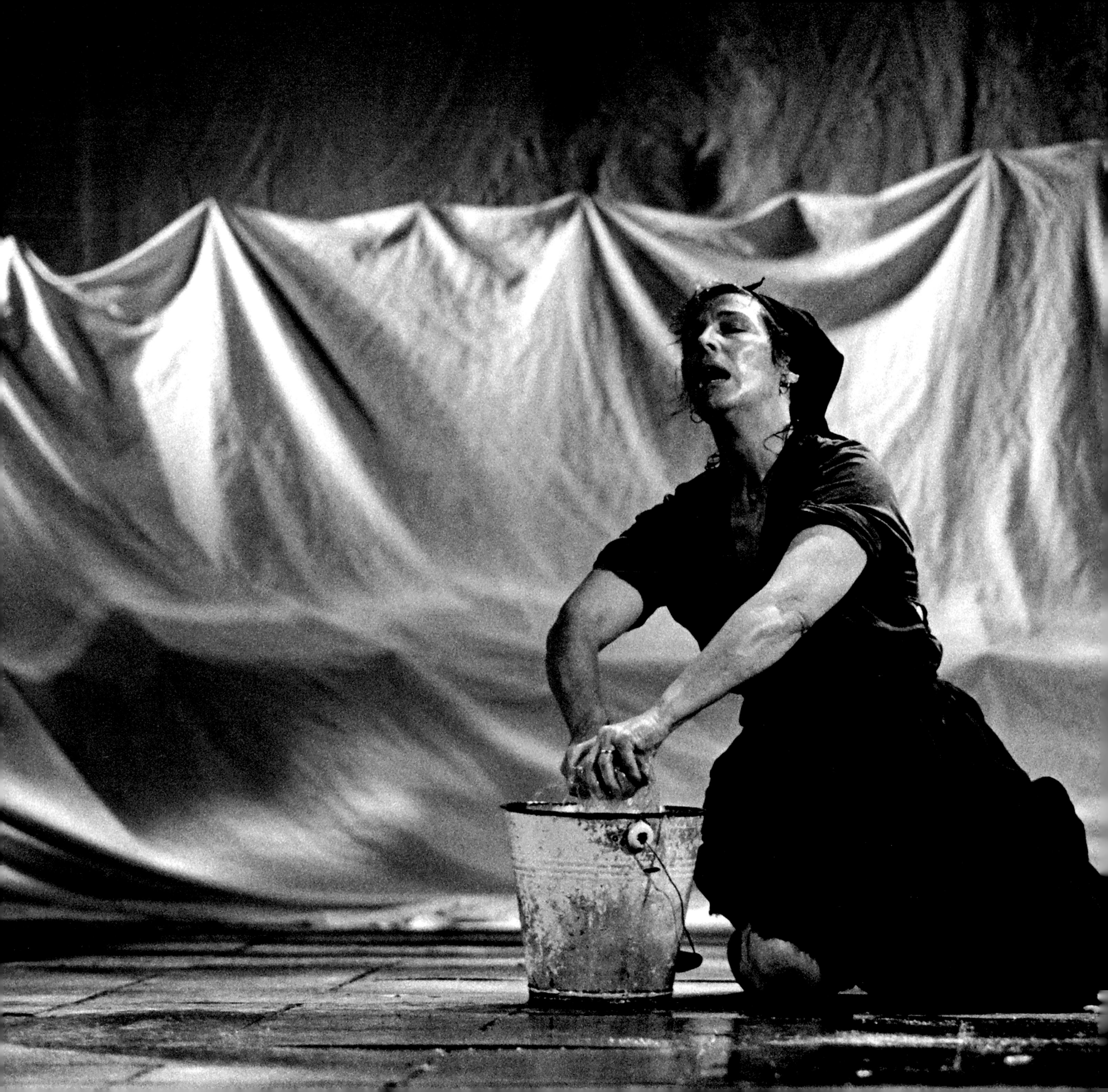

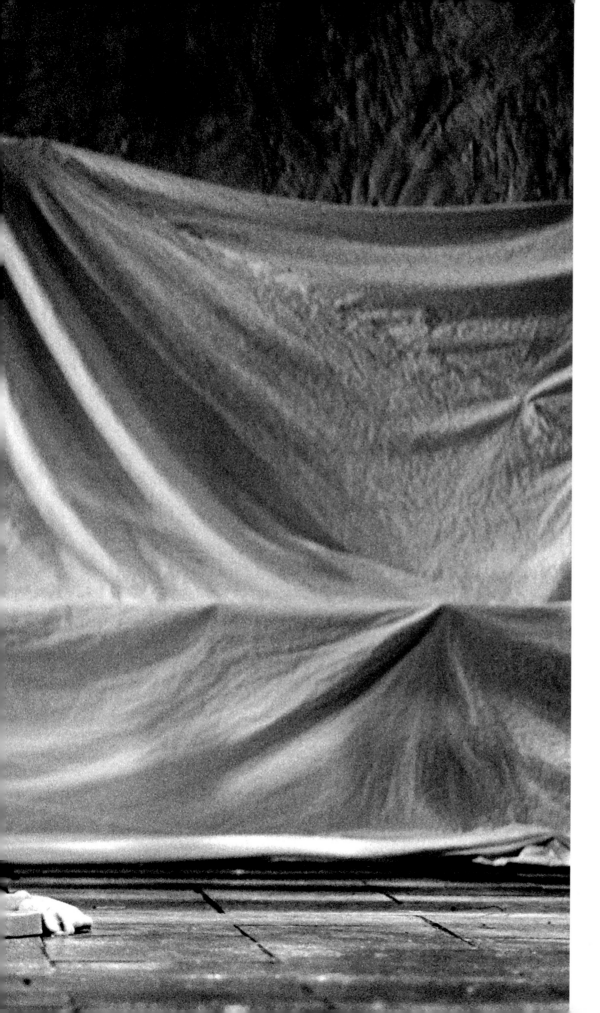

Stella McCusker as the **Maid** in *The House of Bernarda Alba* by **Federico García Lorca** in a translation by **Aidan Mathews**

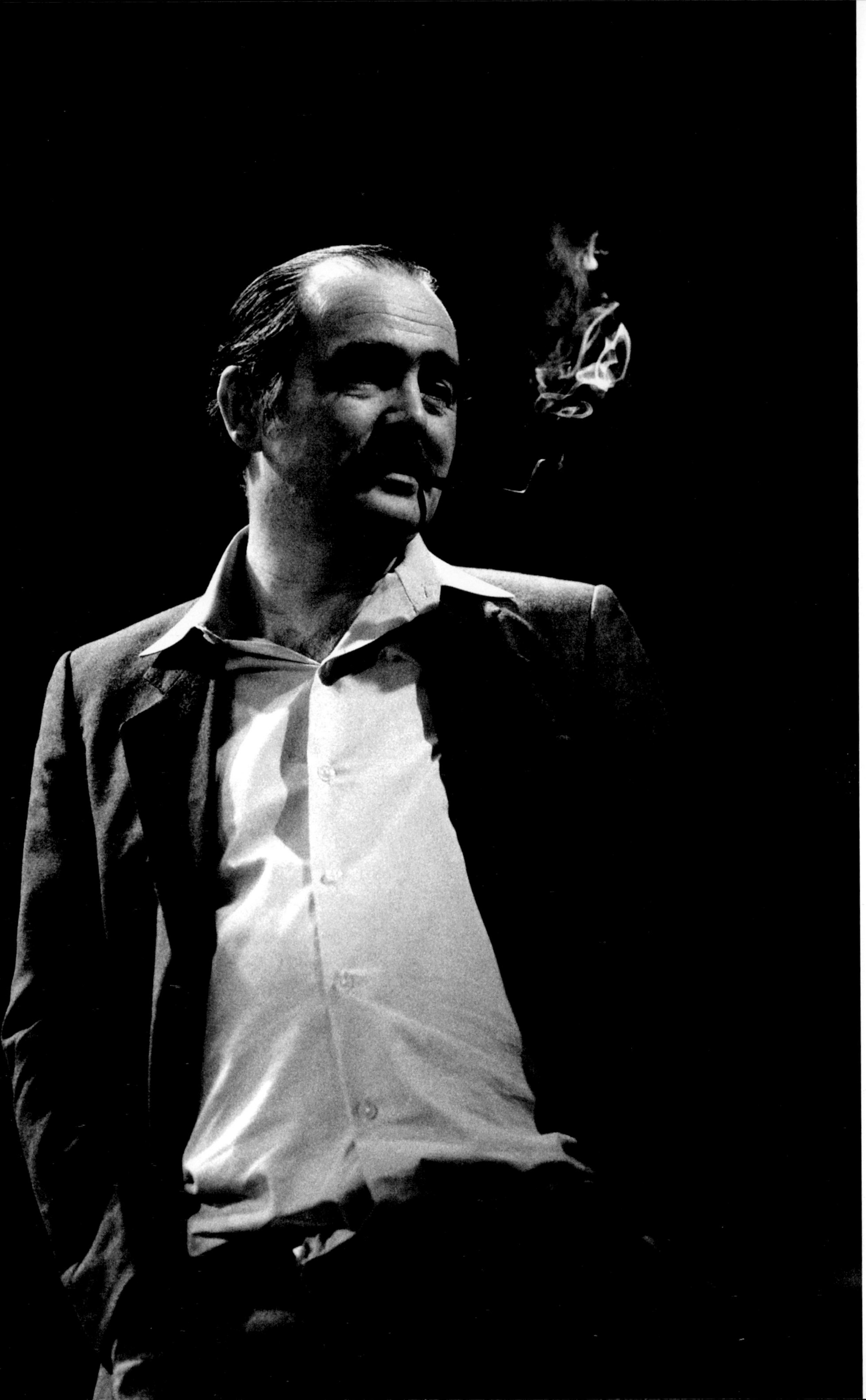

John Olohan as **Willie Diver** in *Aristocrats* by **Brian Friel**

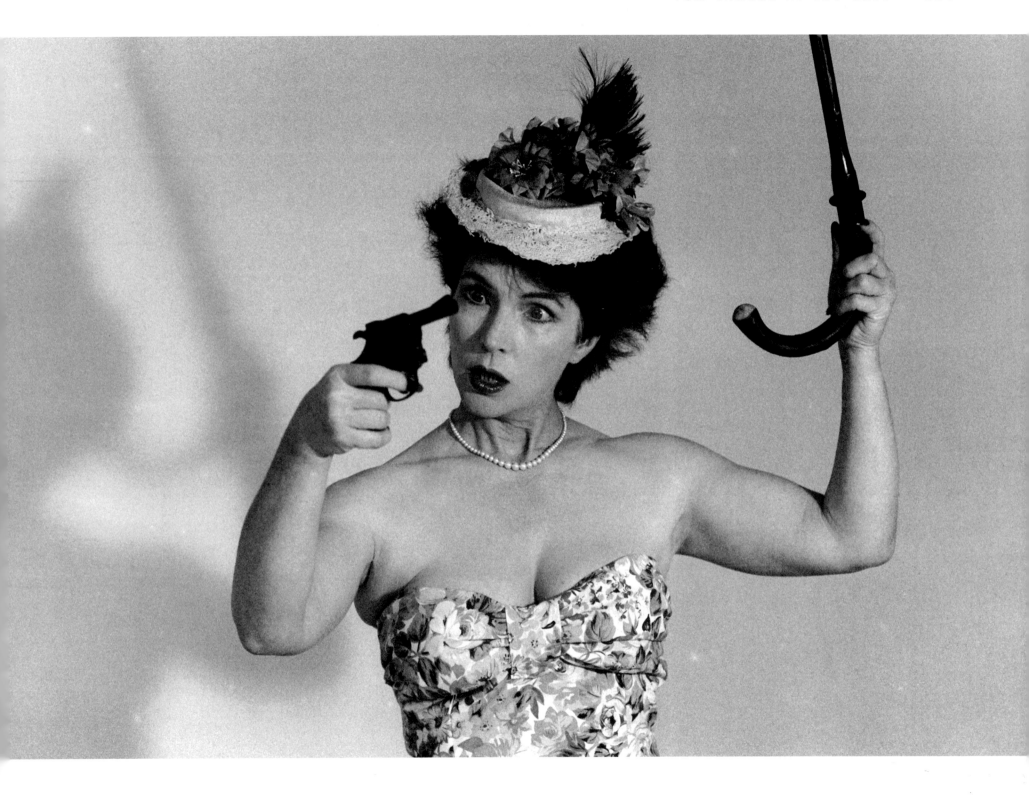

Fionnula Flanagan as **Winnie** in *Happy Days* by **Samuel Beckett**

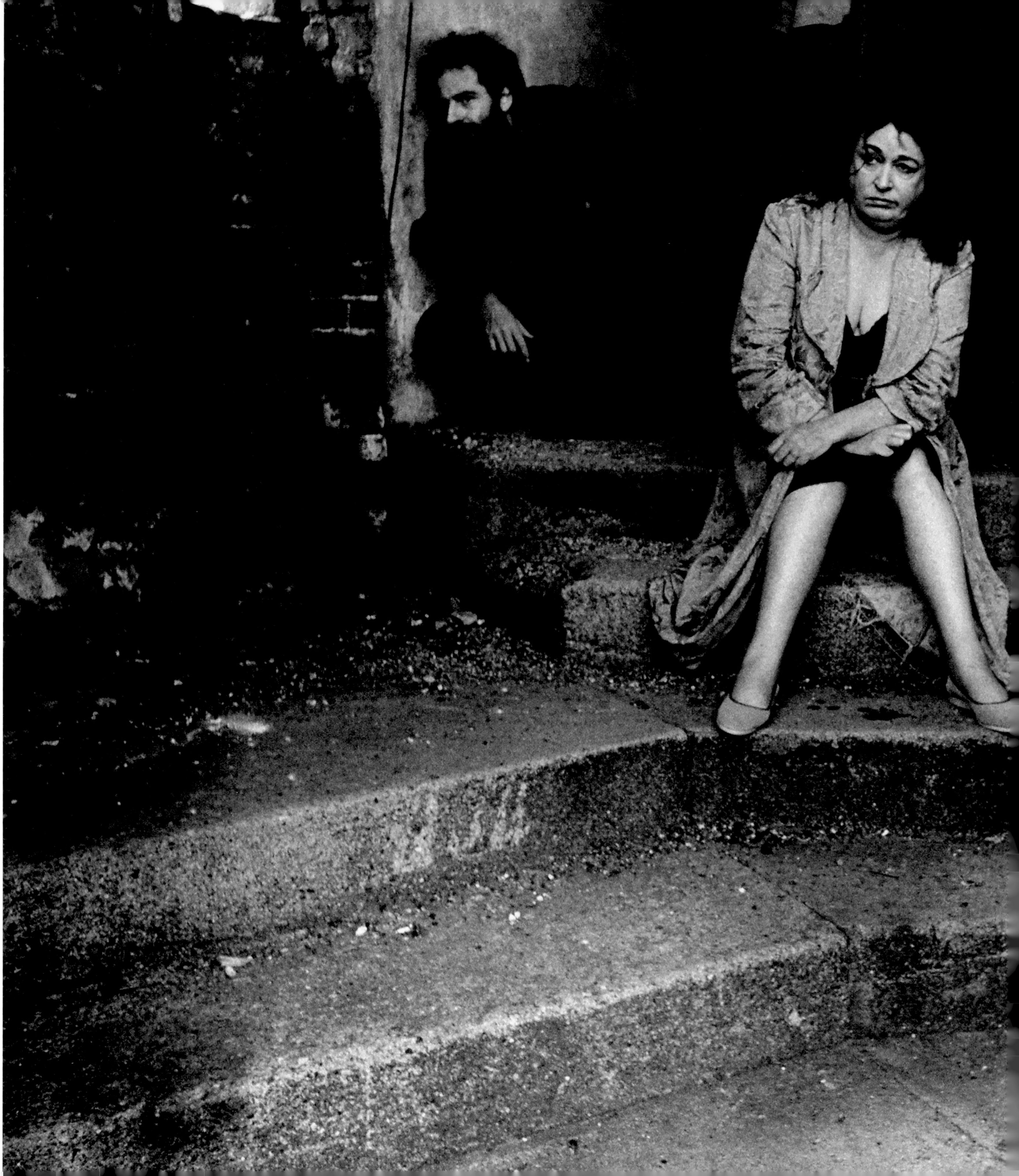

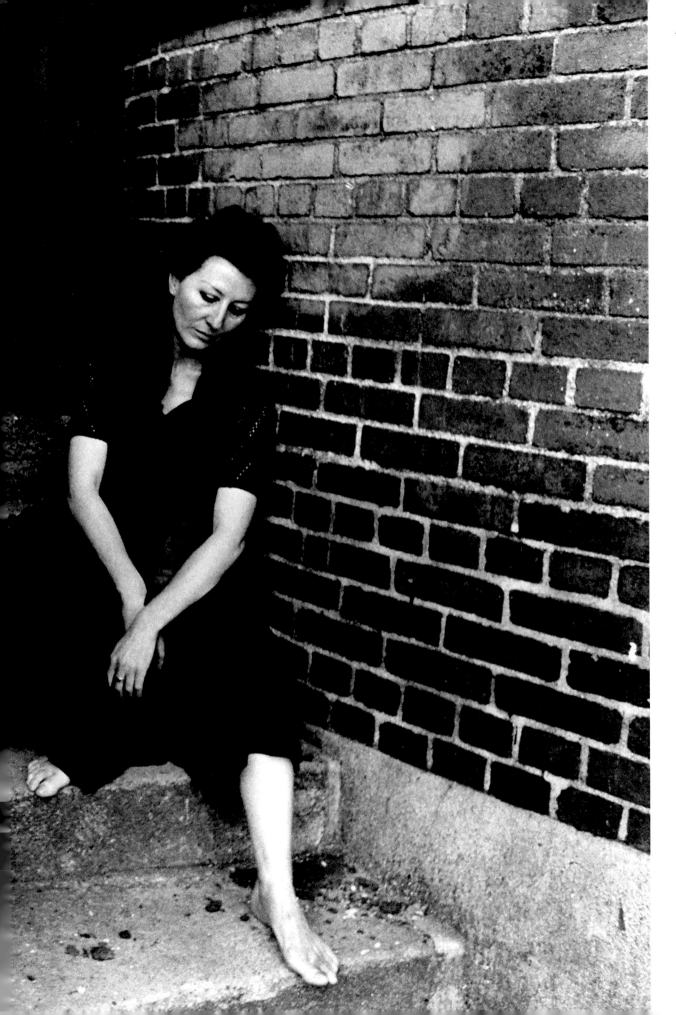

Garrett Keogh as **Caravaggio**, *Pat Leavy* as **the Whore**, *Kate Flynn* as **Lena** in **Innocence**, *The Life of Caravaggio* by **Frank McGuinness**

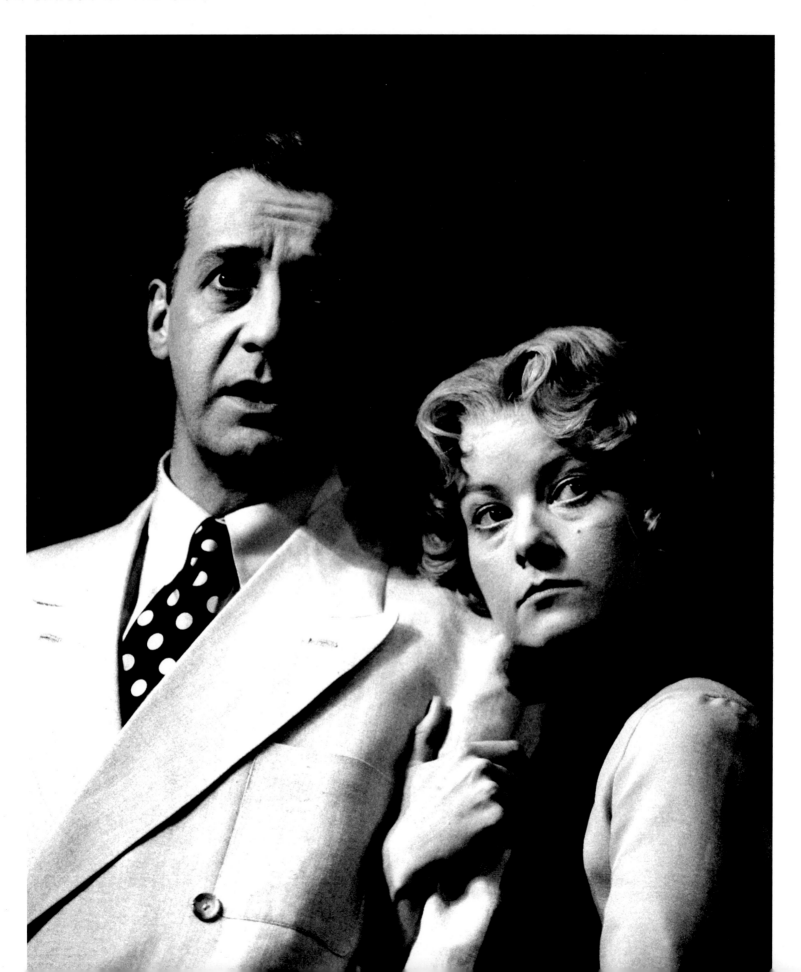

Stephen Brennan as **Elyot Chase**, **Lucy Vigne Welsh** as **Sibyl Chase** in *Private Lives* by **Noël Coward**

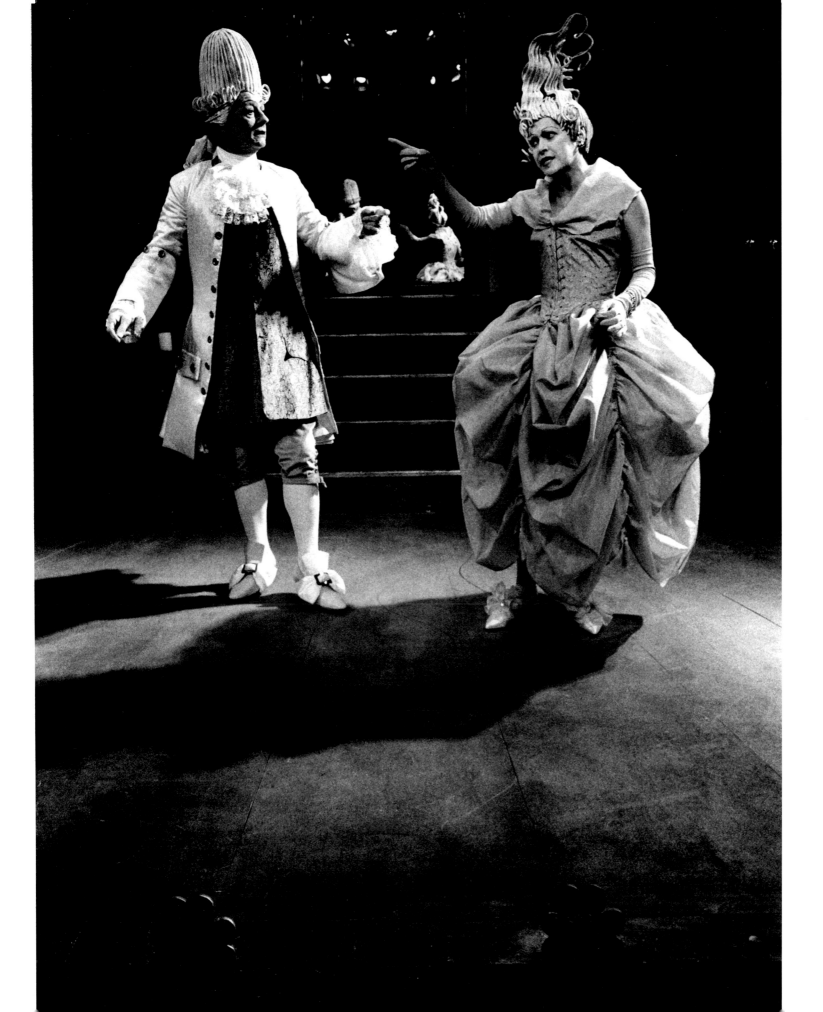

John Hurt as **Count Mushroom**, Gemma Craven as **Mrs Diggerty** in *The London Vertigo* by **Brian Friel** based on a play by **Charles Macklin**

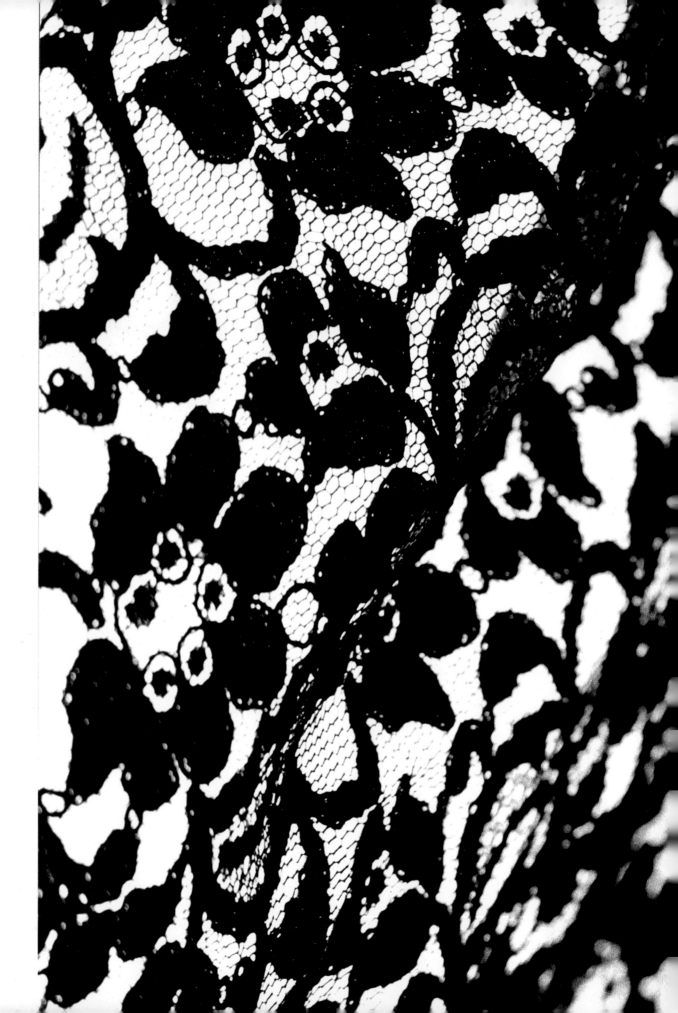

Katherine O'Toole as **Martirio** in *The House of Bernarda Alba* by **Federico García Lorca** in a translation by **Aidan Mathews**

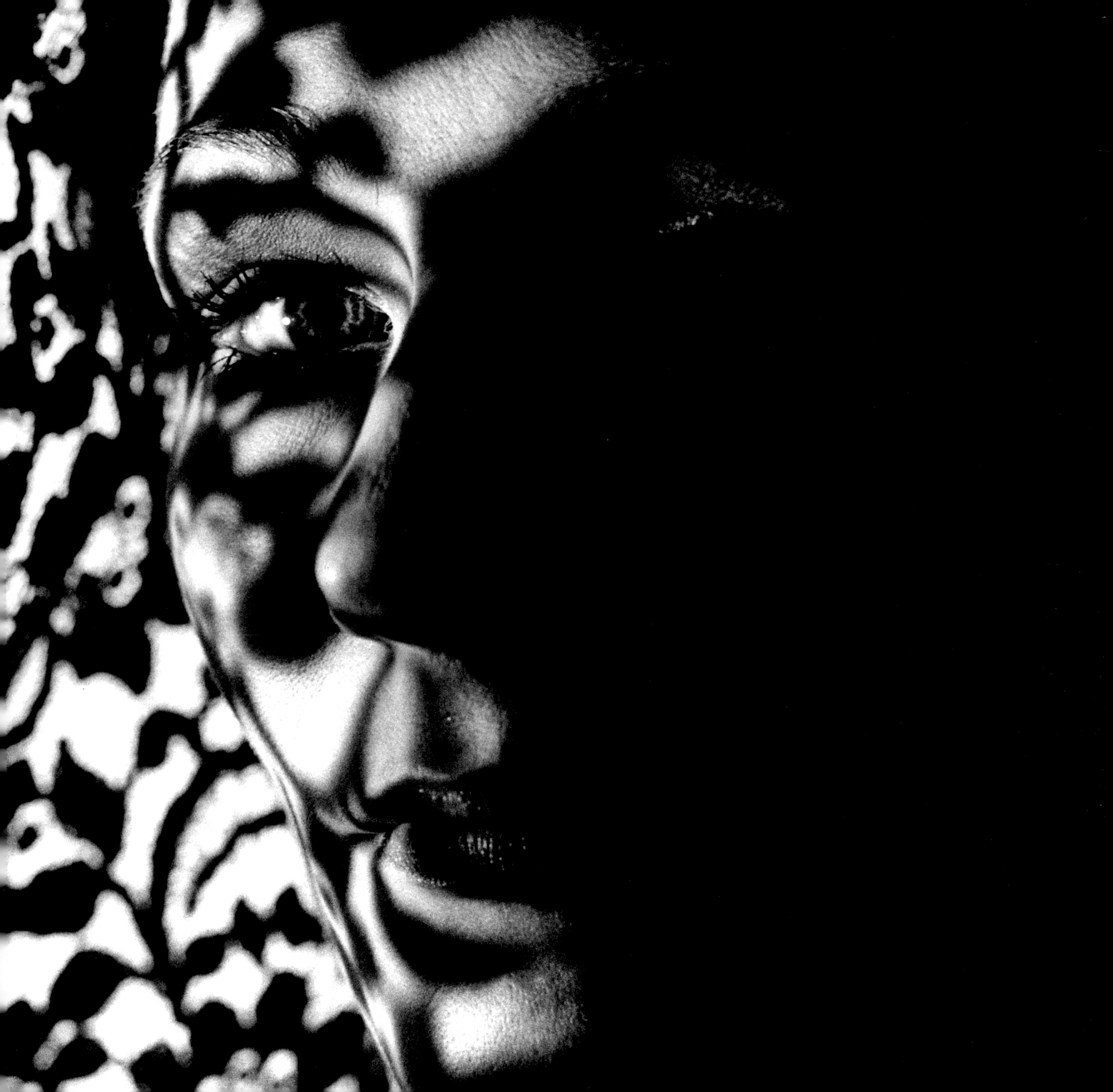

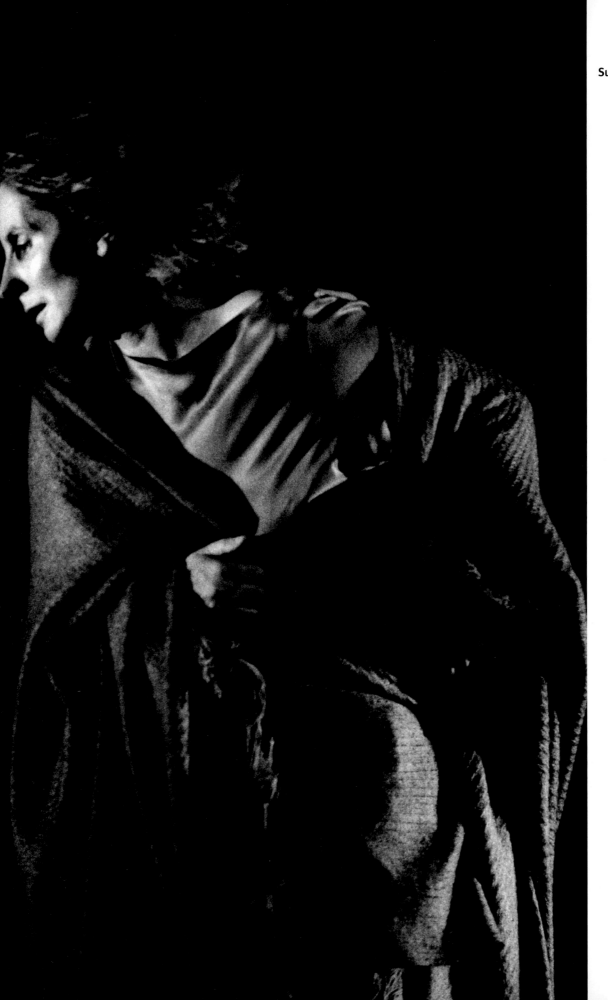

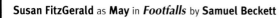

Susan FitzGerald as **May** in *Footfalls* by **Samuel Beckett**

John Kavanagh as Joxer Daly, Donal McCann as Captain Jack Boyle in *Juno and the Paycock* by Sean O'Casey

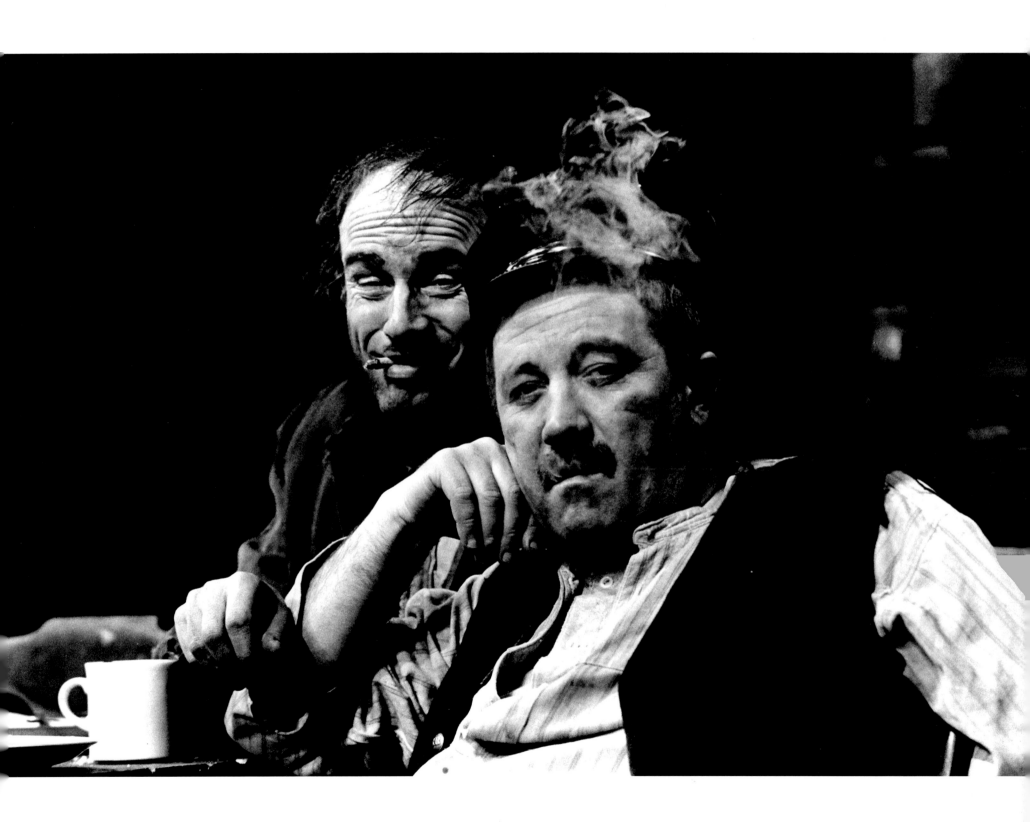

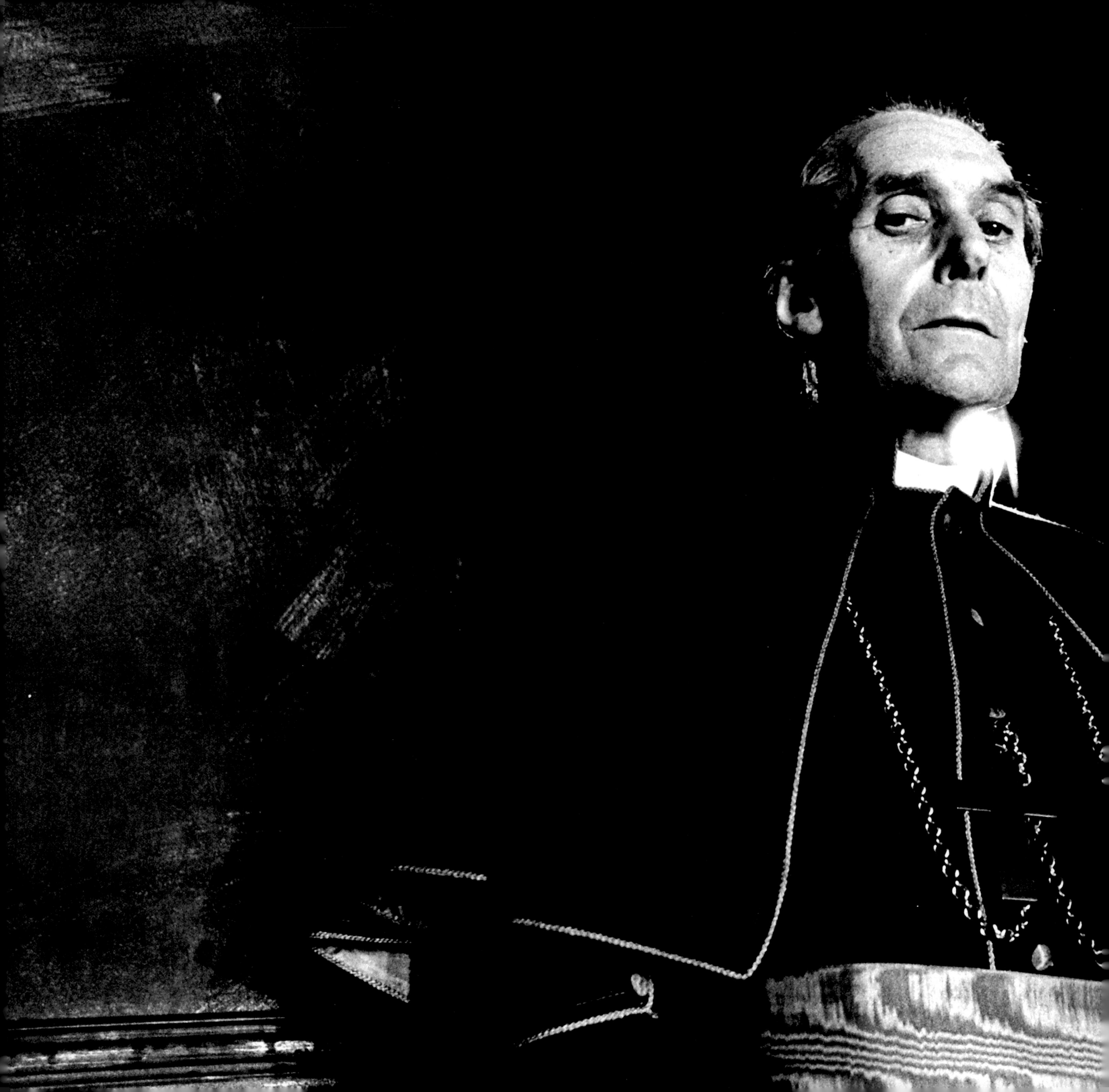

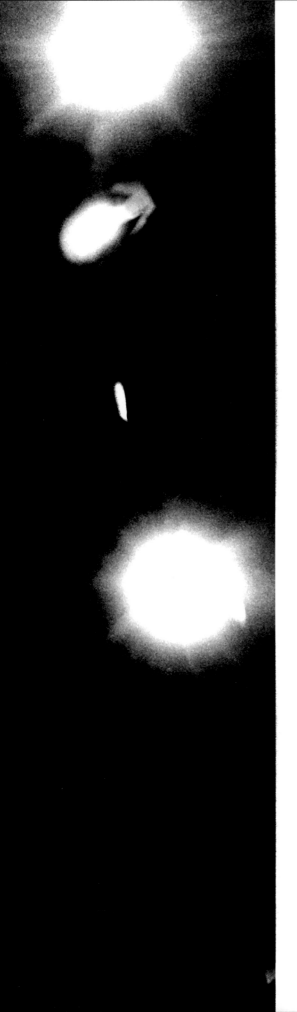

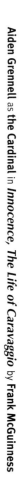

Aiden Grennell as **the Cardinal** in *Innocence, The Life of Caravaggio* by **Frank McGuinness**

Siân Maguire as **Emilie** in *Les Liaisons Dangereuses* by **Christopher Hampton**

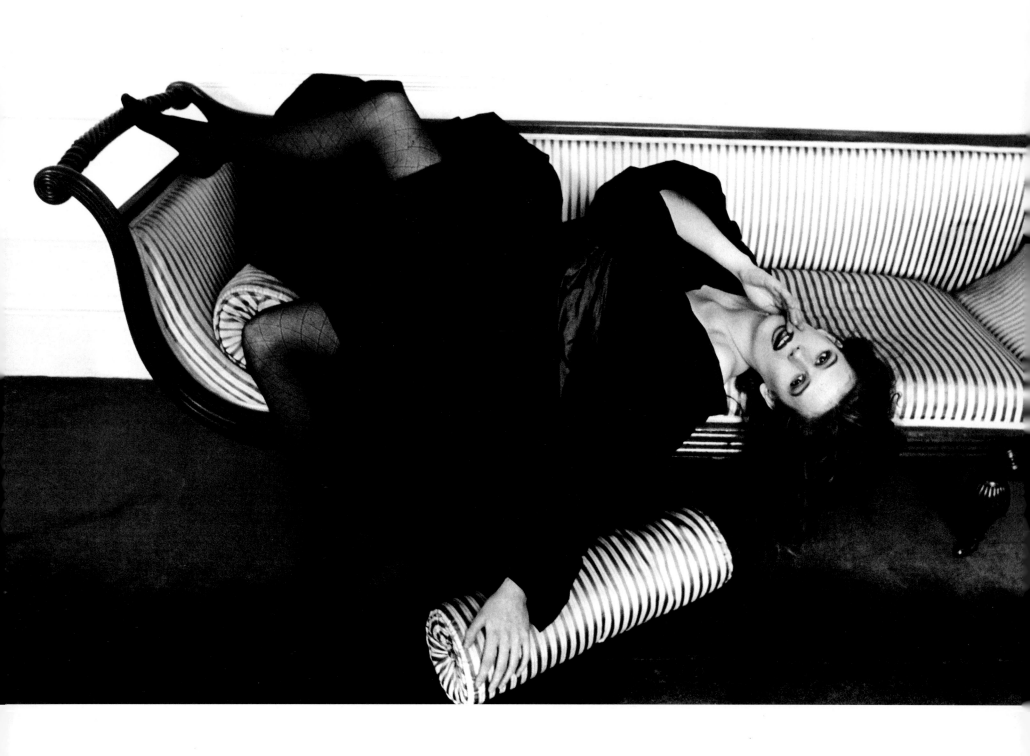

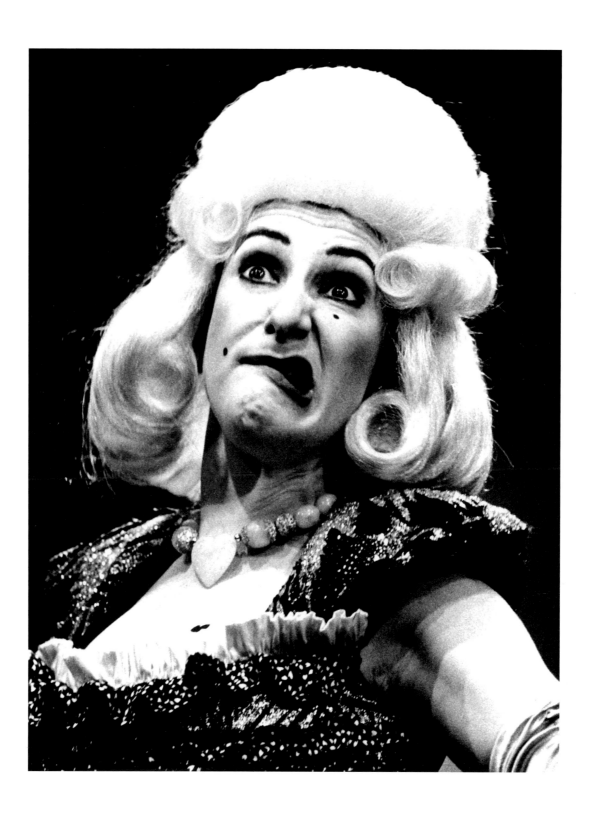

Pauline Mclynn as **Lady Teazle** in *The School for Scandal* by **Richard Brinsley Sheridan**

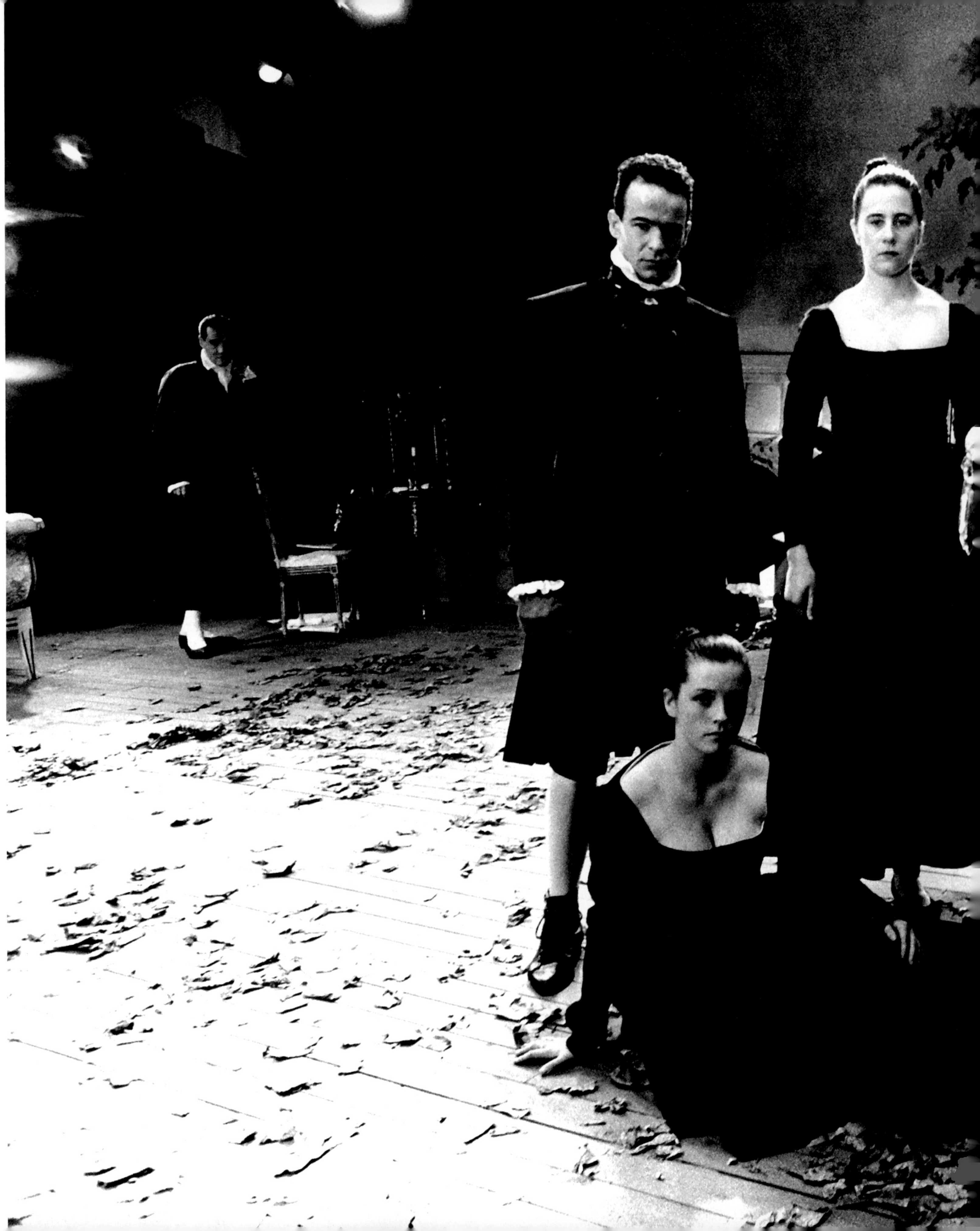

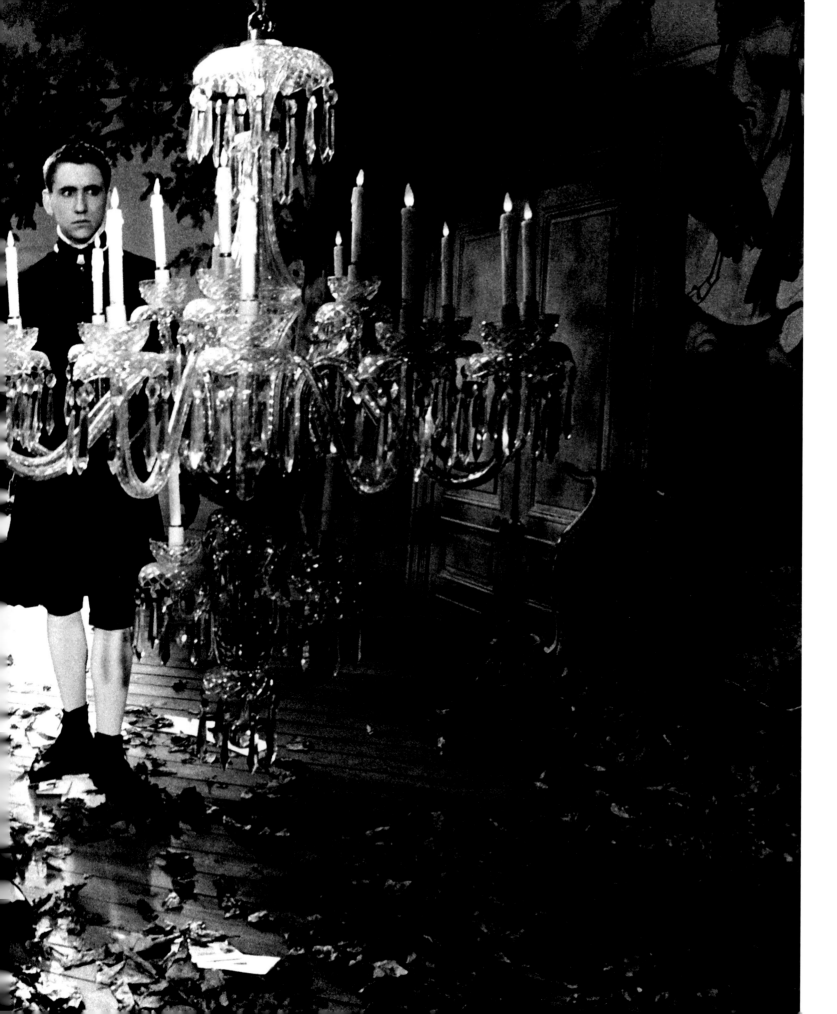

Peter Cooney as **Major-domo**, Catherine Walsh as **Adèle**, Rod Chichignoud as **Georges**, Muireann Kelly as **Sophie** in *Les Liaisons Dangereuses* by Christopher Hampton

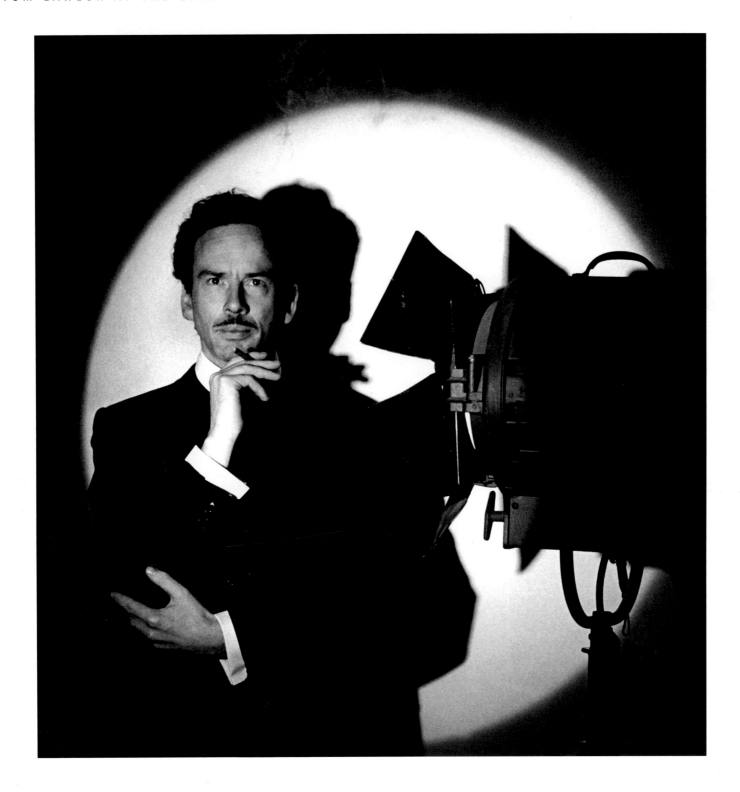

John Kavanagh as **Malvolio** in *Twelfth Night* by **William Shakespeare**

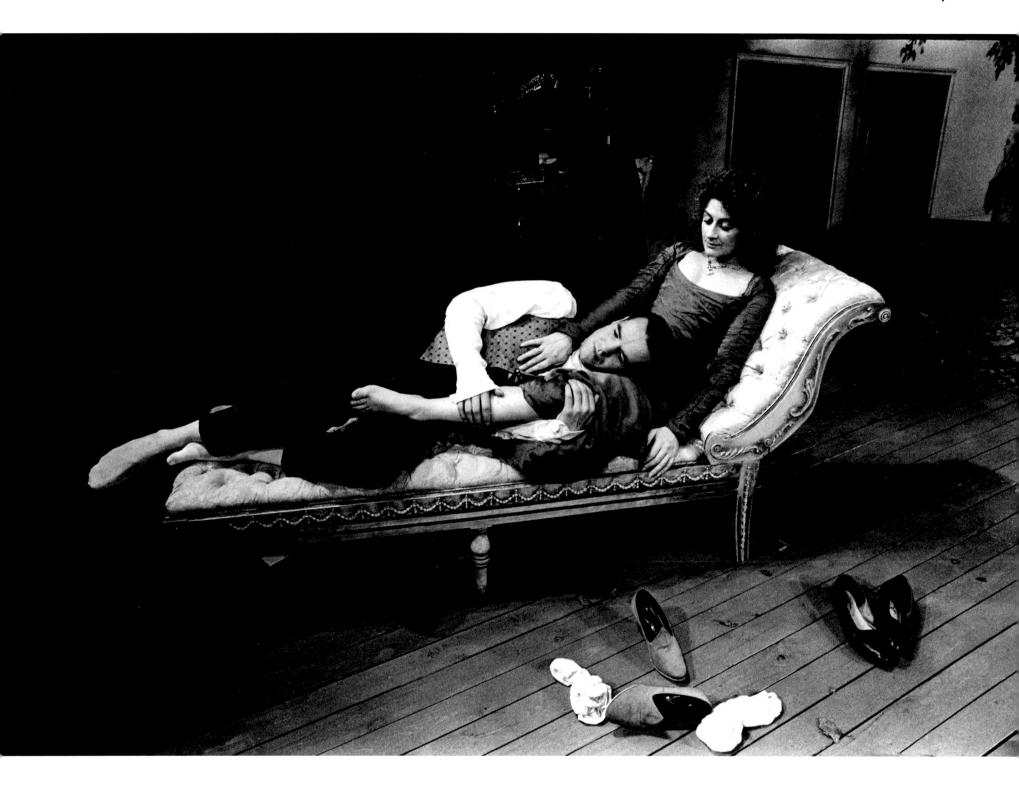

Sorcha Cusack as **La Marquise de Merteuil**, **David Herlihy** as **Danceny** in *Les Liaisons Dangereuses* by **Christopher Hampton**

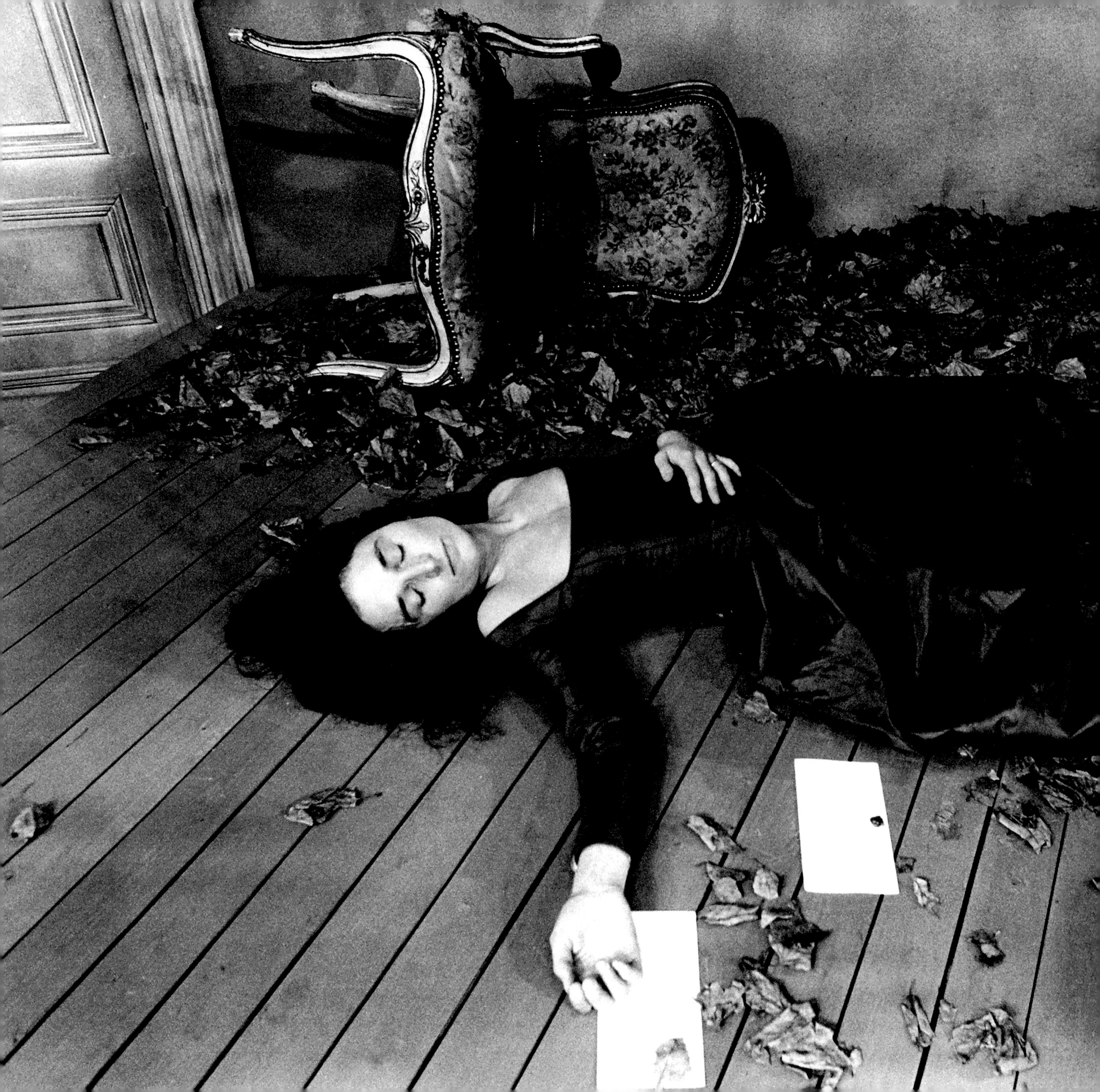

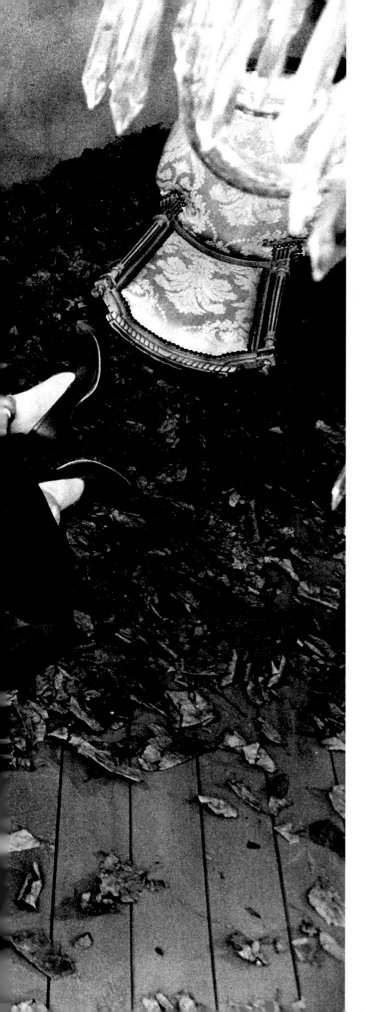

Olwen Fouéré **as** **La Présidente de Tourvel** **in** *Les Liaisons Dangereuses* **by Christopher Hampton**

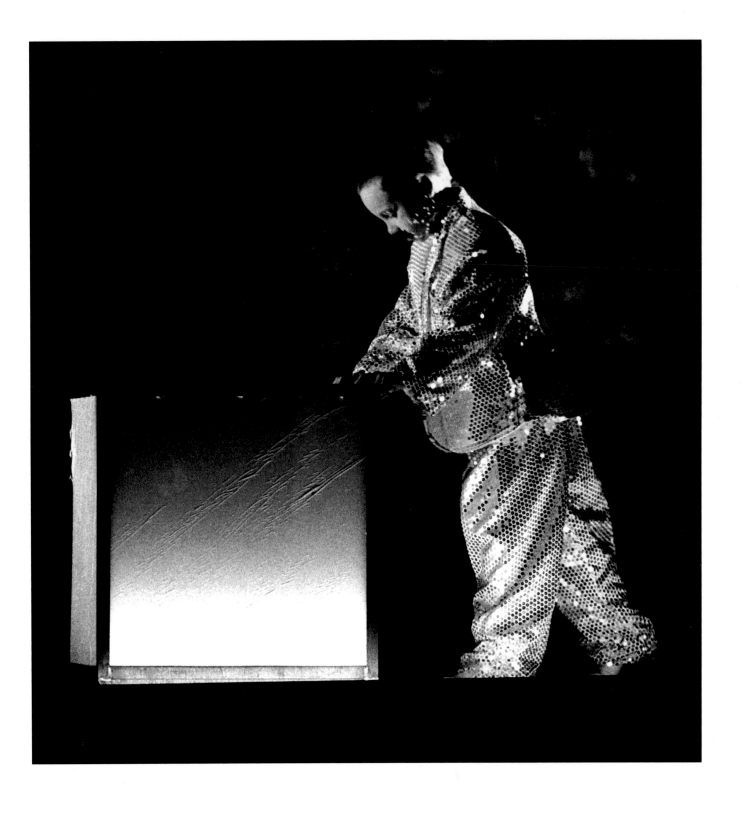

Tomás Killeen as **B** in *Act Without Words II* by **Samuel Beckett**

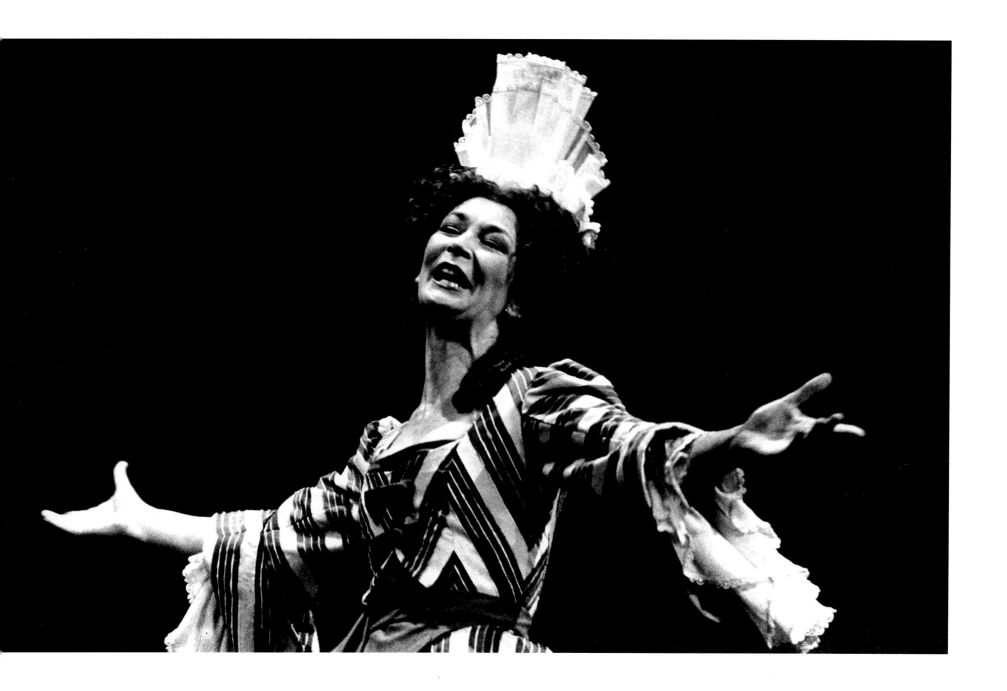

Barbara Brennan as **Silvia** in *The Recruiting Officer* by **George Farquhar**

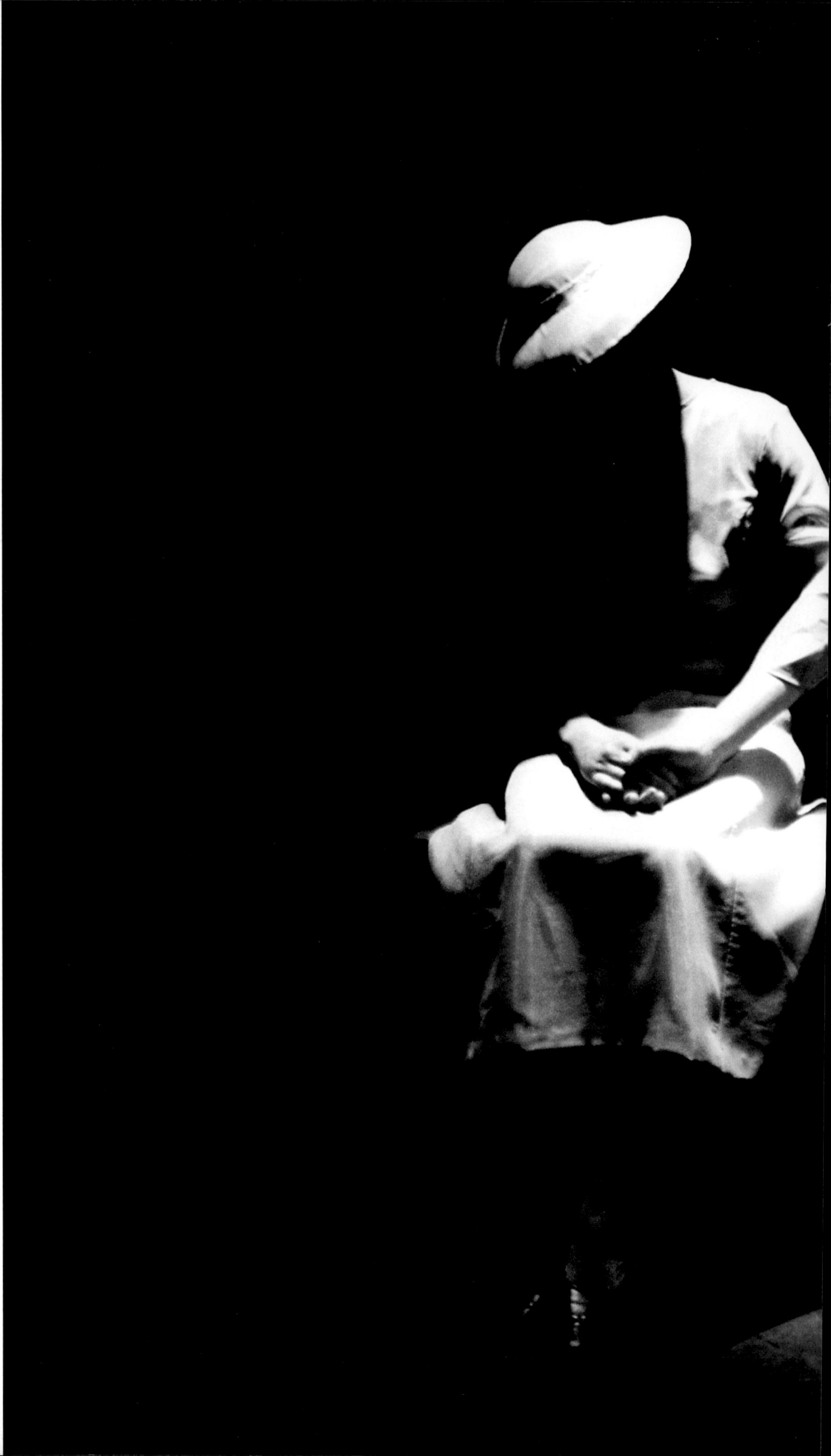

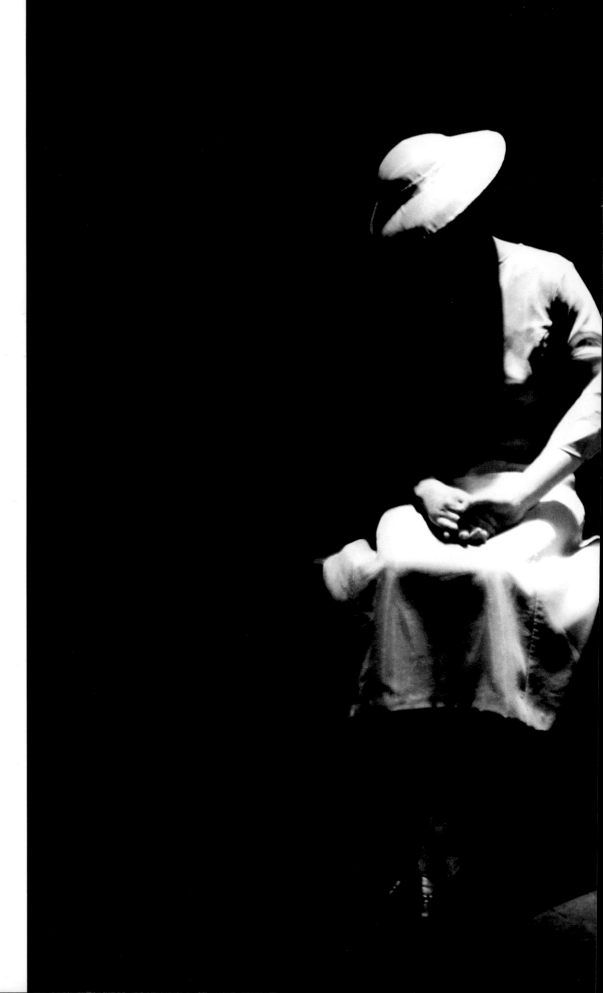

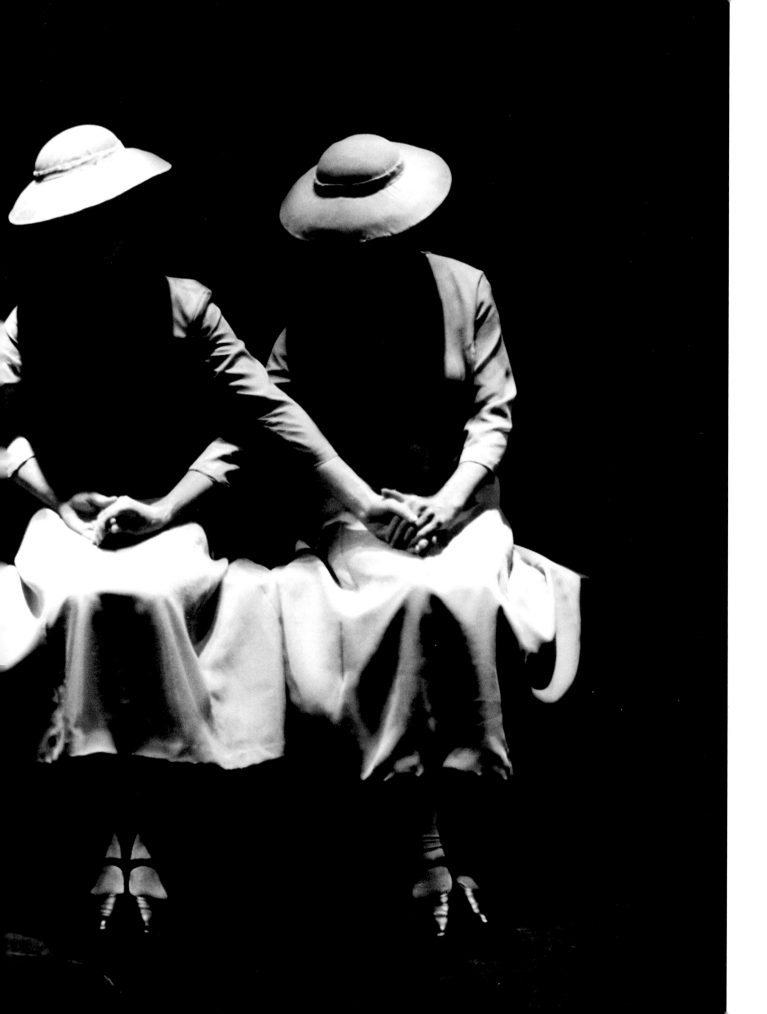

Helene Montague as **Flo**, Bernadette McKenna as **Vi**, Susan FitzGerald as **Ru** in *Come and Go* by **Samuel Beckett**

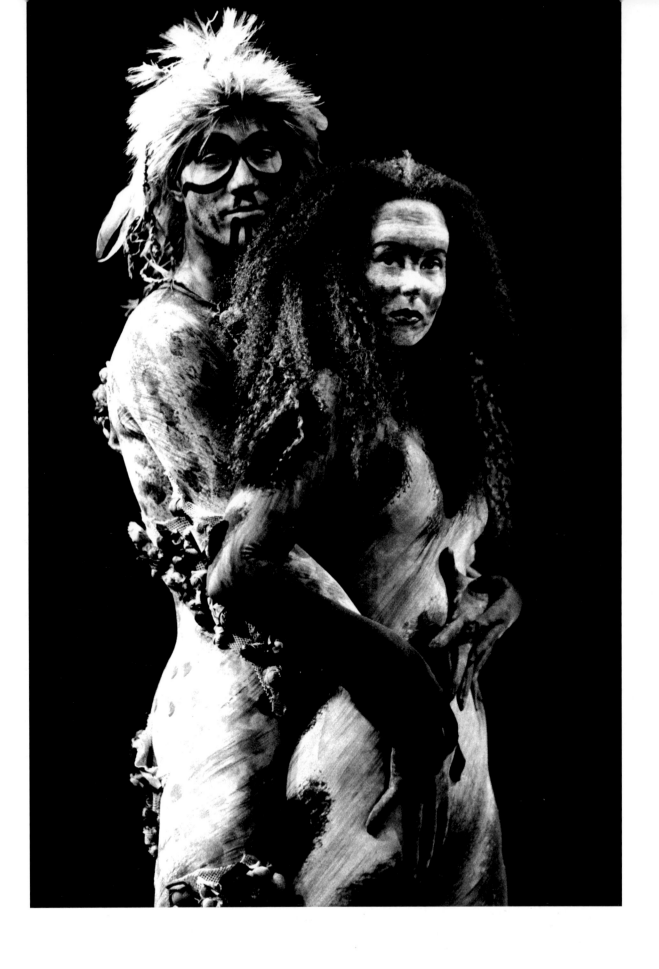

Klaus Hassel as **Mustardseed**, Anne Buckley as **First Fairy** in *A Midsummer Night's Dream* by **William Shakespeare**

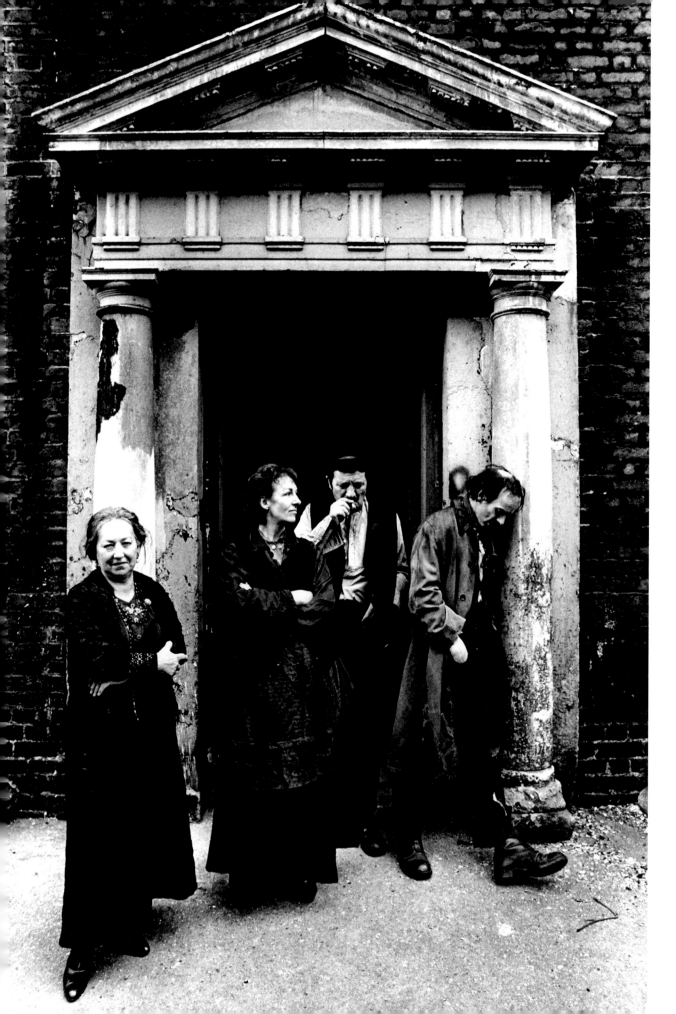

Maureen Potter as Maisie Madigan, Geraldine Plunkett as Juno, Donal McCann as Captain Jack Boyle, John Kavanagh as Joxer Daly in *Juno and the Paycock* by Sean O'Casey

Ingrid Craigie as Gwendolen, Lise-Ann McLaughlin as Cecily in *The Importance of Being Earnest* by Oscar Wilde

Joe Savino as Jokanaan in *Salomé* by Oscar Wilde

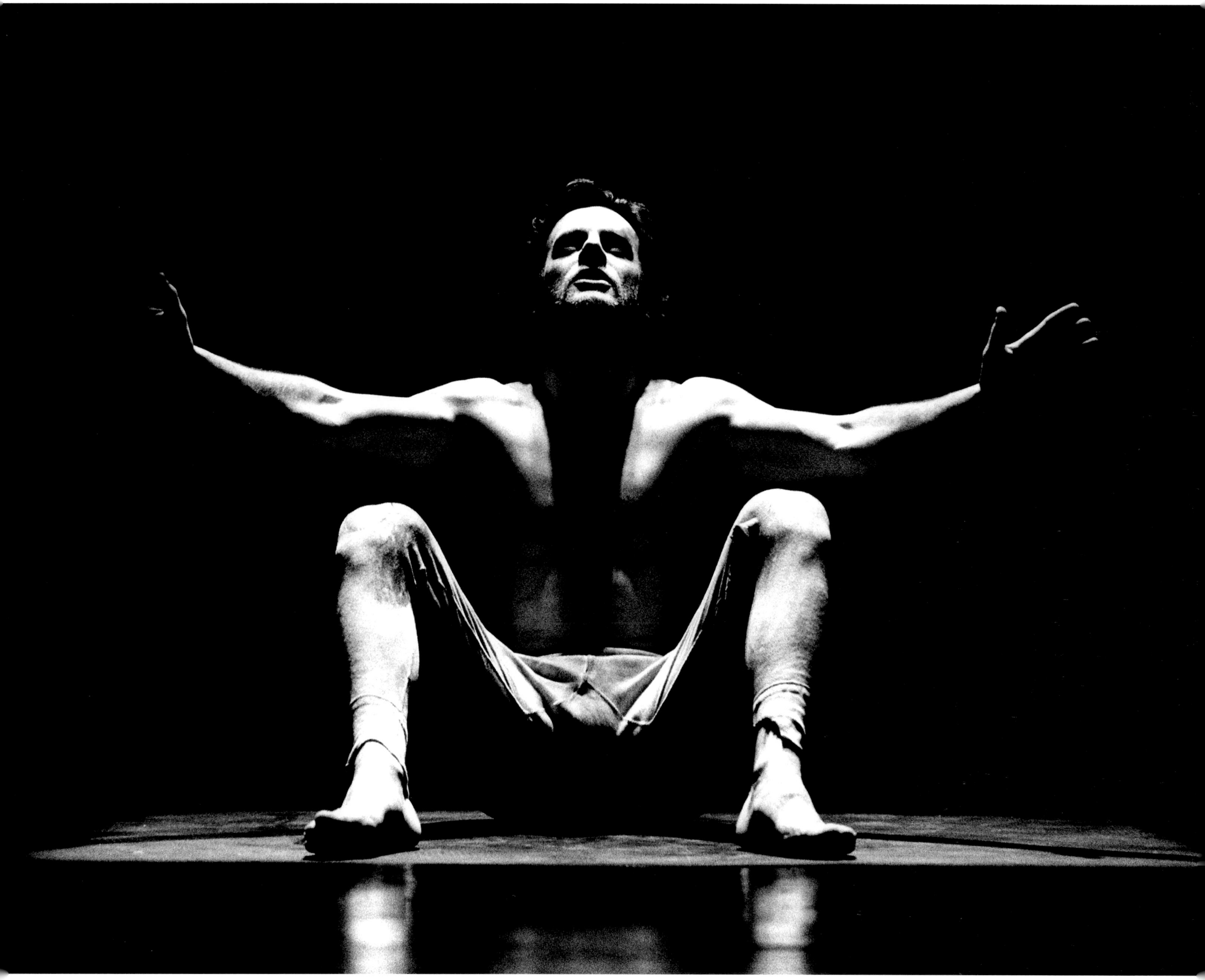

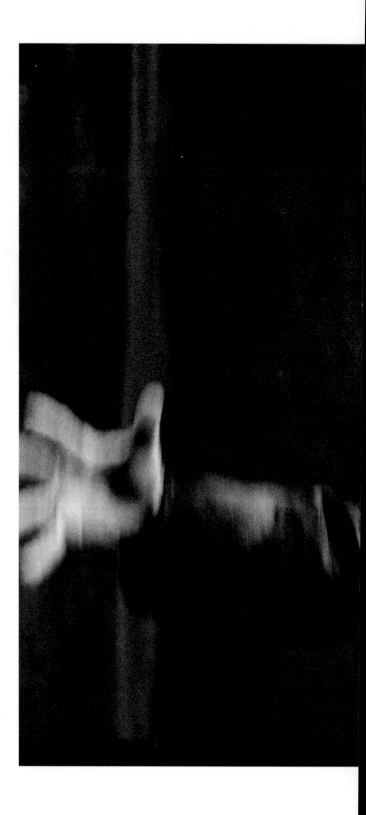

Éanna MacLiam as **Tommy Owens** in *The Shadow of a Gunman* by **Sean O'Casey**

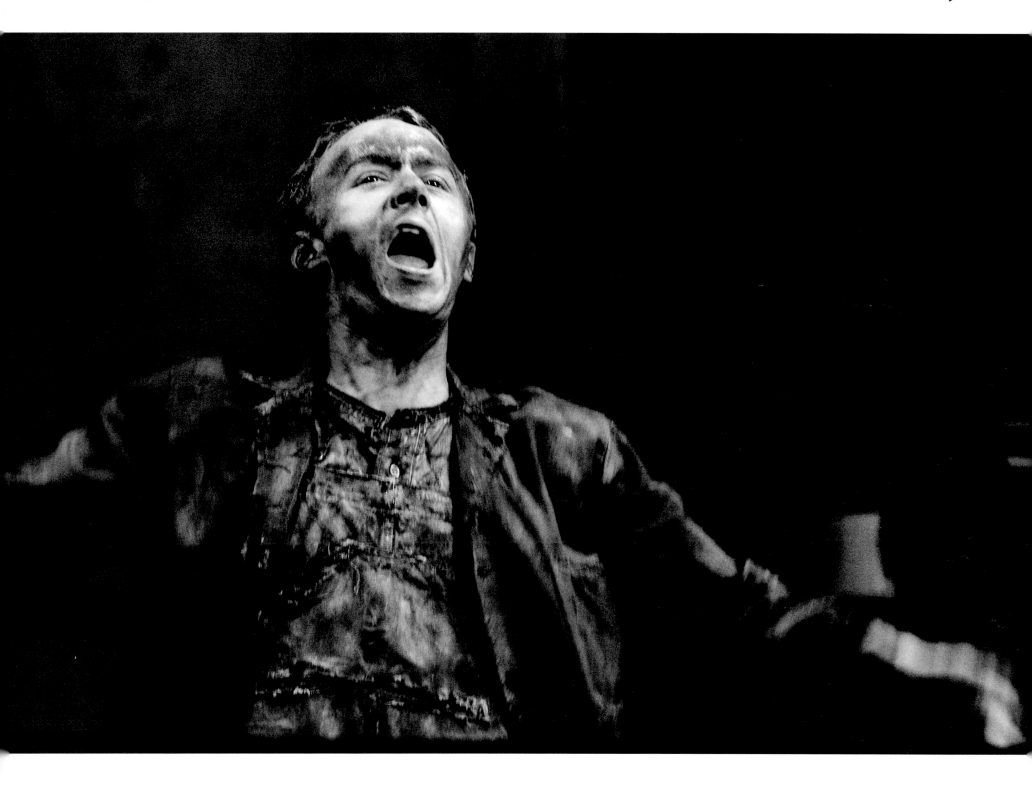

Overleaf: **Tom Murphy** as **Philip Clandon**, **Catherine Cusack** as **Dolly Clandon** in *You Never Can Tell* by **George Bernard Shaw**

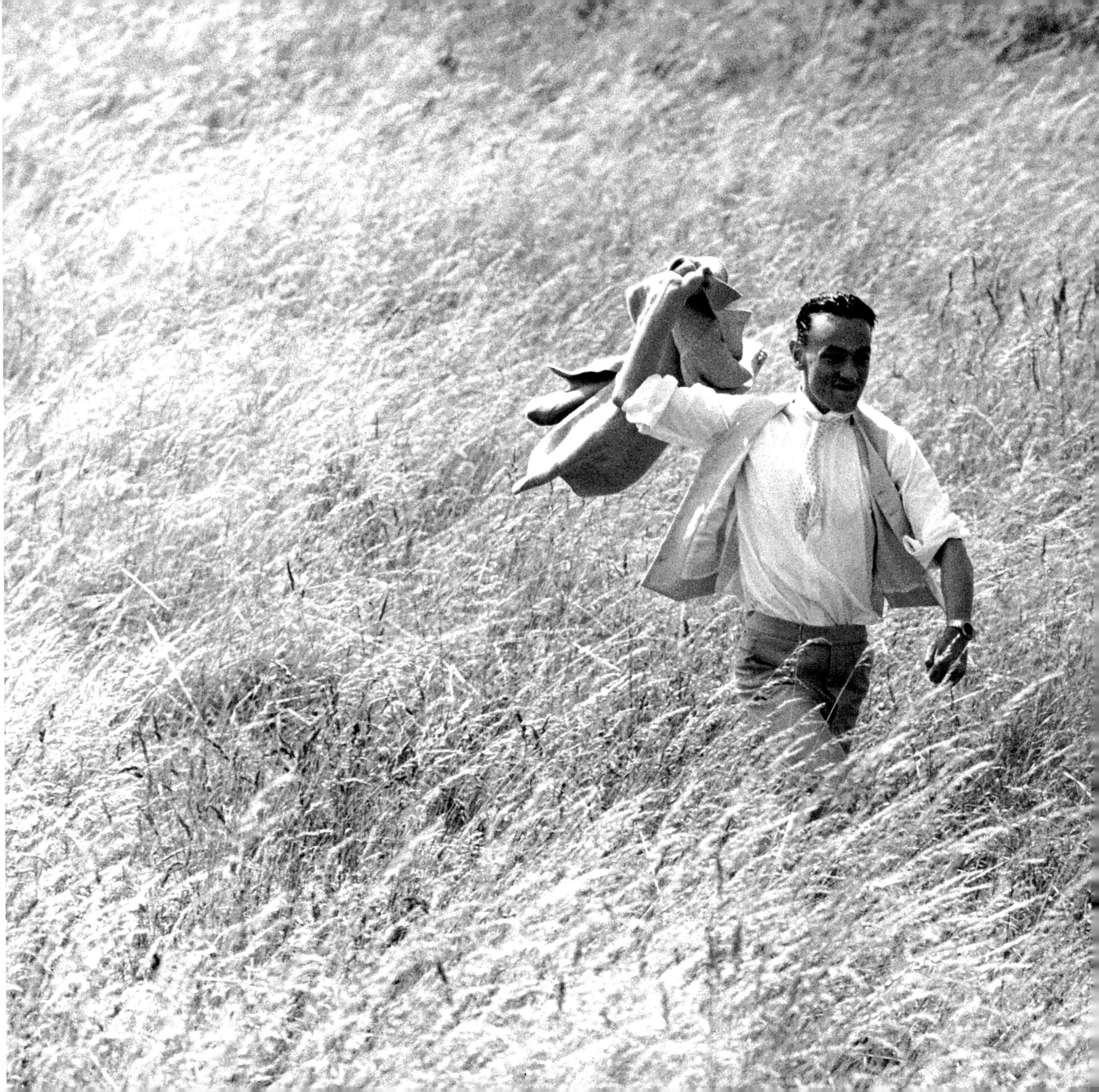

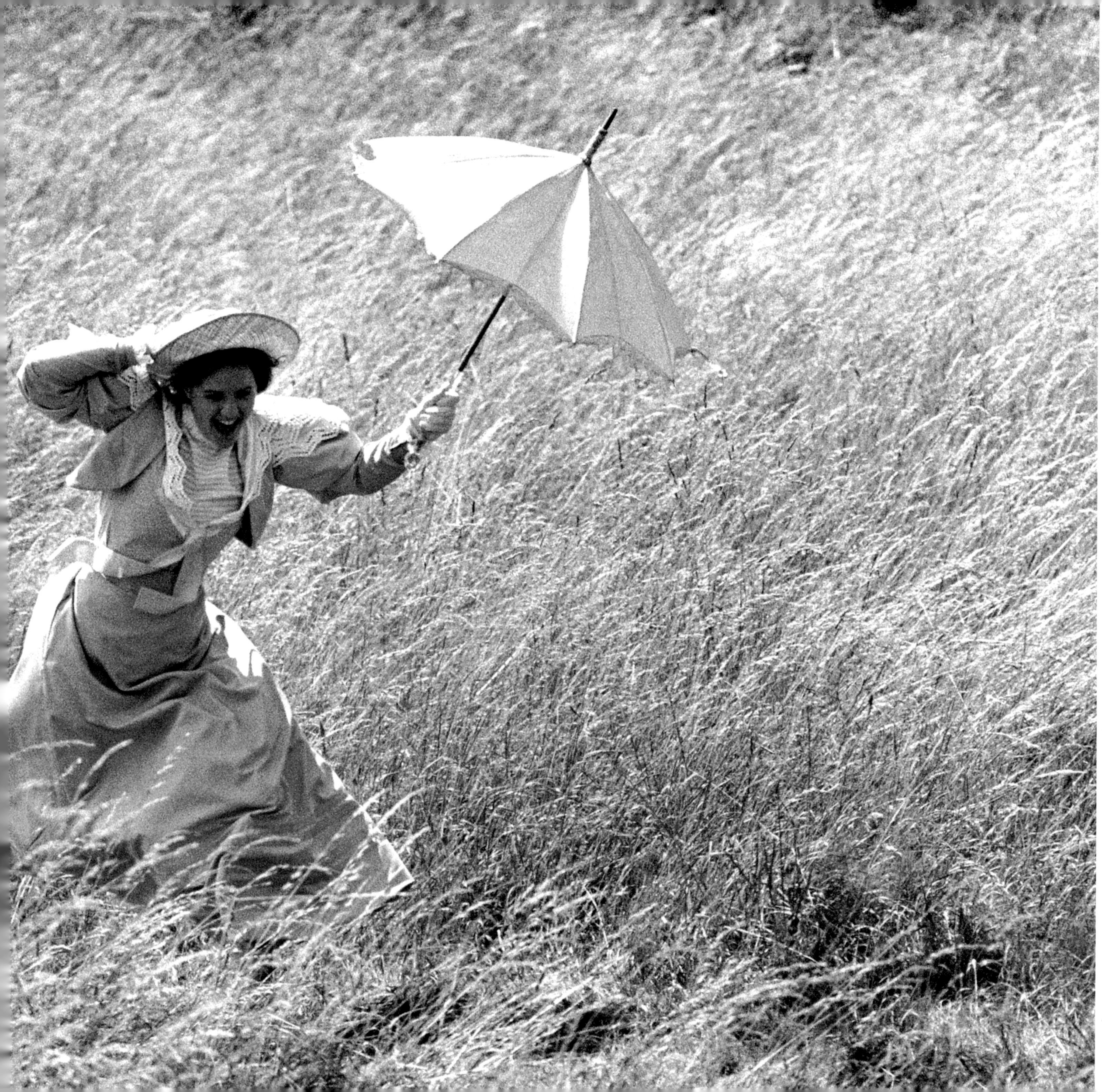

Catherine Byrne as Elmire, Stephen Brennan as Tartuffe in Molière's *Tartuffe* in a version by **Michael West**

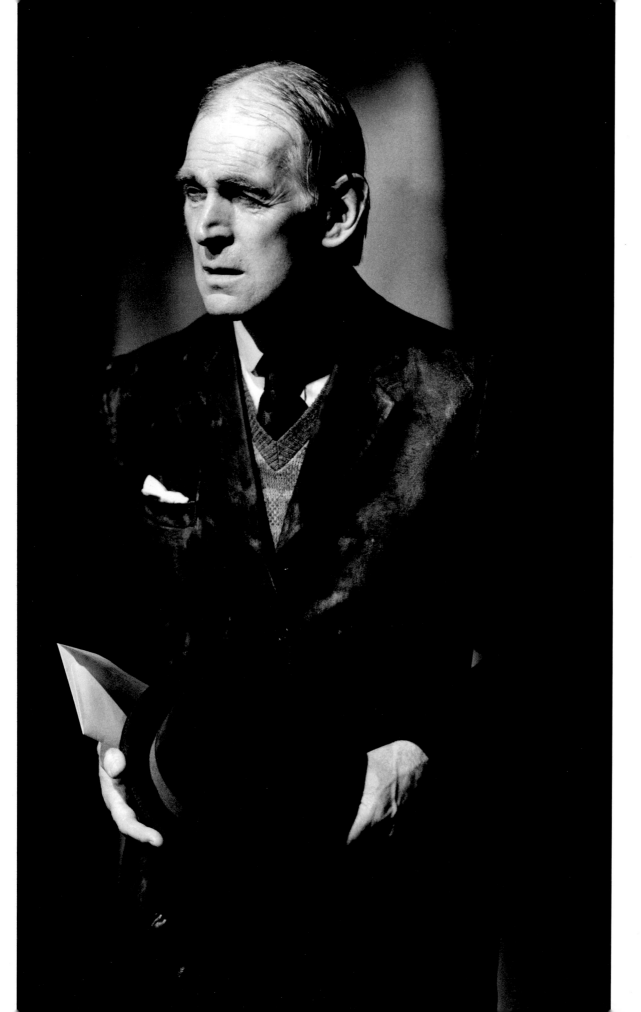

Des Keogh as **Mr Gallogher** in *The Shadow of a Gunman* by **Sean O'Casey**

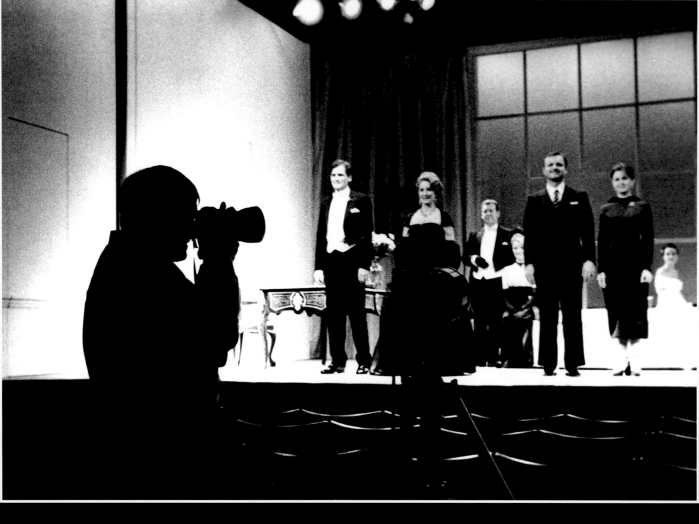

Tom Lawlor photographs the curtain call of *Lady Windermere's Fan* **at the Gate September 1997.** PHOTO: CYRIL BYRNE

1

Johnny Murphy as **Estragon** in *Waiting for Godot* by **Samuel Beckett**

Director: Walter Asmus
Designer: Louis Le Brocquy
Lighting Designer:
Alan Burrett
From the Beckett Festival
OCTOBER 1991

2–3

Sinéad Cusack as **Masha**, Niamh Cusack as **Irina**, Sorcha Cusack as **Olga**, Cyril Cusack as **Chebutykin** in *Three Sisters* by **Anton Chekhov** in a version by **Frank McGuinness**

Director: Adrian Noble
Designer: Bob Crowley
Lighting Designer:
Rupert Murray
MARCH 1990

4

Eamon Morrissey as **Kite** in *The Recruiting Officer* by **George Farquhar**

Director: Patrick Mason
Set Designer: Joe Vanek
Costume Designer:
Nigel Boyd
Lighting Designer:
Trevor Dawson
MAY 1985

5

Donal McCann as **Captain Jack Boyle**, Maureen Potter as **Maisie Madigan** in *Juno and the Paycock* by **Sean O'Casey**

Director: Joe Dowling
Set Designer:
Frank Hallinan Flood
Costume Designer:
Consolata Boyle
Lighting Designer:
Rupert Murray
JULY 1986

6

John Kavanagh as **Joxer Daly** in *Juno and the Paycock* by **Sean O'Casey**

Director: Joe Dowling
Set Designer:
Frank Hallinan Flood
Costume Designer:
Consolata Boyle
Lighting Designer:
Rupert Murray
JULY 1986

7

Barry McGovern as **Estragon**, Tom Hickey as **Vladimir** in *Waiting for Godot* by **Samuel Beckett**

Director: Walter Asmus
Designer: Louis le Brocquy
Lighting Designer:
Rupert Murray
AUGUST 1988

8

Marianne Faithfull as **Pirate Jenny** in *The Threepenny Opera* by **Bertolt Brecht** and **Kurt Weill** in a version by **Frank McGuinness**

Director: Patrick Mason
Designers:
Monica Frawley & Joe Vanek
Lighting Designer:
Mick Hughes
JULY 1991

9

Peter Holmes as **Antonio** in *Innocence, The Life of Caravaggio* by **Frank McGuinness**

Director: Patrick Mason
Set Designer: Joe Vanek
Costume Designer:
Nigel Boyd
Lighting Designer: Mick Hughes
OCTOBER 1986

10–11

David Kelly as **Al Lewis**, Milo O'Shea as **Willie Clark** in *The Sunshine Boys* by **Neil Simon**

Director: John David
Set Designer:
Frank Hallinan Flood
Costume Designer: Joan Bergin
Lighting Designer:
Rupert Murray
JUNE 1996

12

Phelim Drew as **A** in *Rough for Theatre 1* by **Samuel Beckett**

Director: Derek Chapman
Designer: Tim Reed
Lighting Designer:
Alan Burrett
From the Beckett Festival
OCTOBER 1991

13

Olwen Fouéré as **Salomé** in *Salomé* by **Oscar Wilde**

Director: Steven Berkoff
Set Designer: Robert Ballagh
Costume Designer:
Nigel Boyd
Lighting Designer:
Trevor Dawson
APRIL 1988

14

Angela Crowe as **Miss Graham**, Sharon Devlin as **Lady Stutfield** in *Lady Windermere's Fan* by **Oscar Wilde**

Director: Alan Stanford
Set Designer:
Bruno Schwengl
Costume Designer:
Jacqueline Kobler
Lighting Designer:
Rupert Murray
JULY 1997

15

Donal O'Kelly in *Catalpa* by **Donal O'Kelly**

Director: Bairbre Ní Chaoimh
Designer: Giles Cadle
Lighting Designer:
Paul Denby
MARCH 1997

16–17

Barbara Brennan as **Silvia**, Ian McElhinney as **Captain Plume** in *The Recruiting Officer* by **George Farquhar**

Director: Patrick Mason
Set Designer: Joe Vanek
Costume Designer:
Nigel Boyd
Lighting Designer:
Trevor Dawson
MAY 1985

18

Penelope Wilton as **Deborah** in *A Kind of Alaska* by **Harold Pinter**

Director: Karel Reisz
Set Designer:
Frank Hallinan Flood
Costume Designer:
Joan O'Clery
Lighting Designer:
Alan Burrett
From the Pinter Festival
APRIL 1997

19

Niamh Cusack as **Nora** in *A Doll's House* by **Henrik Ibsen** based on the translation by **Joan Tindale**

Director: Karel Reisz
Set Designer:
Assheton Gorton
Costume Designer:
Sue Yelland
Lighting Designer:
Rupert Murray
OCTOBER 1993

20

Lindsay Duncan as **Rebecca**, Stephen Rea as **Devlin** in *Ashes to Ashes* by **Harold Pinter**

Director: Harold Pinter
Set Designer:
Frank Hallinan Flood
Costume Designer: Tom Rand
Lighting Designer:
Alan Burrett
From the Pinter Festival
APRIL 1997

21

Pat Kinevane as **Cecil Graham** in *Lady Windermere's Fan* by **Oscar Wilde**

Director: Alan Stanford
Set Designer:
Bruno Schwengl
Costume Designer:
Jacqueline Kobler
Lighting Designer:
Rupert Murray
JULY 1997

22–23

Geraldine Plunkett as **Juno Boyle**, Donal McCann as **Captain Jack Boyle** (and **James Casey**) in *Juno and the Paycock* by **Sean O'Casey**

Director: Joe Dowling
Set Designer:
Frank Hallinan Flood
Costume Designer:
Consolata Boyle
Lighting Designer:
Rupert Murray
JULY 1986

24

Harold Pinter as **Harry** in *The Collection* by **Harold Pinter**

Director: Alan Stanford
Set Designer:
Frank Hallinan Flood
Costume Designer:
Joan O'Clery
Lighting Designer:
Alan Burrett
From The Pinter Festival
APRIL 1997

25

Ingrid Craigie as **Stella** in *The Collection* by **Harold Pinter**

Director: Alan Stanford
Set Designer:
Frank Hallinan Flood
Costume Designer:
Joan O'Clery
Lighting Designer:
Alan Burrett
From the Pinter Festival
APRIL 1997

26

Gemma Craven as **Mrs Diggerty** in *The London Vertigo* by **Brian Friel** based on a play by **Charles Macklin**

Director: Judy Friel
Designer: Monica Frawley
Lighting Designer:
Rupert Murray
JANUARY 1992

27

David Kelly as **Peter** in *The Seagull* by **Anton Chekhov** in a version by **Thomas Kilroy**

Director: Lindsay Posner
Designer: Mark Bailey
Lighting Designer:
Alan Burrett
MARCH 1994

28

Maureen Potter as **Woman** in *Rockaby* by **Samuel Beckett**

Director: Derek Chapman
Designer: Tim Reed
Lighting Designer:
Alan Burrett
From the Beckett Festival
OCTOBER 1991

29
Ingrid Craigie as **Gwen Mellors** in *The Mask of Moriarty* by **Hugh Leonard**

Director: Brian de Salvo
Set Designer: Poppy Mitchell
Costume Designer:
Joan Bergin
Lighting Designer:
Brian Harris
OCTOBER 1985

30–31
Alan Stanford as **Hamm, Barry McGovern** as **Clov** in *Endgame* by **Samuel Beckett**

Director: Antoni Libera
Designer: Robert Ballagh
Lighting Designer:
Alan Burrett
From the Beckett Festival
OCTOBER 1991

32
Niall Buggy as **Spooner** in *No Man's Land* by **Harold Pinter**

Director: Ben Barnes
Set Designer:
Frank Hallinan Flood
Costume Designer:
Joan O'Clery
Lighting Designer:
Alan Burrett
From the Pinter Festival
APRIL 1997

33
Jane Brennan as **Gila** in *One for the Road* by **Harold Pinter**

Director: John Crowley
Set Designer: Eileen Diss
Costume Designer:
Joan Bergin
Lighting Designer:
Mick Hughes
From the Pinter Festival
MAY 1994

34–35
John Olohan as **B, Phelim Drew** as **A** in *Rough for Theatre I* by **Samuel Beckett**

Director: Derek Chapman
Designer: Tim Reed
Lighting Designer:
Alan Burrett
From the Beckett Festival
OCTOBER 1991

36
Dana Bledsoe as **Carol, Stanley Townsend** as **John** in *Oleanna* by **David Mamet**

Director: Ben Barnes
Set Designer: Eileen Diss
Costume Designer:
Joan O'Clery
Lighting Designer:
Rupert Murray
NOVEMBER 1994

37
Donal McCann as **Captain Jack Boyle, Geraldine Plunkett** as **Juno Boyle** in *Juno and the Paycock* by **Sean O'Casey**

Director: Joe Dowling
Set Designer:
Frank Hallinan Flood
Costume Designer:
Consolata Boyle
Lighting Designer:
Rupert Murray
JULY 1986

38
Seamus Forde as **Nagg** in *Endgame* by **Samuel Beckett**

Director: Antoni Libera
Designer: Robert Ballagh
Lighting Designer:
Alan Burrett
From the Beckett Festival
OCTOBER 1991

39
Helene Montague as **Assistant** in *Catastrophe* by **Samuel Beckett**

Director: Pierre Chabert
Designer: Bláithín Sheerin
Lighting Designer:
Alan Burrett
From the Beckett Festival
OCTOBER 1991

40–41
O Z Whitehead as **Bem, Barry Cassin** as **Bam, Seamus Forde** as **Bim, Micheál Ó Briain** as **Bom** in *What Where* by **Samuel Beckett**

Director: Colm Ó Bríain
Designer: Ian McNicholl
Lighting Designer:
Alan Burrett
From the Beckett Festival
OCTOBER 1991

42
Michael Pennington as **Nicolas, Nicholas Grennell** as **Victor** in *One for the Road* by **Harold Pinter**

Director: John Crowley
Set Designer: Eileen Diss
Costume Designer:
Joan Bergin
Lighting Designer:
Mick Hughes
From the Pinter Festival
MAY 1994

43
Stephen Brennan as **Tartuffe** in **Molière's** *Tartuffe* in a version by **Michael West**

Director: Alan Stanford
Set Designer:
Robert Ballagh
Costume Designer:
Annena Stubbs
Lighting Designer:
Alan Burrett
OCTOBER 1992

44
Flo McSweeney as **Titania, Stephen Brennan** as **Oberon** in *A Midsummer Night's Dream* by **William Shakespeare**

Director: Joe Dowling
Designer: Hayden Griffin
Lighting Designer:
Rupert Murray
JULY 1993

45
Bairbre Ní Chaoimh as **a guest at the dinner, Michael James Ford** as **the page of Herodias** in *Salomé* by **Oscar Wilde**

Director: Steven Berkoff
Set Designer: Robert Ballagh
Costume Designer:
Nigel Boyd
Lighting Designer:
Trevor Dawson
APRIL 1988

46
David Kelly as **Krapp** in *Krapp's Last Tape* by **Samuel Beckett**

Director: Pat Laffan
Designer: Ian McNicholl
Lighting Designer:
Alan Burrett
OCTOBER 1991

47
Alan Stanford as **Herod** in *Salomé* by **Oscar Wilde**

Director: Steven Berkoff
Set Designer: Robert Ballagh
Costume Designer:
Nigel Boyd
Lighting Designer:
Trevor Dawson
APRIL 1988

48–49
Michael Pennington as **Nicolas, Ciarán Fitzgerald** as **Nicky** in *One for the Road* by **Harold Pinter**

Director: John Crowley
Set Designer: Eileen Diss
Costume Designer:
Joan Bergin
Lighting Designer:
Mick Hughes
From the Pinter Festival
MAY 1994

50
David Herlihy as **Gus** in *The Dumb Waiter* by **Harold Pinter**

Director: Joe O'Byrne
Set Designer: Eileen Diss
Costume Designer:
Joan Bergin
Lighting Designer:
Mick Hughes
From the Pinter Festival
MAY 1994

51
Ian McElhinney as **Ben** in *The Dumb Waiter* by **Harold Pinter**

Director: Joe O'Byrne
Set Designer: Eileen Diss
Costume Designer:
Joan Bergin
Lighting Designer:
Mick Hughes
From the Pinter Festival
MAY 1994

52
Jeananne Crowley as **Lady Touchwood** in *The Double Dealer* by **William Congreve**

Director: Jonathan Miller
Designer: Mark Bailey
Lighting Designer:
Robert Bryan
DECEMBER 1992

53
Derek Chapman as **Man** in *Act Without Words I* by **Samuel Beckett**

Director: Colm Ó Bríain
Designer: Ian McNicholl
Lighting Designer:
Alan Burrett
From the Beckett Festival
OCTOBER 1991

54–55
Alan Stanford as **Marc, Mark Lambert** as **Yvan, Stephen Brennan** as **Serge** in *Art* by **Yasmina Reza** translated by **Christopher Hampton**

Director: Robin Lefevre
Set Designer: Robert Ballagh
Costume Designer:
Michael Mortell
Lighting Designer:
Rupert Murray
MAY 1997

56
T P McKenna as **Hirst** in *No Man's Land* by **Harold Pinter**

Director: Ben Barnes
Set Designer:
Frank Hallinan Flood
Costume Designer:
Joan O'Clery
Lighting Designer:
Alan Burrett
APRIL 1997

57
Tom Baker as **Sherlock Holmes** in *The Mask of Moriarty* by **Hugh Leonard**

Director: Brian de Salvo
Set Designer: Poppy Mitchell
Costume Designer:
Joan Bergin
Lighting Designer:
Brian Harris
OCTOBER 1985

58–59
Cinzia Hardy as
**Methylated Mary, David
Henry** as **Herbert Travesty**
in *The Mask of Moriarty*
by **Hugh Leonard**

Director: Brian de Salvo
Set Designer: Poppy Mitchell
Costume Designer:
Joan Bergin
Lighting Designer:
Brian Harris
OCTOBER 1985

60
Thom McGinty as **Naaman**
in *Salomé* by **Oscar Wilde**

Director: Steven Berkoff
Set Designer: Robert Ballagh
Costume Designer:
Nigel Boyd
Lighting Designer:
Trevor Dawson
APRIL 1988

61
Catherine Byrne as
**Molly Sweeney,
Mark Lambert** as
Frank Sweeney in
Molly Sweeney by
Brian Friel

Director: Brian Friel
Set Designer: Joe Vanek
Costume Designer:
Joan Bergin
Lighting Designer:
Mick Hughes
AUGUST 1994

62
Rosaleen Linehan as **Feste**
in *Twelfth Night* by
William Shakespeare

Director: Joe Dowling
Set Designer: Frank Conway
Costume Designer:
Consolata Boyle
Lighting Designer:
Rupert Murray
DECEMBER 1988

63
Rosaleen Linehan as
Mrs Malaprop in
The Rivals by
Richard Brinsley Sheridan

Director: John David
Designer: Annena Stubbs
Lighting Designer:
Trevor Dawson
DECEMBER 1987

64
Jane Brennan as **Gila,
Michael Pennington** as
Nicolas in *One for the
Road* by **Harold Pinter**

Director: John Crowley
Set Designer: Eileen Diss
Costume Designer:
Joan Bergin
Lighting Designer:
Mick Hughes
From the Pinter Festival
MAY 1994

65
Barry Lynch as **Sebastian,
Catherine Byrne** as
Cesario in *Twelfth Night*
by **William Shakespeare**

Director: Joe Dowling
Set Designer: Frank Conway
Costume Designer:
Consolata Boyle
Lighting Designer:
Rupert Murray
Double exposure–
One negative
DECEMBER 1988

66
Phelim Drew as **Roland
Maule** in *Present Laughter*
by **Noël Coward**

Director: Alan Stanford
Designer: Bruno Schwengl
Lighting Designer:
Rupert Murray
JUNE 1994

67
Claudia Carroll as **Caroline
Bingley, Christopher
Casson** as **Sir William
Lucas** in **Jane Austen's**
Pride and Prejudice
adapted for the stage by
James Maxwell

Director: Alan Stanford
Designer: Bruno Schwengl
Lighting Designer:
Rupert Murray
DECEMBER 1994

68
Stanley Townsend as
Maskwell in *The Double
Dealer* by **William
Congreve**

Director: Jonathan Miller
Designer: Mark Bailey
Lighting Designer:
Robert Bryan
DECEMBER 1992

69
Alison McKenna as **Lydia
Bennet** in **Jane Austen's**
Pride and Prejudice
adapted for the stage by
James Maxwell

Director: Alan Stanford
Set and Costume Designer:
Bruno Schwengl
Lighting Designer:
Rupert Murray
DECEMBER 1994

70
Barry McGovern as
Estragon in *Waiting for
Godot* by **Samuel Beckett**

Director: Walter Asmus
Designer: Louis le Brocquy
Lighting Designer:
Alan Burrett
AUGUST 1988

72
Garrett Keogh as
Caravaggio in *Innocence,
The Life of Caravaggio* by
Frank McGuinness

Director: Patrick Mason
Set Designer: Joe Vanek
Costume Designer:
Nigel Boyd
Lighting Designer:
Mick Hughes
OCTOBER 1986

73
Kate Flynn as **Lena** in
*Innocence, The Life of
Caravaggio* by
Frank McGuinness

Director: Patrick Mason
Set Designer: Joe Vanek
Costume Designer:
Nigel Boyd
Lighting Designer:
Mick Hughes
OCTOBER 1986

74-75
James Laurenson as
Mr Aston, Gillian Barge as
Isobel Desmond in *The
Seagull* by **Anton Chekhov**
in a version by
Thomas Kilroy

Director: Lindsay Posner
Designer: Mark Bailey
Lighting Designer:
Alan Burrett
MARCH 1994

76
Brendan Gleeson as
Epikhovdov in *The Cherry
Orchard* by **Anton
Chekhov** in a version by
Michael Bogdanov

Director: Michael Bogdanov
Designer: Chris Dyer
Lighting Designer:
Mark Pritchard
MAY 1992

77
John Cowley as
Bolshintsov in
Brian Friel's version of
A Month in the Country
by **Ivan Turgenev**

Director: Joe Dowling
Set Designer: Eileen Diss
Costume Designer:
Dany Everett
Lighting Designer:
Mick Hughes
AUGUST 1992

78
Donal McCann as
Shpigelsky, Karen Ardiff
as **Vera** in **Brian Friel's**
version of *A Month in
the Country* by **Ivan
Turgenev**

Director: Joe Dowling
Set Designer: Eileen Diss
Costume Designer:
Dany Everett
Lighting Designer:
Mick Hughes
AUGUST 1992

79
Ian Holm as **Duff,
Penelope Wilton** as **Beth** in
Landscape by **Harold
Pinter**

Director: Harold Pinter
Set Designer: Eileen Diss
Costume Designer:
Joan Bergin
Lighting Designer:
Mick Hughes
From the Pinter Festival
MAY 1994

80
Garrett Keogh as
Caravaggio in *Innocence,
The Life of Caravaggio* by
Frank McGuinness

Director: Patrick Mason
Set Designer: Joe Vanek
Costume Designer:
Nigel Boyd
Lighting Designer:
Mick Hughes
OCTOBER 1986

81
Bill Golding as
Sir Peter Teazle in
The School for Scandal by
Richard Brinsley Sheridan

Director: Patrick Mason
Designer: Joe Vanek
Lighting Designer:
Mick Hughes
JULY 1989

82–83
Orla Brady as **Adela,
Katherine O'Toole** as
Martirio, Barbara Brennan
as **Magdalena, Jane
Brennan** as **Amelia,
Bernadette McKenna** as
Angustias in *The House
of Bernarda Alba* by
Federico García Lorca in a
translation by **Aidan
Mathews**

Director: Ben Barnes
Set Designer: Tim Reed
Costume Designer:
Nigel Boyd
Lighting Designer:
Rupert Murray
SEPTEMBER 1989

84
Marion O'Dwyer as **Lucy**
in *The Threepenny Opera*
by **Bertolt Brecht** and
Kurt Weill in a version by
Frank McGuinness

Director: Patrick Mason
Designers:
Monica Frawley & Joe Vanek
Lighting Designer:
Mick Hughes
JULY 1991

85
John Kavanagh as
Malvolio in *Twelfth Night*
by **William Shakespeare**

Director: Joe Dowling
Set Designer: Frank Conway
Costume Designer:
Consolata Boyle
Lighting Designer:
Rupert Murray
DECEMBER 1988

86
Patricia Hayes as
Maria Josefa in *The House of Bernarda Alba* by
Federico García Lorca in a
translation by
Aidan Mathews
Director: Ben Barnes
Set Designer: Tim Reed
Costume Designer:
Nigel Boyd
Lighting Designer:
Rupert Murray
SEPTEMBER 1989

87
Anna Healy as **Dunyasha**
in *The Cherry Orchard* by
Anton Chekhov in a version
by **Michael Bogdanov**
Director: Michael Bogdanov
Designer: Chris Dyer
Lighting Designer:
Mark Pritchard
MAY 1992

88
Susan FitzGerald as **La Marquise de Merteuil** in
Les Liaisons Dangereuses
by **Christopher Hampton**
from the novel by
Choderlos de Laclos
Director: Ben Barnes
Designer: Antony McDonald
Lighting Designer:
Rupert Murray
JULY 1988

89
Deirdre Donnelly as **Judith**
in *Aristocrats* by **Brian Friel**
Director: Joe Dowling
Set Designer:
Bláithín Sheerin
Costume Designer:
Consolata Boyle
Lighting Designer:
Rupert Murray
FEBRUARY 1990

90–91
Jane Brennan as
Lydia Languish,
Rosaleen Linehan as
Mrs Malaprop,
Barry Lynch as **Captain**
Absolute in *The Rivals* by
Richard Brinsley Sheridan
Director: John David
Designer: Annena Stubbs
Lighting Designer:
Trevor Dawson
DECEMBER 1987

92
Doreen Hepburn as **Ase,**
Joe Dowling as **Peer Gynt**
in *Peer Gynt* by **Henrik**
Ibsen in a version by
Frank McGuinness
Director: Patrick Mason
Designer: Joe Vanek
Lighting Designer:
Mick Hughes
OCTOBER 1988

93
Pauline McLynn as **Jane** in
Absurd Person Singular
by **Alan Ayckbourn**
Director: John David
Designer: Martin Sutherland
Lighting Designer:
Trevor Dawson
DECEMBER 1989

94–95
Corinne Jaber as **Woman,**
Bruce Myers as **Man** in
Dybbuk by **Bruce Myers**
adapted from the play
by **Anski**
Director: Bruce Myers
Lighting Designer:
Stephen McManus
NOVEMBER 1989

96
Barry Lynch as **Peer Gynt**
in *Peer Gynt* by **Henrik**
Ibsen in a version by
Frank McGuinness
Director: Patrick Mason
Designer: Joe Vanek
Lighting Designer:
Mick Hughes
OCTOBER 1988

97
Máire Hastings as
Mrs Brocklehurst,
Anna Healy as
Mrs Rochester in *Jane*
Eyre by **Charlotte Brontë**
adapted for the stage by
Fay Weldon
Director:
Helena Kaut-Howson
Designer: Lez Brotherston
Lighting Designer:
Nick Beadle
DECEMBER 1990

98–99
Stella McCusker as
the Maid in *The House of*
Bernarda Alba by **Federico**
García Lorca in a translation
by **Aidan Mathews**
Director: Ben Barnes
Set Designer: Tim Reed
Costume Designer:
Nigel Boyd
Lighting Designer:
Rupert Murray
SEPTEMBER 1989

100
John Olohan as **Willie**
Diver in *Aristocrats* by
Brian Friel
Director: Joe Dowling
Set Designer:
Bláithín Sheerin
Costume Designer:
Consolata Boyle
Lighting Designer:
Rupert Murray
MAY 1991

101
Fionnula Flanagan as
Winnie in *Happy Days* by
Samuel Beckett
Director: Caroline FitzGerald
Designer: Tim Reed
Lighting Designer:
Alan Burrett
From the Beckett Festival
OCTOBER 1991

102–103
Garrett Keogh as
Caravaggio, Pat Leavy as
the Whore, Kate Flynn as
Lena in *Innocence, The*
Life of Caravaggio by
Frank McGuinness
Director: Patrick Mason
Set Designer: Joe Vanek
Costume Designer:
Nigel Boyd
Lighting Designer:
Mick Hughes
OCTOBER 1986

104
Stephen Brennan as
Elyot Chase,
Lucy Vigne Welsh as
Sibyl Chase in *Private*
Lives by **Noël Coward**
Director: Robin Lefevre
Set Designer: Eileen Diss
Costume Designer:
Nigel Boyd
Lighting Designer:
Rupert Murray
MARCH 1992

105
John Hurt as
Count Mushroom,
Gemma Craven as **Mrs**
Diggerty in **The London**
Vertigo by **Brian Friel**
based on a play by
Charles Macklin
Director: Judy Friel
Designer: Monica Frawley
Lighting Designer:
Rupert Murray
JANUARY 1992

106–107
Katherine O'Toole as
Martirio in *The House of*
Bernarda Alba by **Federico**
García Lorca in a translation
by **Aidan Mathews**
Director: Ben Barnes
Set Designer: Tim Reed
Costume Designer:
Nigel Boyd
Lighting Designer:
Rupert Murray
SEPTEMBER 1989

108
Susan FitzGerald as
May in *Footfalls* by
Samuel Beckett
Director: Derek Chapman
Designer: Tim Reed
Lighting Designer:
Alan Burrett
From the Beckett Festival
OCTOBER 1991

109
John Kavanagh as
Joxer Daly,
Donal McCann as
Captain Jack Boyle in
Juno and the Paycock by
Sean O'Casey
Director: Joe Dowling
Set Designer:
Frank Hallinan Flood
Costume Designer:
Consolata Boyle
Lighting Designer:
Rupert Murray
JULY 1986

110–111
Aiden Grennell as **the**
Cardinal in *Innocence,*
The Life of Caravaggio by
Frank McGuinness
Director: Patrick Mason
Set Designer: Joe Vanek
Costume Designer:
Nigel Boyd
Lighting Designer:
Mick Hughes
OCTOBER 1986

112
Siân Maguire as **Emilie** in
Les Liaisons Dangereuses
by **Christopher Hampton**
from the novel by
Choderlos de Laclos
Director: Ben Barnes
Designer: Antony McDonald
Lighting Designer:
Rupert Murray ·
OCTOBER 1987

113
Pauline McLynn as
Lady Teazle in
The School for Scandal by
Richard Brinsley Sheridan
Director: Patrick Mason
Designer: Joe Vanek
Lighting Designer:
Mick Hughes
JULY 1989

114–115
Peter Cooney as
Major-domo,
Catherine Walsh as **Adèle,**
Rod Chichignoud as
Georges, Muireann Kelly
as **Sophie** in *Les Liaisons*
Dangereuses by
Christopher Hampton
from the novel by
Choderlos de Laclos
Director: Ben Barnes
Designer: Antony McDonald
Lighting Designer:
Rupert Murray
OCTOBER 1987

116
John Kavanagh as
Malvolio in *Twelfth Night*
by **William Shakespeare**
Director: Joe Dowling
Set Designer: Frank Conway
Costume Designer:
Consolata Boyle
Lighting Designer:
Rupert Murray
DECEMBER 1988

117

Sorcha Cusack as
La Marquise de Merteuil,
David Herlihy as
Danceny in *Les Liaisons Dangereuses* by
Christopher Hampton from
the novel by **Choderlos de Laclos**

Director: Ben Barnes
Designer: Antony McDonald
Lighting Designer:
Rupert Murray

OCTOBER 1987

118–119

Olwen Fouéré as **La Présidente de Tourvel** in
Les Liaisons Dangereuses
by **Christopher Hampton**
from the novel by
Choderlos de Laclos

Director: Ben Barnes
Designer: Antony McDonald
Lighting Designer:
Rupert Murray

OCTOBER 1987

120

Tomás Killeen as **B** in
Act Without Words II by
Samuel Beckett

Director: Lucy Bailey
Designer: Simon Vincenzi
Lighting Designer:
Alan Burrett
From the Beckett Festival

OCTOBER 1991

121

Barbara Brennan as **Silvia**
in *The Recruiting Officer*
by **George Farquhar**

Director: Patrick Mason
Set Designer: Joe Vanek
Dostume Designer:
Nigel Boyd
Lighting Designer:
Trevor Dawson

MAY 1985

122–123

Helene Montague as **Flo,**
Bernadette McKenna as
Vi, Susan FitzGerald as
Ru in *Come and Go* by
Samuel Beckett

Director: Lucy Bailey
Designer: Simon Vincenzi
Lighting Designer:
Alan Burrett
From the Beckett Festival

OCTOBER 1991

124

Klaus Hassel as
Mustardseed, Anne
Buckley as **First Fairy** in
A Midsummer Night's
Dream by **William**
Shakespeare

Director: Joe Dowling
Designer: Hayden Griffin
l ighting Designer:
Rupert Murray

JULY 1993

125

Maureen Potter as
Maisie Madigan,
Geraldine Plunkett as
Juno Boyle,
Donal McCann as
Captain Jack Boyle,
John Kavanagh as
Joxer Daly in *Juno and the*
Paycock by **Sean O'Casey**

Director: Joe Dowling
Set Designer:
Frank Hallinan Flood
Costume Designer:
Consolata Boyle
Lighting Designer:
Rupert Murray

JULY 1986

126

Ingrid Craigie as
Gwendolen, Lise-Ann
McLaughlin as **Cecily** in
The Importance of Being
Earnest by **Oscar Wilde**

Director: Patrick Mason
Set Designer: Robert Ballagh
Costume Designer:
Nigel Boyd
Lighting Designer:
Trevor Dawson

JULY 1987

127

Joe Savino as **Jokanaan** in
Salomé by **Oscar Wilde**

Director: Steven Berkoff
Set Designer: Robert Ballagh
Costume Designer:
Nigel Boyd
Lighting Designer:
Trevor Dawson

APRIL 1988

128–129

Éanna MacLiam as
Tommy Owens in *The*
Shadow of a Gunman by
Sean O'Casey

Director: Lynne Parker
Designer: Kathy Strachan
Lighting Designer:
Tina MacHugh

JULY 1996

130–131

Tom Murphy as
Philip Clandon,
Catherine Cusack as
Dolly Clandon in
You Never Can Tell by
George Bernard Shaw

Director: John David
Set Designer:
Bláithín Sheerin
Costume Designer:
Annena Stubbs
Lighting Designer:
Stephen McManus

AUGUST 1990

132

Catherine Byrne as **Elmire,**
Stephen Brennan as
Tartuffe in **Molière's**
Tartuffe in a version by
Michael West

Director: Alan Stanford
Set Designer:
Robert Ballagh
Costume Designer:
Annena Stubbs
Lighting Designer:
Alan Burrett

OCTOBER 1992

133

Des Keogh as
Mr Gallogher in *The*
Shadow of a Gunman by
Sean O'Casey

Director: Lynne Parker
Designer: Kathy Strachan
Lighting Designer:
Tina MacHugh

JULY 1996

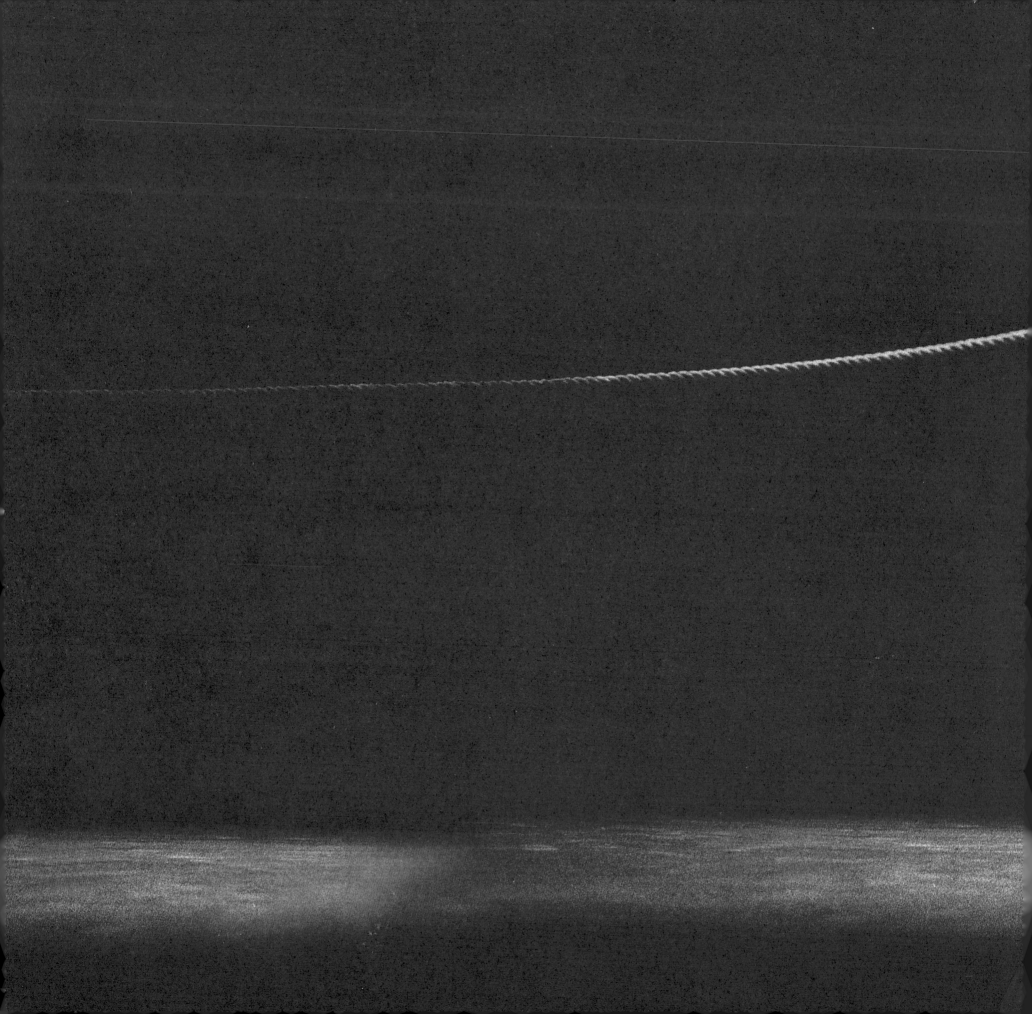